the Unofficial Guide® to Getting Pregnant

*Joan Liebmann-Smith, Ph.D.,
Jacqueline Nardi Egan, and
John J. Stangel, M.D.*

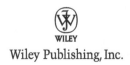

WILEY

Wiley Publishing, Inc.

Library of Congress Control Number: 2005923063

ISBN-10: 0-7645-9550-4

ISBN-13: 978-0-7645-9550-9

10 9 8 7 6 5 4 3 2 1

Book design by Melissa Auciello-Brogan
Page creation by Wiley Publishing, Inc. Composition Services

To my daughter, Rebecca, upon her graduation from Barnard College, Columbia University. May she achieve all her goals, wishes, and dreams in life, as she fulfilled ours for a longed-for child.

—Joan Liebmann-Smith, Ph.D.

To my late husband, Edward, who always provided unfailing support and strength; and to our daughter, Elizabeth, for her continued encouragement and enthusiasm.

—Jacqueline Nardi Egan

To Lois, Eric , Liz, Justin, Lara, and Emily with greatest love and appreciation. To my patients, who have shared their problems and feelings with me, who have taught me more than any textbook, and who have allowed me the privilege of treating them. To those who yearn to have a child of their own, I wish you the fulfillment of your dreams.

—John J. Stangel, M.D.

Acknowledgments

We would like to thank our editors at Wiley, especially Roxane Cerda, for suggesting that we write this book; Pam Mourouzis, for her guidance and encouragement each step of the way; and Lynn Northrup, who helped us get through this project as smoothly—and painlessly—as possible. Not only was Lynn a terrific editor, she rose to the challenge of dealing with three authors with the patience of a saint and the skills of a therapist.

Joan and Jacqueline would like to thank their colleague, co-author, and friend, Dr. John Stangel, not only for his invaluable contributions to this book, but also for providing us with many of the illustrations from his book, *The New Fertility and Conception.*

We all would like to acknowledge three pioneers of IVF—Dr. Robert Edwards of Bourn Hall, Cambridge, England; and Doctors Carl Wood and Alan Trounson of Monash University, Melbourne, Australia—for their contributions to this book as well as for their contributions to the field of assisted reproductive technology.

Thanks to the following doctors (in alphabetical order) for each of his or her unique and expert contributions: Dr. Sami David, Dr. Loren Greene, Dr. Mark Leondires, Dr. Larry Lipshultz, Dr. Harris Nagler, Dr. Spencer Richlin, Dr. Richard Scott, and Dr. Mac Talbot. And thanks to Dr. Lucinda Veeck Gosden for her wonderful photographs.

We would like to acknowledge the American Society for Reproductive Medicine (ASRM), especially Jennifer Price for her help with many of the illustrations for this book; and Joyce Zeitz, Sean Tipton, and Eleanor Nicoll, who provided us with invaluable information, data, and other resources. And special thanks to Dana Pylilo, of Serono; Laurie Reyes, of Organon; and Timothy Glynn, of Ferring. We also appreciate the help of Richard Liebmann-Smith, who generously donated his skills as a science editor.

Julie Greenstein of RESOLVE was extremely helpful in getting us information about insurance coverage at a moment's notice. We also want to thank RESOLVE itself for being there as a terrific resource not only for us writers, but—more importantly—for the one-in-six couples struggling with infertility. And we would like to thank those women and men who anonymously—and very generously—shared with us their stories about their struggles with infertility.

Special thanks to Amy Alton-Primrose, RPA-C, Genny Delannoy, and Anne Morabito for their assistance in gathering information and materials. This book couldn't have been written without their help and the help of the rest of Dr. Stangel's staff: Lisa Burke, Cheryl Daly, Ronnie Guarente, Carol Holden, Geri Lewis, Audrey Loveridge, Pat Mazzola, Sue Salvo, Lisa Viskup, Pat Walsh, and Kathleen York. Additionally, thanks to Vicki Baldwin and Robin Mangieri.

And last but not least, we'd like to thank our immediate and extended families, who remind us each day of the importance and true meaning of family.

About the Authors

Joan Liebmann-Smith, Ph.D., is a medical sociologist and an award-winning medical writer. Her articles have appeared in such publications as *American Health, Ms., Newsweek, Redbook, Self,* and *Vogue.* She is the author of *In Pursuit of Pregnancy* and co-author of *The Unofficial Guide to Overcoming Infertility.* She has also written a book on women and substance abuse to be published in 2006. Dr. Liebmann-Smith is a consultant at the Strang Cancer Prevention Center and is on the board of the National Council on Women's Health. She was a member of the board of directors of RESOLVE, INC. and co-president of RESOLVE, NYC.

Jacqueline Nardi Egan is a medical journalist and editor. She specializes in writing educational programs for physicians, allied health professionals, patients, and consumers. She has been the editor of several specialty medical publications and a contributor to national consumer magazines. She is co-author of *The Unofficial Guide to Overcoming Infertility.*

John J. Stangel, M.D., a board certified specialist in Reproductive Medicine, is the Westchester County Medical Director of Reproductive Medicine Associates of Connecticut, and has a private practice in Rye, New York.

Dr. Stangel has also been the Medical Director of the Westchester Affiliate of the Institute for Reproductive Medicine and Science at Saint Barnabas Medical Center; the Clinical Director of Reproductive Medicine at Montefiore Medical Center; and the Medical Director of IVF America.

Dr. Stangel is a charter member of the Society of Reproductive Endocrinologists (SART) and the Society of Reproductive Surgeons. He is the editor and contributing author of the textbook *Infertility Surgery*, has published numerous scientific papers and articles, and has contributed to many textbooks. Dr. Stangel is the author of *Fertility and Conception* and co-author of *The Unofficial Guide to Overcoming Infertility.*

Contents

The decision to start a family is one of the most important—and in some cases, most difficult—decisions a couple will make. There is so much to consider: the relationship with your partner, your career goals, your biological clock, the size of your home, and the size of your savings account. But there's one important issue that many couples tend to overlook, and that is the state of their health.

If you've been basically healthy, there's probably no reason to think that this should be an issue when you decide to start a family. However, there is a lot you can and should do to be in the best state of health before trying to conceive. Both you and your partner should have a preconception exam early on to rule out a variety of conditions that you may not be aware of—but that can prevent you from conceiving or cause you or your baby problems during or after pregnancy.

But being in the best shape to procreate involves more than just being free from disease; it includes such factors as eating the right foods, maintaining a healthy weight, and being physically active—but not overdoing it. It also involves being free from sexually transmitted diseases (STDs), which are more common than most people suspect. And speaking of sex, there are myriad myths about when and how to have sex. Some may be true, but many are not. While most couples certainly know what's normally involved in getting pregnant, they often don't know what they can do to maximize their chances of success. One thing is certain: There's a lot more to making babies than making love!

Once they make a decision to start a family, most couples think it will happen pretty quickly, if not the first time they have unprotected sex. The reality, however, is that it takes the average, healthy, *young* couple six months to a year to conceive. Age is an especially important fertility factor; the older you are, the longer it's likely to take you to conceive and have a successful pregnancy.

Unfortunately, it will take many couples—even young, healthy ones—considerably longer than a year to conceive. For some, it may just be a matter of time. But for others—about one in six couples—it may require fertility drugs, surgery, or even in-vitro fertilization (IVF) to have their own children.

While many people associate infertility treatment with IVF and the other assisted reproductive technologies (ARTs), the fact is only 3 percent of all infertile couples who enter treatment go through in-vitro fertilization. This means that many other effective—and often less expensive—forms of treatment, such as fertility drugs for hormonal problems and surgical correction of structural problems, are available for both men and women. As you'll read in this book, the good news is that with the proper medical diagnosis and treatment, more than half of all infertile couples will ultimately conceive their own biological children. Many of the others will become parents through third-party reproduction procedures such as sperm donation, egg donation, surrogacy, or adoption.

Getting Pregnant in the 21st Century

It's been a quarter century since Louise Brown, the world's first test-tube baby, was born. Since then, tremendous strides have been made in the understanding of fertility and the treatment of infertility. More infertile—and even previously sterile—men and women are now having children. Over a million babies worldwide have been born through IVF and the other assisted reproductive technologies (ARTs). At the other end of the spectrum, alternative medicine is being more widely researched, used—and recognized as useful—for enhancing fertility than in past decades.

Research has uncovered new factors, such as race, that affect success rates. Prenatal diagnoses techniques have improved, and couples who undergo IVF can rule out major defects while their embryos are still in the Petrie dish. There is also new data on the effects of ARTs on babies, children, and adolescents.

You can hardly turn on your TV without seeing a story on infertility, the ARTs, multiple births, stem cell research, and cloning. In 2005, a 66-year-old Romanian woman gave birth after using donor eggs and sperm. Also to hit the news was a report that Korean scientists reported the first therapeutic cloning of human embryos and the successful extraction of stem cells from those embryos. And just as this book went to press, there was another medical first: A woman who had gone through premature menopause in her 20s gave birth after an ovarian transplant from her identical twin sister.

Along with new treatment techniques, new problems and challenges have emerged. As success rates have increased, multiple births—and multiple ethical dilemmas—have as well. While considered a blessing by most parents, multiple births can cause serious problems for pregnant women and their babies. IVF patients are also confronted with ethical dilemmas they never anticipated, such as whether or not to donate their extra frozen embryos for stem cell research. This book will provide you with the very latest information on these and other key issues related to your pursuit of pregnancy.

What This Book Offers You

The Unofficial Guide to Getting Pregnant will help you get in the best possible shape *before* you even start trying to get pregnant to maximize your chances of conceiving quickly. We'll give you the inside scoop on how weight, exercise, nutrition, vitamins, herbs, stress, and sex positions affect fertility. Those women and men who have to delay childbearing because they must undergo chemotherapy or radiation for cancer treatment or other reasons will find invaluable information on fertility preservation so they can maximize the chances of having their own children in the future.

If you're concerned that you might have problems conceiving—or if you've been trying for awhile to no avail—this *Unofficial Guide* will give you the latest information on home ovulation and sperm tests, and diagnostic tests. And, if you are among the one in six couples who do turn out to have fertility problems, you will find the most current and comprehensive information available to help you in your quest for a child. By reading this *Unofficial Guide,* you will get:

- Information on the effect of age and ethnicity on fertility treatment.

- The inside scoop on the newest fertility drugs to hit the market.

- Details about the latest microsurgical techniques.

- A description of the newest assisted reproductive techniques.

- The latest data on the health of children born through IVF.

- Important information about third-party reproduction.

- A clear explanation of embryonic stem cell research and cloning and their implications for you.

- Recent research on alternative treatments that might work...or might be a waste of money.

- Detailed information on the costs of different treatments.

- The very latest state mandates on insurance coverage for infertility treatment.

You will also find a glossary; reading list; comprehensive list of useful resources that deal with the medical, emotional, and other aspects of fertility and infertility; a sample genetic testing flow sheet; and a state-by-state chart of infertility insurance coverage.

First and foremost, by reading *The Unofficial Guide to Getting Pregnant* you maximize your chances of getting pregnant. It will also help you and your partner navigate the complex worlds of fertility and infertility; it covers the medical, interpersonal, emotional, ethical, and financial issues related to getting pregnant. Reading this book can help you avoid unnecessary, unsuccessful, or unproven treatments. You will learn how to choose and work with a qualified fertility specialist and, if necessary, an IVF program. We will also help you become an informed patient so that you can make the best medical decisions for you and your partner. And last but not least, it will also help you maximize your chances of being reimbursed for the costs of your journey to parenthood.

A Personal Message from John J. Stangel, M.D.

This is a "how-to" book. But, unlike most books in this category that tell you how to build an object or acquire a skill, this book will guide you through the many reproductive treatment choices to maximize your chances of having a child of your own. This may be one of the most important "how-to" books you will ever read.

If it does turn out that you have a fertility problem, you will need the most accurate, up-to-date information available. This book is a complete and current source written in an easy-to-read format. It covers everything from the initial work-up to the assisted reproductive technologies (ARTs). Our knowledge of human reproduction has progressed so rapidly in the last few years—and even months—that even if you have read extensively in the field you will still benefit by reading this *Unofficial Guide*. This is the state of the art—and the ARTs—as of this very afternoon.

If you think you have an infertility problem, you need to have a way of checking your concerns. If you find your concerns are real, what do you do? To whom do you go? What questions do you ask? What should your evaluation involve? How long should it take? Are there further tests that should be done?

What are the treatment choices? What are the risks and benefits of each? How successful are they, and are there alternatives? How much will all this cost? Will your insurance plan cover this? These are some of the questions that create the maze through which an infertile couple must travel.

Some people are fearful of being in a doctor's office. Others are overcome by a paralyzing anxiety just going through the evaluation steps. These feelings may make it hard to absorb the information presented by your physician. If this describes you, you may find that when you get home to review your discussion with your doctor and the information provided to you, you may remember nothing. This book can provide the missing information helping you to fill in the gaps. It can also help you formulate some questions for your doctor. In these ways, this book can help you use your time more efficiently and make the whole experience gentler.

The nightmare of every infertile couple is seeing a physician and being told: "I am sorry. There's nothing that can be done for you." It is the fear of hearing these words that keeps many people from seeking help.

The good news is that it is rare for there to truly be no hope. For the vast majority of couples, a physician can find a way to help them achieve a successful pregnancy. And for those rare occasions when the words are, "I'm sorry. We can't help you," remember, don't give up. The field of reproductive medicine is changing and progressing so quickly that what was not doable one moment is reality six months later and commonplace a year after. If having a child is important to you, do not give up. Pursue this goal aggressively. Find the right doctor. Find the right treatment and stay with it until it works. This book can guide you through the maze of diagnosis and treatment and invisibly stand by your side offering information and support.

All three of us who have worked on this book want you to succeed in your quest to have a child.

Special Features

Every book in the *Unofficial Guide* series offers the following four special sidebars that are devised to help you get things done cheaply, efficiently, and smartly.

1. **Moneysaver:** Tips and shortcuts that will help you save money.

2. **Watch Out!:** Cautions and warnings to help you avoid common pitfalls.

3. **Bright Idea:** Smart or innovative ways to do something; in many cases, the ideas listed here will help you save time or hassle.

4. **Quote:** Anecdotes from real people who are willing to share their experiences and insights.

We also recognize your need to have quick information at your fingertips, and have provided the following comprehensive sections at the back of the book:

1. **Glossary:** Definitions of complicated terminology and jargon.

2. **Recommended Reading List:** Suggested titles that can help you get more in-depth information on related topics.

3. **Resource Guide:** Lists of relevant agencies, associations, institutions, websites, and so on.

4. **Sample Genetic Testing Flow Sheet:** Questions to help you decide whether to have pre-pregnancy genetic testing.

5. **State-by-State Infertility Insurance Coverage:** RESOLVE's state guide to insurance coverage of infertility treatment.

6. **Index.**

Preparing for Pregnancy

PART I

GET THE SCOOP ON...
The importance of the preconception exam ▪
Making healthy choices ▪ Fertility considerations
for older men and women ▪ What you can do
to preserve your fertility ▪ Pregnancy after
cancer treatment

A Healthy Start

Chapter 1

You and your partner most likely have spent a good deal of time discussing if you'd like to have children, and if so, when to start your family. Many couples believe that choosing when to start trying to become pregnant is the most difficult decision they will make, and in some ways, they're right. But deciding to have children is just the beginning; there are many other key choices you should make now that can help improve your chances of conceiving, having a healthy pregnancy, and most importantly, a healthy baby.

The preconception checkup

Everyone is aware of the importance of prenatal checkups, but a preconception checkup is equally important. Both partners should be in good physical condition before starting a family. Therefore, it makes sense for both of you to get a physical exam before attempting a pregnancy. The main purpose of the preconception exam is to rule out diseases that can interfere with your chances of conceiving and carrying a healthy baby to full term. A routine

3

physical exam might turn up a condition or conditions that can reduce your fertility, such as diabetes, thyroid disorders, or sexually transmitted diseases (STDs). Although the woman is the one who becomes pregnant and gives birth, both parents can pass on genetic disorders. And because medical conditions, both past and present, affect the development of sperm and their ability to fertilize eggs and produce a healthy embryo, men must ensure that they too are healthy.

The preconception exam goes well beyond specific reproductive issues and encompasses general health and lifestyle considerations that can affect you before, during, and long after a pregnancy. Most primary care providers—such as family physicians, general practitioners, internists, physician assistants, and nurse practitioners—can conduct preconception exams on both men and women. Because many women use their OB/GYN (obstetrician/gynecologist) as their primary care physician, they may want to see him or her for the preconception exam as well. But not all OB/GYNS will fill the role of a primary care physician, since they are trained specifically in female reproduction. Be sure to ask your OB/GYN if he or she is willing to act in this capacity and screen you for nonreproductive health problems that can also interfere with your becoming pregnant and carrying a healthy baby to term.

You'll want to bring your partner along when you go for a preconception checkup. It's important for both partners to be aware of the medical issues related to conception, pregnancy, and childbearing. The preconception checkup should take place at least three months before you start trying to conceive.

 Watch Out!

Women who take birth control pills should stop taking them at least three months before trying to conceive. It might take at least that long for a woman's reproductive hormones to get back to normal.

If you need certain immunizations, you will have to postpone attempting a pregnancy for at least three months.

Reproductive health

Obviously, reproductive health is of prime importance. Before a woman even attempts to become pregnant, her doctor should be aware of her reproductive history, including menstrual disorders; past and current contraceptive use; past pregnancies, abortions, and miscarriages; and past and current STDs.

Sexually transmitted diseases (STDs)

It's essential that both partners be screened for STDs before attempting to become pregnant. STDs have been on the increase and can have serious adverse effects on fertility, pregnancy, delivery, and offspring. STDs can lead to pelvic inflammatory disease (PID), which is the major cause of infertility.

The most common STDs—and those most responsible for PID and its aftermath, infertility or ectopic pregnancy—are chlamydia and gonorrhea (which we'll discuss in more detail in a moment). When recognized and treated promptly, these infections are usually easily treated with appropriate antibiotics. If left unchecked, these organisms can travel from the vagina and cervix up the reproductive tract. However, the organisms are not found in nearly one third of women with PID, although they might have been present in the early stages of the infection.

Because STDs often don't cause symptoms, they can be passed unknowingly countless times between partners, causing extensive damage. It's often not until you're trying to conceive or you suffer an ectopic pregnancy that their damage is discovered. Although a history of STDs or multiple sexual partners increases the chances of having a current STD, virtually any sexually active man or woman can be infected. It's therefore important that both partners are tested for the following STDs prior to attempting a pregnancy.

Moneysaver

A preconception dental exam might spare you the cost and pain of expensive dental work after pregnancy. Pregnancy can cause or exacerbate dental problems, so a visit to the dentist before you conceive may help preserve your teeth and gums.

Chlamydia

Chlamydia is one of the most prevalent STDs in the United States, with almost three million new cases every year. Because it rarely produces symptoms in either men or women, it's known as the "silent infection." If untreated, chlamydia can cause PID and damage the reproductive system. Not only can chlamydia interfere with conception and pregnancy, it can also have serious consequences for newborns. Babies born to women with active chlamydial infection are subject to infection during passage through the birth canal. If they pick up the organism, it can cause serious eye infection and pneumonia. Chlamydia does not affect men as seriously as it does women, although some severe cases can lead to sterility. Antibiotics can easily and inexpensively cure chlamydial infection in both men and women.

Gonorrhea

Approximately 700,000 men and women contract gonorrhea, a bacterial infection, each year. Gonorrhea can cause tubal damage in women and scarring and obstruction of the epididymis—the long tube attached to the testicle in which sperm mature before being released—in men. Gonorrhea often does not produce symptoms in men and women, but can cause pain, burning when urinating, and vaginal or penile discharge. If untreated, gonorrhea can cause infertility in men and PID in women, thus increasing a woman's risk of infertility, ectopic pregnancy, and miscarriage. Babies born to mothers infected with gonorrhea can be born blind, with serious joint infections, or with life-threatening blood infections.

HIV/AIDS

STD screening would be incomplete without testing for HIV/AIDS. Indeed, the American College of Obstetricians and Gynecologists (ACOG) recommends that the HIV antibody test be offered to all women seeking preconception care. It's critical to make sure you and your partner do not carry the AIDS virus not only for your own sakes, but also for the sake of your future child. Having AIDS is no longer the death sentence it once was, thanks to antiviral agents that can successfully control the virus. But without proper treatment and special precautions during pregnancy and childbirth, the AIDs virus can be passed from the mother to the fetus.

HPV

Human papillomavirus (HPV) is the most common STD in the United States, with more than six million new cases each year. An astonishing 80 percent of American women will have acquired the virus by the time they reach 50. Although some people get genital warts from the virus, most have no symptoms. Although HPV has not been directly linked to infertility, genital warts, if large, can cause problems during pregnancy and delivery. The virus can also be transmitted to a baby during childbirth, and there is a small chance that the infant can develop a rare but serious condition called laryngeal papillomatosis (warts on the throat).

One of the biggest concerns about HPV is that it can cause cervical cancer. In fact, virtually all women with cervical cancer have HPV. The good news is that only one in a thousand women with the virus develops invasive cervical cancer. HPV is typically diagnosed by a Pap smear in women, but there is no test yet

 Watch Out!

Don't douche when you're trying to conceive. Douching kills sperm and it may increase your risk of PID.

available for men. When abnormal cervical cells are found, it's recommended that women undergo treatment to remove the precancerous cells. Unfortunately, the treatments themselves occasionally impair fertility or prevent the woman from carrying a baby to term. If left untreated, however, a woman can develop cervical cancer and need a hysterectomy.

HPV can also cause other cancers in the female and male reproductive systems, such as cancer of the vulva, vagina, and penis. Cancer treatment can result in infertility or sterility, a topic discussed later in this chapter. Although there is no known cure for HPV, it can—and should—be treated.

Genital herpes

Genital herpes is caused by the herpes simplex virus (HSV). While one form of herpes, HSV-1, typically causes blisters or cold sores around the lips, the other form (HSV-2) usually causes blisters or sores in the genital region. Approximately 45 million Americans (20 percent) over the age of 12 are infected with HSV-2. It's more common in women than men; one in four women has this virus compared with one in five men. Most of the time people have no symptoms and they may be unaware of having the virus until they break out in painful blisters or sores. Although genital herpes doesn't normally interfere with conception, it increases the risk of premature delivery. HSV can also be transmitted to the fetus during pregnancy or the baby during delivery. Half of the babies who are infected either die or suffer nerve damage. If a woman has an active case of genital herpes at the time of delivery, a Caesarian section is usually performed to protect the baby. Although the painful symptoms of HSV can be treated, there is no cure for the virus. Unfortunately, HSV increases the risk of acquiring HIV and AIDS.

General health issues

It's important for your health-care professional to know if you or your partner has now or has had in the past any illness that could have serious reproductive consequences. A variety of disorders can cause fertility problems, miscarriages, or other problems during pregnancy or delivery, and even birth defects. In the following section we discuss just a few of the more common conditions that may be of concern, and that are easily screened for during a preconception exam.

High blood pressure

High blood pressure (hypertension) can cause serious medical and pregnancy complications for both mother and fetus. A blood pressure reading of greater than 140/90 mmHg should alert you and your health-care provider. If you're already being treated for high (or low) blood pressure, consult your doctor to make certain the drug or drugs you're taking are safe to use during pregnancy and breastfeeding.

Diabetes

If you or your partner have diabetes and you are thinking about trying to conceive, be certain to get your blood sugar (glucose) under control. Uncontrolled diabetes can have serious adverse effects on fertility in both men and women. For example, diabetes in women can prevent ovulation or implantation. And women whose blood sugar is not under control have an increased risk of miscarriage, stillbirth, and giving birth to a baby with birth defects. Men with diabetes may suffer from erectile dysfunction (impotence) as well as a condition called *retrograde ejaculation,* the backward movement of semen into the bladder instead of forward out the urethra.

 Bright Idea

If you have any medical problem, make sure you get treated before attempting to get pregnant. But because your condition may cause problems with conception, pregnancy, or your future child, it's a good idea to also consult a fertility specialist before attempting a pregnancy.

Moneysaver

Make sure you get and keep copies of your preconception exam and test results. If you see a fertility specialist, he or she will need the information. Having your own records can help you avoid repeating costly tests. Be sure to bring them to your first appointment.

Thyroid disease

Both hypo- and hyperthyroidism can lead to infertility and miscarriage. If you are being treated for thyroid disease, check with your doctor to make sure your medication is safe to use during pregnancy and nursing.

Other medical considerations

A pregnant woman may contract any number of diseases that can adversely affect her pregnancy or cause birth defects. A preconception exam should include testing for immunity against the following diseases. (There's some controversy about how long you should wait to conceive after vaccinations, ranging from a minimum of one month to three months. To be on the safe side, it would be prudent to wait.)

Rubella (German measles)

Even if a woman has had German measles or was previously vaccinated, she should be tested for her current immune status. If she is not immune, she should receive a rubella vaccination at least three months before attempting a pregnancy. Contracting German measles early in a pregnancy can be devastating to the fetus. It can cause deafness and serious eye, heart, and neurological problems; it can also lead to fetal death, miscarriage, or premature delivery.

Chickenpox

Women who never had chickenpox are probably not immune and should be immunized against this disease. As with rubella, pregnancy should be postponed for three months after the vaccination. If a pregnant woman gets chickenpox in the first or early second trimester of pregnancy, the fetus is at risk for serious neurological and eye problems or limb deformities.

Toxoplasmosis

Women should be screened for toxoplasmosis, a mild, common parasitic infection that can cause serious birth defects, especially during the first trimester. The infection is commonly transmitted through undercooked meat and animal feces, and there is no immunization available. Women who are found not to be immune should make sure any meat they eat is well done and wear rubber gloves when emptying cat litter or working in the garden, where animal feces may be hidden.

Hepatitis B

This liver infection can be contracted through sexual contact or exposure to infected feces, or blood, urine, saliva, or other bodily fluids. It is the only form of hepatitis that can cause serious harm to newborns. Women should be screened for hepatitis B and those found not immune should be vaccinated at least three months before attempting to conceive.

Rh incompatibility

It's important for you and your partner to know both your blood type and Rh or *Rhesus* factor before you become pregnant. This information is, of course, necessary in the event a blood transfusion is needed. But there are other reasons for couples to have this information before they attempt a pregnancy. Of special concern for a future pregnancy is Rh incompatibility.

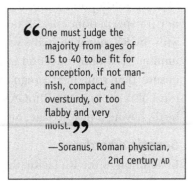

66 One must judge the majority from ages of 15 to 40 to be fit for conception, if not mannish, compact, and oversturdy, or too flabby and very moist. 99

—Soranus, Roman physician, 2nd century AD

There are four blood types (A, B, AB, or O) and each blood type can have one of two Rh factors (Rh positive or Rh negative). Rh is a protein that coats the surface of red blood cells. Most people—85 percent of white Americans and an even larger percentage of African-Americans and Asians—are Rh positive. The remaining 15 percent are Rh negative. Having a different blood type from your partner isn't a problem. Nor is there a problem if the mother is Rh positive and the father Rh negative. But if the future mother is Rh negative and the future father is Rh positive there could be a problem. To be more precise, if the woman is A-, B-, AB-, or O- and her male partner is A+, B+, AB+, or O+, the baby has a 50 percent chance of being Rh positive, and your pregnancy would be Rh incompatible. If, however, the mother is Rh positive and the father Rh negative, there would be no problem.

Rh incompatibility is not usually a problem in a first pregnancy, but can be deadly to the fetus in a subsequent pregnancy. When a pregnant Rh negative mother carries an Rh positive fetus, the baby's blood can leak into the mother's circulatory system. Her immune system may react to the baby's blood as if it were a foreign substance, and to protect itself, creates antibodies to destroy the baby's blood.

The good news is that this problem is entirely preventable when proper precautions are taken. If an Rh negative woman has ever had a pregnancy, abortion, miscarriage, amniocentesis, or blood transfusion, there is a possibility that she has been exposed to Rh positive blood and will be sensitized. If your partner (or sperm donor) is Rh negative and you become pregnant with an Rh negative baby, you must receive a RhoGAM (Rh immune globulin) injection in the 28th week of pregnancy. To ensure that your next pregnancy will not be a problem, you must also get another RhoGAM shot within 72 hours of giving birth, having a miscarriage, or stillbirth.

Genetic disorders

In addition to the Rh factor, there are some other serious, often deadly, genetic conditions that run in families and can be passed on to your offspring. These diseases include cystic fibrosis, Thalassemia, Tay-Sachs, sickle cell anemia, Huntington's disease, and hemophilia. If you or your partner have any family members with these or other genetic diseases you both should go for genetic counseling and screening before attempting a pregnancy. Also, some genetic disorders tend to occur more often in certain nationalities or racial groups. For example, cystic fibrosis is most prevalent among people of Irish and Northern European descent; Tay-Sachs, a fatal brain disorder, primarily affects Eastern European Jews and French Canadians; Thalassemia, a serious blood disorder, primarily affects those of Mediterranean, South Asian, or African descent; and sickle cell anemia, another serious blood disease, predominately affects African-Americans. It's important to know what your chances are of passing on a serious genetic disorder to your future child and what impact that will have on his or her life—and yours. There are ways to screen for certain genetic disorders prior to conception as well as during pregnancy (see Chapter 9 and Appendix D).

> ❝When we finally made up our minds to get pregnant, we were roaring to go. But we had to put everything on hold for over a month because I had to get a rubella shot and had to go for genetic testing. When we discovered that I was a Tay-Sachs carrier, we were not only devastated, we had to put everything on hold again while my husband got tested. Luckily everything turned out okay, but the waiting had been very hard on us. ❞
>
> —Susan, 35

Bright Idea

If you or your partner were adopted and/or don't know your biological families' medical histories, you may be at risk for passing on certain genetic disorders. It makes good sense, therefore, to go for genetic screening prior to trying to get pregnant.

Healthy choices

Although your immediate goal is getting pregnant, we assume that your ultimate goal is parenthood and that you want to be there for your children as they grow up. The same health issues that apply to all adults are especially salient when it comes to pregnancy and parenthood. Choosing to live a healthy lifestyle is one of the best things you can do to maximize your chances of having a healthy pregnancy and baby. Most of the following lifestyle choices apply to both women and men. But because women are the ones who become pregnant and give birth, it's especially important that they choose a healthy lifestyle and avoid hazardous substances and behaviors.

A previous pregnancy doesn't mean a woman will easily conceive again—or at all. And just because a man previously got a woman—or even his current partner—pregnant doesn't guarantee he can impregnate her now. Many things can cause a previously fertile man or woman to experience infertility. Secondary infertility, as this is known, can be the result of many of the same factors that cause primary infertility. The causes of fertility problems are discussed in Chapters 4 and 6.

Avoid smoking and tobacco smoke

More than one in four women of reproductive age smoke. If you're one of those women, now is the time to stop! It's fairly well known that cigarette smoking increases the risk of spontaneous abortion and low-birth-weight babies. But did you know that smoking can increase the time to conception as well? Researchers aren't sure why, but they think that cigarette smoking reduces some types of estrogen production and depletes egg supply.

 Moneysaver

Make sure you and your future family are not only covered by health insurance, but that you are covered for pre- and postnatal care, childbirth, and fertility treatments, should you need them.

Smoking interferes with Fallopian tube motility (movement), embryo cleavage, blastocyst formation, and implantation, which we'll discuss in Chapter 2; it has also been linked to a whole host of problems from ectopic pregnancies to miscarriages. Smoking can also cause premature menopause, thus shortening the amount of time you have to conceive.

If you do conceive, stopping smoking is one of the best things you can do to help ensure having a healthy pregnancy and baby. Astonishingly, 17 percent of pregnant women continue to smoke! They are putting not only themselves and their pregnancies at risk, but their babies as well. Babies born to mothers who smoke are at increased risk of being born prematurely, having low birth weight, having birth defects, and dying from Sudden Infant Death Syndrome (SIDS). Pregnant women should also make every effort to avoid secondhand smoke; research has shown that the chemicals in the smoke can reach the mother's blood and be passed on to her unborn child. It goes without saying that once the baby is born, it should be protected from exposure to all tobacco smoke.

Smoking also interferes with male fertility. It can decrease sperm production, motility, and morphology (shape). Men who smoke have sperm counts that are 15 percent lower than those of nonsmokers. Indeed, a small study published in the journal *Fertility and Sterility* found that sperm counts rose dramatically— at least 50 percent and as high as 800 percent—in men who stopped smoking. The sperm of smokers are also more likely to be abnormal and less likely to be able to fertilize an egg. Other studies confirm that quitting smoking appears to improve the sperm of men who have low sperm counts or poor quality sperm.

Avoid alcohol

Most people know by now that it's important to avoid alcohol during pregnancy because it can cause fetal alcohol syndrome. Drinking during pregnancy can also cause miscarriages, stillbirths, and preterm deliveries.

But drinking while trying to conceive can also be risky. In fact, the Surgeon General, the U.S. Department of Agriculture, the U.S. Department of Health and Human Services, the American College of Obstetricians and Gynecologists, and the American Academy of Pediatrics all recommend that women not only abstain from drinking alcohol during pregnancy but while trying to conceive as well. Some studies have found that the chances of conceiving in any given cycle decrease with increasing alcohol consumption. In one recent study in Denmark, women who drank 10 alcoholic drinks a week took significantly longer to conceive than those who drank from 1 to 5 drinks a week. Another Danish study, however, found that moderate drinking did not affect the time it takes to conceive. Moderate drinking is defined as no more than one glass of alcohol a day for women and no more than two glasses a day for men. A drink is typically defined as 5 ounces of wine, 12 ounces of beer, or 1.5 ounces of spirits.

If you do decide to drink while trying to conceive, fertility experts recommend that you drink no more than four drinks a week. Also, only drink in the first part of your menstrual cycle before you ovulate and abstain from alcohol during the second part until you menstruate. Because most women don't know precisely when they conceive, if they do drink when trying to become pregnant, they may unknowingly be putting their pregnancies and babies at risk.

Alcohol can interfere with male fertility as well. Heavy drinking in men can cause a reduction in testosterone and a decrease in the volume and density of sperm. In addition, men who drink excessively often suffer from reduced libido and erectile dysfunction. Moderate drinking, however, has not been shown to negatively affect fertility.

Do not use illicit drugs

Everyone is aware that illicit drugs such as marijuana, cocaine, amphetamines, and LSD can be dangerous to both the mother and her developing fetus. But you may not be aware that many

Watch Out!

It is estimated that as many as 60 percent of pregnant women do not discover that they are pregnant until after the first trimester. That means they are unwittingly exposing their fetuses to harm if they smoke, drink, and use certain drugs.

illicit drugs can also interfere with fertility. Marijuana, for example, can shorten a woman's menstrual cycle, thus decreasing the chances of conception.

In men, marijuana and other illicit drugs can lower sperm counts and impair sperm quality, upset hormonal balance, and even cause impotence. Anabolic steroids, especially when used nonmedically, can have serious negative effects on male fertility, causing a decrease in sperm production and sperm quality.

Limit caffeine

Most American adults consume approximately 200 mg of caffeine a day in the form of coffee, tea, soft drinks, or chocolate. There is some evidence that more than 250 mg of caffeine a day increases a woman's risk of endometriosis and tubal-factor infertility. (There are approximately 300 mg of caffeine in three cups of coffee.) Women who consume more than 500 mg of caffeine take longer to conceive than women who don't. And an intake of more than 500 mg of caffeine has also been reported to increase the risk of miscarriage. Fertility experts recommend that women who are trying to conceive limit their caffeine intake to a maximum of 250 mg a day; that is, fewer than about three 8-ounce cups of coffee a day. A cup of black or green tea typically contains less caffeine than coffee. Black tea contains the most caffeine—from 40 to 100 milligrams per cup if you steep it for five minutes—but if you steep it for three minutes it contains about half that amount. Drinking tea in moderation may actually help a woman conceive; a recent California study of 210 women found that drinking a half a cup or more of black or green tea a day doubled the rate of conception per cycle.

Bright Idea

If you steep the tea for 45 minutes, discard the water and add fresh boiling water to eliminate most of the caffeine.

Caffeine has not been found to have a detrimental effect on male fertility. On the contrary, there is some evidence that caffeine may increase sperm motility, thus increasing the chance of conception.

Be cautious when taking prescription or over-the-counter (OTC) drugs

You may have heard the horrible story of thalidomide—a sleeping pill that was also prescribed for morning sickness that caused severe birth defects in the 1960s. Other drugs also caused serious problems for pregnant women and women trying to conceive.

Diethylstilbestrol (DES), a synthetic estrogen, was prescribed until 1971 to prevent miscarriages in women who were prone to them. Some daughters of women who took DES developed vaginal or cervical cancer, and some of their sons also developed various cancers. Ironically, both the male and female offspring of DES mothers are also at increased risk of having fertility problems themselves. Some DES daughters have suffered from a wide range of cervical, uterine, and tubal abnormalities. Any one of these can prevent conception or lead to ectopic pregnancy, miscarriage, or premature labor. And some DES sons have had undescended testes, a condition in which the testes have not descended normally into the scrotum during fetal development. They have also had diminished sperm production, and cysts and obstructions in their reproductive organs that cause fertility problems. If you think your mother may have taken DES while pregnant, be sure to tell your doctor.

Some currently used drugs have been linked to severe birth defects; these include Accutane, an acne medicine; Tegison;

and Soriatane. The last two drugs—which are used to treat psoriasis—can even be harmful in women if taken up to three years *before* conception.

Many of the drugs used to treat hypertension—including calcium channel blockers and beta-blockers—can have a negative impact on male fertility, causing a decrease in sperm production, libido, and erectile function. Other prescription drugs, especially those used to treat depression, other psychiatric problems, and seizures—such as lithium, Compazine, and Dilantin—have also caused erectile and ejaculatory problems, or other fertility problems. If these or any other drugs are prescribed to you, be sure to tell your doctor that you are trying to start a family. With your doctor's assistance, you can weigh the risks and benefits of the prescribed medication.

OTC drugs may also be risky to take if you're trying to conceive (or are pregnant). Drugs such as NoDoz, Excedrin, and Anacin contain caffeine, and as mentioned earlier, caffeine can cause problems with conception and pregnancy. Since there are many other drugs that can be risky to take, be sure to read the labels and patient materials carefully. Be sure to tell your doctor at your preconception exam what prescription and OTC drugs you are taking.

Be careful about using herbal teas or supplements

Plants and herbs form the basis of many of the traditional prescription and over-the-counter medicines. But just because they're natural doesn't mean they're safe. Some of these plants or herbs—which are also sold as herbal teas and supplements—have been found to interfere with conception and/or be harmful to a pregnancy or developing fetus. Herbal supplements and medicines are not tested for safety nor regulated in the same way as prescription and over-the-counter drugs. Nor are the doses and formulations standardized. And while you may assume herbal teas are safe and better for you than black tea, that's not always true. Drinking a lot of peppermint or red raspberry leaf tea, for example, may cause miscarriages and other problems, while black tea may actually enhance fertility.

A recent study found evidence that taking large amounts of gingko biloba, echinacea, and St. John's Wort could cause damage to reproductive cells and hinder the ability of sperm to fertilize eggs. Also, St. John's Wort was shown to cause mutations in sperm cells.

In addition, more than 500 plants have been linked to miscarriages or birth defects. Approximately 50 are commonly consumed in the United States. Some of the more popular ones that have been linked to problems in pregnancy include the following (for a more complete list, check the March of Dimes website at: www.modimes.org):

Barberry	Golden seal
Black cohosh	Juniper
Blue cohosh	Mandrake
Donq quai	Pennyroyal
Ephedra	Peppermint
Feverfew	Senna
Kava kava	Uva-ursi
Ginseng	Wormwood

Unfortunately, the precise amounts of these herbs that cause problems are either unknown or unavailable. So, to be on the safe side, it's probably best to avoid them altogether. If you do want to take herbs or drink herbal tea, be sure to discuss it with your doctor first—and definitely avoid taking or drinking large amounts.

 Bright Idea

Make a list of all prescription drugs, over-the-counter drugs, herbal teas, and supplements you are taking or would like to take. Bring the list to your doctor and write down his or her comments about each drug.

Eat a healthy diet

Two of the key ingredients in disease prevention are eating a healthy diet and maintaining a healthy weight. The U.S. government has just issued new dietary guidelines. Following these guidelines can help ensure that you eat nutritious meals and either maintain or achieve a healthy weight.

Maintain a healthy weight

Being either overweight or underweight can interfere with fertility. One of the best ways to determine if you are over- or underweight is by evaluating your Body Mass Index (BMI). BMI is your weight in kilograms divided by your height in meters squared (kg/m^2). If math is not your thing, don't panic! Check out the BMI tables at www.asrm.org/Patients/FactSheets/weightfertility.pdf and www.consumer.gov/weightloss/bmi.htm; they've already done the math and metric conversions for you.

Another good measure is body fat or skinfold thickness, but it requires the use of a caliper by a health-care provider or in a gym. Body fat is measured in percentages; normal body fat is between 22 and 25 percent for women, and 15 to 18 percent for men.

If you're overweight, lose weight

Extra weight in a woman can increase insulin levels, which may cause the ovaries to overproduce male hormones and stop releasing eggs. Being overweight also contributes to the development of diabetes, a risk factor for infertility. Fat can also

Table 1.1: Interpreting BMI	
BMI	**Weight Status**
Below 18.5 kg/m^2	Underweight
18.5 - 24.9 kg/m^2	Normal
25.0 - 29.9 kg/m^2	Overweight
30.0 and above kg/m^2	Obese

Dietary Guidelines for Americans, 2005

- Consume a sufficient amount of fruits and vegetables while staying within energy needs. Two cups of fruit and 2½ cups of vegetables per day are recommended for a reference 2,000-calorie intake, with higher or lower amounts depending on the calorie level.

- Choose a variety of fruits and vegetables each day. In particular, select from all five vegetable subgroups (dark green, orange, legumes, starchy vegetables, and other vegetables) several times a week.

- Consume three or more ounce-equivalents of whole-grain products per day, with the rest of the recommended grains coming from enriched or whole-grain products. In general, at least half the grains should come from whole grains.

- Consume three cups per day of fat-free or low-fat milk or equivalent milk products.

FATS

- Consume less than 10 percent of calories from saturated fatty acids and less than 300 mg/day of cholesterol, and keep trans fatty acid consumption as low as possible.

produce hormone changes, which can affect ovulation in women and sperm production in men.

Women with a BMI over 27 kg/m² or those whose body fat levels are 10 to 15 percent above normal may be at increased risk of anovulatory infertility and miscarriage. Those with a BMI of over 30 may have polycystic ovarian syndrome, a serious risk factor for infertility. Obese women are at high risk for many serious pregnancy complications such as gestational diabetes

- Keep total fat intake between 20 and 35 percent of calories, with most fats coming from sources of polyunsaturated and monounsaturated fatty acids, such as fish, nuts, and vegetable oils.

- When selecting and preparing meat, poultry, dry beans, and milk or milk products, make choices that are lean, low-fat, or fat-free.

- Limit intake of fats and oils high in saturated and/or trans fatty acids, and choose products low in such fats and oils.

CARBOHYDRATES

- Choose fiber-rich fruits, vegetables, and whole grains often.

- Choose and prepare foods and beverages with few added sugars or caloric sweeteners, such as amounts suggested by the USDA Food Guide and the DASH Eating Plan.

- Reduce the incidence of dental caries by practicing good oral hygiene and consuming sugar- and starch-containing foods and beverages less frequently.

and preeclampsia, a potentially deadly condition that is one of the leading causes of maternal and infant mortality. Obesity during pregnancy can also increase the risk of miscarriage and birth defects in babies. Do not, however, crash diet! Sudden weight loss can cause hormonal imbalances, which may in turn cause infertility.

A recent study found that men who have high BMIs (over 25) are at increased risk of infertility due to DNA fragmentation in their sperm. The higher the weight, the greater the reduction in sperm quality. The study found that the partners of overweight men not only had a decreased chance of conception, those who did become pregnant were at increased risk of miscarriage. The problems were most pronounced in men with a BMI of over 30.

If you're underweight, try to put on some weight

Women with BMIs under 17 kg/m² or whose body fat levels are 10 to 15 percent below normal are at increased risk of anovulatory infertility. Anorectic and bulimic women are at especially high risk of having fertility problems.

Exercise in moderation

Everyone knows that exercise and being physically fit is good for you. Exercise and maintaining a healthy weight go hand in hand. As we've seen, being overweight can hinder your chance of conceiving, and exercise is one of the best ways to keep weight down. While exercise itself won't help you conceive, it will keep your heart healthy and your blood pressure down, both especially important for a healthy pregnancy.

On the other hand, too much exercise can interfere with fertility. For example, women athletes and women who engage in very vigorous sports or activities such as marathon running are predisposed to menstrual irregularities and may have trouble conceiving.

Take appropriate vitamins and supplements

Folic acid—one of the B vitamins—is not only important for the health of the mother, it is essential to the health of the developing fetus. Folic acid contributes to the neural tube development in early pregnancy and inadequate amounts can lead to serious neurological and spinal birth defects. It's recommended, therefore, that women of childbearing age have a minimum of 400 micrograms (.4mg) of folic acid daily. Although many foods contain folic acid—such as whole wheat grains, brown rice, fortified cereals, oranges, spinach, and beans—it's often difficult to get an adequate amount through diet. To be safe, it's recommended that all women who are planning to conceive start talking folic acid supplements three months before they start trying to conceive and for at least the first three months of pregnancy.

Other essential vitamins and minerals include iron and vitamin A. But make certain you do not take more that 5,000 units of vitamin A each day.

Vegetarians should be especially careful to make certain they are receiving adequate nutrition from their diet or supplements. If they don't have adequate amounts of zinc, iron, vitamin B-12, and folic acid, they may have trouble conceiving or increase their chances of having a baby with birth defects. A recent pilot study, published in the *Journal of Reproductive Medicine,* found a nutritional supplement containing green tea extracts, chasteberry, folic acid, and other vitamins and minerals to be promising in improving fertility in women. Larger studies are needed to definitively determine if this supplement does indeed enhance fertility.

Men should also consider taking vitamin supplements, especially zinc. However, too much zinc can be toxic. Between 15 and 30 mg is considered safe for both men and women; anything above that amount can be dangerous.

 Moneysaver

Rather than take separate supplements, look for a multivitamin that contains all you need in one pill. Some companies make prenatal vitamins, which may or may not be less expensive than regular multivitamins. Compare prices and ingredients. You might also think about buying these at warehouse stores that usually have cheaper prices.

Watch Out!

Men should avoid wearing jockey shorts and tight pants because they can overheat the testes and interfere with sperm production. Boxer shorts and loose-fitting pants are better choices for future fathers.

Avoid hot tubs, saunas, and Jacuzzis

Excessively high temperatures can cause neural tube defects in the developing fetus during the first trimester, when many women don't realize they're pregnant. The high temperatures can also interfere with sperm production. STDs have also been linked to hot tubs, saunas, and Jacuzzis.

Avoid hazardous chemicals and radiation

There are many toxic chemicals and environmental hazards in the home and workplace that can interfere with fertility, as well as cause miscarriages and birth defects. Solvents, pesticides, and heavy metals (such as lead and cadmium) have all been linked to reproductive problems in men and women. Exposure to these substances should be avoided if possible. Nurses who mix chemotherapeutic agents, for example, have almost a twofold increase in the chance of having a miscarriage. If you must use chemicals, make certain you're in a well-ventilated area. Exposure to radiation can also reduce fertility in both sexes and can be hazardous to a growing fetus. If you must have dental or any other X-rays, be sure to tell your doctor, dentist, or radiologist that you're trying to conceive. Make sure he or she gives you a lead apron to wear to protect your reproductive organs.

Age and fertility

Age has adverse effects on fertility in both sexes, but more so in women. In general, the longer a woman waits to try to become pregnant, the longer it will take her. The optimal time for a woman to conceive is from her mid to late 20s. However, many women in their 20s may not be married, or they may be busy pursuing their education or careers, or they just may not yet feel ready to start their families.

Fertility in older women

Fertility in women starts declining significantly after age 30, and even more rapidly after 35. A woman under 30 has about a 20 percent chance of conceiving each month. By the time she reaches 40, her chances of conceiving drop to only 5 percent each month. Approximately one in three women aged 35 or older will have a fertility problem. By age 40, two out of three women will be infertile. Older women are also significantly more likely to have miscarriages, as well as babies with birth defects.

Why is this? After age 30, hormone levels start declining and egg production starts to deteriorate. At birth, a female has as many eggs as she will ever have in her lifetime—over a million. By the time a girl reaches puberty, she has about 300,000 left, and only 300 of those will ever be ovulated. The older a woman is, the older her eggs, and older eggs are not as fertilizable as young eggs. Because they've been around for a lifetime, they've had decades of exposure to various adverse elements—viruses, X-rays, drugs, and environmental toxins. As a result, older eggs are much more likely to carry chromosomal abnormalities that can cause such disorders as Down syndrome. In addition, older

Table 1.2: How Maternal Age Affects Pregnancy Rate		
Age	**Cumulative Pregnancy Rate**	**Monthly Pregnancy Rate**
Under 30	74	10.5
31 to 35	61	9.1
Over 35	54	6.5

Source: E. H. Illinions, M. T. Valley, and A. M. Kaunitz, "Infertility: A Clinical Guide For The Internist." *Med Clin N. Am.* 1998; 82(2): 271-291.

Table 1.3: Percentage of Pregnancies Ending in Miscarriage, by Age

Age of Woman at Pregnancy	Percentage Ending In Miscarriage
Under 35 years	10 to 12
Between 35 and 39	18
Between 40 and 44	34
45 or over	>50

Source: P. R. Gindoff and R. Jewelewicz. "Reproductive Potential in the Older Woman." *Fertility and Sterility.* 1986; 46: 989.

women may not be in as good physical health as younger women. The older you are, the greater the chance that you've had a serious illness—such as an STD, diabetes, thyroid disease, or hypertension—that can interfere with your fertility and your ability to carry the child to full term.

Fertility in older men

Fertility in men also decreases with age, although not as dramatically as for women. Starting at about age 25, sperm cell production starts decreasing. And the sperm that are produced tend to have decreased mobility, thus hindering their ability to reach and fertilize an egg. Men over the age of 35 are twice as likely as men under 25 to take more than a year to impregnate their partners.

One reason may be that older couples tend to have sex less often than younger couples. As men grow older, they tend to have lower levels of testosterone. This in turn affects their sexual drive as well as their ability to achieve and maintain an erection, which, of course, can affect their ability to impregnate their partners. Older men are also more likely to have medical conditions, such as atherosclerosis (hardening of the arteries) or diabetes, which can impair sexual ability.

Age and problem pregnancies

Aging can cause genetic mutations in the sperm cells, potentially leading to genetic defects in their offspring as well as miscarriages. Indeed, pregnant women who are 35 or older with male partners over the age of 40 have a significantly increased risk of miscarriages.

Regardless of the age of the father, if conception does occur, the age of the mother has serious implications for the outcome of a pregnancy. Not only does the chance of conceiving decrease the older one gets, the chance of miscarriage increases as well. This may be due to the various medical conditions such as those mentioned earlier, or to genetic problems in the embryo. Miscarriage is a relatively common occurrence, as you can see from the previous table.

> 66 One of the reasons for getting married was because we both wanted to have children...but it was very important for me...to really have my career in place. It was a question of priorities and doing things that I felt were very important before I really became serious about being a mother. 99
>
> —Diane, 38

Older women are also at increased risk of having stillborn babies, low-birth-weight babies, premature deliveries, and Caesarian sections. As a result, their babies are at increased risk for serious health problems. Babies of older women are also at risk for having genetic or congenital problems. But if you're older, don't despair. The good news is that the majority of older women who do carry a pregnancy to full term give birth to healthy babies.

 Bright Idea

If you're over 35, you and your partner should make appointments as soon as possible for your preconception checkups. You should also start your search for an OB/GYN who is experienced in working with older pregnant women.

Preserving your fertility

If you're in your 20s or 30s and for some reason you must delay childbearing, you need to do everything you can now to preserve your fertility. Doing so involves following all the earlier advice in this chapter about being screened for medical disorders, being immunized against potentially serious diseases, and choosing a healthy lifestyle. There are also other options available such as embryo freezing, which we'll touch on in an upcoming section.

Cancer and fertility preservation

Approximately 100,000 women and men of reproductive age are diagnosed with cancer each year. Many of these men and women want to start families or have more children. They may be concerned that their cancer and cancer treatment will affect their ability to procreate. The bad news is that chemotherapy, radiation therapy, and some surgical treatments for cancer (and some other serious medical conditions) can cause temporary infertility or permanent sterility. Even if their fertility is unaffected by cancer or its treatment, especially chemotherapy, women may be advised to delay getting pregnant for several years, when the greatest chance of recurrence will have passed. The good news is that there are steps that can be taken prior to and even after treatment to enhance a cancer patient's chance of becoming a biological mother or father.

If you have been diagnosed with cancer and will be undergoing surgery, chemotherapy, or radiation, talk to your oncologist about your concerns regarding your future fertility. Also, make an appointment with a reproductive endocrinologist or fertility specialist (also called an "infertility specialist"; see Chapter 5) who can work with you and your oncologist and other doctors you will be seeing over the course of your treatment.

There are many things both men and women can do to preserve their fertility.

Moneysaver

If you have to have extensive abdominal surgery for any reason, consider harvesting your eggs for use at a future time. It may save you the cost of infertility treatment.

Embryo freezing (cryopreservation)

Before cancer treatment, a woman can undergo *in-vitro fertilization* (IVF); this involves removing her eggs and having them fertilized by her partner's or donor's sperm. The resulting embryos are then frozen and stored until the woman is ready to have them implanted in her, or in a surrogate's uterus, if necessary.

Oocyte (egg) freezing

Still considered experimental, oocyte (egg) freezing is similar to embryo freezing except that the eggs are frozen before they're fertilized. Theoretically, the frozen unfertilized eggs can be thawed at a later date and subsequently fertilized by a partner's or donor's sperm. Unfortunately, previously frozen and thawed eggs are not easily fertilizable and, to date, very few pregnancies have resulted from this technology.

Ovarian transplantation

The only other option currently available for women who want to preserve their eggs before cancer or other medical treatment involving surgery, chemotherapy, or radiation therapy is ovarian transplantation. This is a new but experimental technology in which ovarian tissue is transplanted to another part of the body. Recently, the *Journal of the American Medical Association* (JAMA) reported a study of two women; one had to undergo pelvic radiation and the other had to have her ovaries removed. Prior to treatment, they both had strips of their ovarian tissue removed and transplanted to their forearms! Ten weeks after the transplants, these women resumed production of ovarian hormones and development of egg follicles in their forearms. Indeed, one of the women actually ovulated from her upper arm! This past year, the journal *Cancer* reported another successful case of ovarian autotransplantation to the upper arm. And in June 2005, *JAMA* reported the first successful case of a woman who gave birth after receiving an ovarian tissue transplant from her identical twin sister.

Sperm freezing

Cancer or its treatment can cause infertility or sterility in men. Unlike eggs, sperm can be successfully frozen and thawed for future use. Any man undergoing cancer treatment who wants to father a child should have his sperm frozen unless there is some medical, personal, or religious reason not to do so.

Laparoscopic radical vaginal trachelectomy (LRVT)

This is a new fertility-preserving technique for women with early-stage cervical cancer who have very small tumors confined to the cervix. In LRVT, only part of the cervix is removed, thus increasing the woman's chances of conceiving. However, the surgeon can't determine which women are appropriate candidates for LRVT until surgery is underway. Also, this technique is not available in all medical centers. Still, LRVT holds great promise for young women with cervical cancer. Previously the only options for these women were hysterectomies, radiation, and/or chemotherapy—all of which have typically resulted in sterility.

Some of these techniques, which are also used to treat infertile patients who do not have cancer, and how to find a fertility specialist are described in greater detail in upcoming chapters.

If you have or had cancer, you may want to check out www.fertilehope.org. Fertile Hope is a nonprofit organization that provides information about issues related to fertility and cancer. The American Society for Reproductive Medicine (ASRM) at www.asrm.org and the American Cancer Society (ACS) at www.cancer.org are also good sources of information about cancer treatment and pregnancy.

Moneysaver

Check to see if either of your employers offers pregnancy and adoption benefits such as maternity and paternity leave. Also, it's a good idea that you both have life and disability insurance, and a will.

Pursuing pregnancy after cancer treatment

Many cancer patients also fear that if they do conceive, it will cause the cancer to recur or even spread. Most studies, however, demonstrate that pregnancy after cancer treatment is not detrimental to the mother. Indeed, one study published in *The American Journal of Obstetrics and Gynecology* found the risk of death for women under the age of 40 treated for breast cancer was almost five times *lower* in women who became pregnant compared with cancer patients who did *not* become pregnant. The researchers attributed these results to the "healthy mother effect," a phenomenon in which only the healthiest breast cancer survivors become pregnant and give birth. Other more recent studies published in *The Journal of Clinical Oncology* and *Cancer* also found increased survival rates and a reduced risk of breast cancer recurrence in women who had become pregnant compared with those who did not experience a pregnancy. Some of the researchers speculated these results may not only reflect "healthy mother effect," but also the protective, antitumor effect that pregnancy is believed to confer.

Cancer patients may also be worried that if they have their own biological child, they may have a problem pregnancy or their child will be born with serious problems, including cancer. Breast cancer survivors, in fact, do have an increased risk of miscarriage. This may be the result of hormonal changes caused by the cancer treatment rather than the cancer. However, the good news is there appears to be no increase in birth defects in the children of male or female cancer patients who have undergone treatment for cancer.

If there are any reasons why a cancer patient should avoid a pregnancy, she always has the option of pursuing third-party reproduction including embryo-, egg-, and sperm donation as well as surrogacy and adoption. These options are discussed in Chapters 11 and 12.

The road to pregnancy

Starting a family is a big decision. As with many things in life, taking the time to prepare will be enormously worthwhile in the end. These have been just a few of the steps you should take on the road to pregnancy and a healthy baby. Now the fun—or some may say work—begins. The next chapter explains what is physiologically necessary for conception to take place, and what some of the hurdles are that you and your partner might encounter along the way.

Just the facts

- Both women and men should have preconception exams at least three months before trying to conceive.
- Commit to a healthy lifestyle before you try and conceive a baby.
- Men as well as women become less fertile as they grow older.
- Older women who are able to conceive have a higher risk of miscarriages and other problems.
- There are several options available to men and women who wish to preserve their fertility.
- Many cancer patients can have healthy pregnancies and babies following treatment.

Conception and Misconceptions

Chapter 2

U nderstanding human reproduction and the process of conception will be extremely helpful to you in your pursuit of pregnancy. A knowledge of the male and female reproductive systems will not only help you be better able to talk more confidently and comfortably with your doctor about fertility-related issues, it can save you lots of confusion, anxiety, time, and even money. You'll also be in a better position to dispel the common myths and misconceptions you're likely to be bombarded with from well-meaning friends and family members.

Reproduction 101

Contrary to what you might think, most couples do not conceive the minute they start trying. In fact, the average healthy young couple who has regular sexual intercourse has only about a 20 percent chance of conceiving each month. That's why it takes most young couples about five or six months to conceive their first child, and why it takes older couples—who have a lower chance of conceiving each month—even longer.

Bright Idea

Go over this section on male and female reproduction with your partner. It's important for both of you to understand each other's reproductive system.

Although having sex at the right time of the month is a prerequisite for getting pregnant, there's a lot more that must happen at the right time and in the right manner for conception to occur. You may think you learned everything there is to know about making babies from those late night chats with your highschool girlfriends or from your locker-room buddies. If you're like most of us, you learned more myth than reality—and probably more about how *not* to get pregnant than about getting pregnant. If you've forgotten what you learned in high school biology class—or just didn't pay much attention—it's a good idea to review the facts about what it really takes to conceive. Conception is not a simple process but a multiple-step, multifaceted process. At any point, one or more elements may not be working up to par—or may not be functioning at all.

For conception to occur, three key factors must be in place:

1. A well-functioning female reproductive system

2. A well-functioning male reproductive system

3. Effective sexual practices

The female reproductive system

Visualized from the lower portion of the female body, the main parts of a woman's reproductive system are the *vagina* (the lowermost segment), *cervix, uterus, Fallopian tubes,* and *ovaries* (the uppermost segment). These highly specialized structures have some common features:

▪ Some structures—such as the vagina and cervix—produce mucus, a substance that—depending on its consistency— can either facilitate or interfere with conception.

■ Some—such as the uterus and Fallopian tubes—contract or undulate rhythmically, serving to move cells and tissues along the reproductive tract.

■ Others—such as the ovaries—release hormones at specific times during a woman's menstrual cycle, as well as produce eggs.

Vagina

This lower structure of the female reproductive system is a long, tube-like vault. The vaginal membranes secrete a mucus that keeps the vaginal tissue soft and slippery, facilitating intercourse.

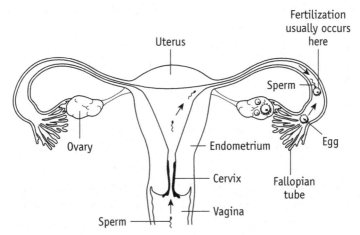

The female reproductive system after sexual intercourse. On entering the female reproductive system, sperm follow the direction of the arrows shown in the figure.

Cervix

At the end of the vagina is a small, circular area called the cervix, which leads into the uterus, or womb. The cervix has several purposes:

■ It helps protect the uterus and other reproductive organs against invasion by bacteria, fungi, and viruses.

- During menstruation, the endometrial lining of the uterus is shed and expelled through the cervix.

- It's through the cervix that sperm enter the uterus as they try to swim up to the Fallopian tubes.

- During childbirth, the cervix dilates to allow the fetus to pass through its uppermost portion, the birth canal.

The cervix also produces mucus, which, as you will learn more about later, changes consistency throughout the menstrual cycle. During most of the cycle, when a woman's not fertile, a small amount of very thick cervical mucus is present. This consistency tends to trap sperm, blocking them from entering the uterus easily. But that's okay. No eggs are yet available to be fertilized anyway. In contrast, cervical mucus becomes watery and abundant during ovulation. This helps sperm swim more easily through it and up into the uterus and Fallopian tubes, on their journey to a mature egg.

Uterus

Located within the protection of the woman's pelvis, the uterus is thick-walled and muscular. It resembles an inverted sack. It is here that a fertilized egg normally implants itself in the uterine lining, is nourished, and matures for nine months until labor and delivery. During labor, the uterus contracts rhythmically and powerfully to move the fetus out of the womb into the birth canal and out through the dilated cervix and vagina. During menstruation, the uterus also contracts, though less violently, to expel the unfertilized egg and shed endometrial tissue.

 Moneysaver

If you have attempted pregnancy more than three months without success, at mid-cycle you can use Robitussin or another similar over-the-counter cough syrup that contains expectorants. Expectorants can improve the quality of your cervical mucus at a fraction of the cost of fertility drugs. But make certain the expectorant doesn't contain an antihistamine that can dry out the mucus, making matters worse. A good rule: If it dries out your nose, it will dry out your vagina.

The position of the uterus is described by the direction in which it leans inside the pelvis. In 80 percent of women, the uterus leans forward—this is called an *anteverted* uterus. If the uterus leans forward but bends in upon itself, it is called *antiflexed.* Sometimes a woman is told she has a *tipped* uterus. This merely means that her uterus tends to tilt backward toward her spine. A tipped uterus is also known as a *retroverted* uterus. When it is tipped backward but bends in upon itself, it's called *retroflexed.* It's not unusual to have a tipped uterus, and it doesn't necessarily mean that you can't conceive, as some old wives' tales suggest.

> **❝**I'm very voluptuous and I got my period when I was eleven. I never skipped a period. Everything about my biological system seemed to work according to the textbook. So that the concept of it not obeying me...never entered my mind. **❞**
>
> —Bonnie, 29

The walls of the uterus are lined with tissue called the *endometrium,* which responds to hormone changes throughout the menstrual cycle. It is the endometrium that sheds and sloughs off during menstruation.

Fallopian tubes

On each side of the uterus is a long, muscular structure called the Fallopian tube or oviduct, which serves as a conduit for the passage of eggs to the uterus. Each part of the Fallopian tube is lined with cells covered with microscopic hairlike projections—called *cilia*—that move in a wavelike manner to help guide the eggs through the tubes. The ends of the Fallopian tubes are delicate, funnel-shaped structures called *fimbria* that catch the eggs as they are expelled from the ovaries.

The Fallopian tube lining itself produces a nutritive medium to nourish the eggs. Both the contractions of the Fallopian wall and the beating of the cilia move a fertilized egg to the uterus for implantation.

Ovaries

Last but certainly not least are the all-important ovaries. These olive-sized and -shaped structures, found just beneath the Fallopian tubes and to each side of the uterus, contain eggs, each called an *ovum.* Every egg is actually housed in a bubble-like structure called a follicle. Each month, several eggs mature and normally one is released from its follicle. Most women have two ovaries, but if a woman only has one, the other takes over the monthly menstrual cycle functions.

Female hormones

Menstruation, ovulation, fertilization, conception, and, if successful, labor, are elegantly orchestrated by the rise and fall of hormone levels. The human body, whether male or female, houses many different glands that produce a wide variety of hormones. Traveling through the bloodstream to special target tissues, hormones act as chemical messengers to regulate the myriad bodily functions, from blood pressure control and thyroid function to urine output, and, of course, fertility. If you aren't already, you should become knowledgeable about the different female and male hormones.

GnRH

The menstrual cycle begins as signals are sent from the *hypothalamus,* a specialized area just above the *pituitary gland* at the base of the brain. Every 60 to 90 minutes, the hypothalamus pumps out a hormone called *gonadotropin-releasing hormone (GnRH)* for about one minute. GnRH stimulates the pituitary glands above it to release two more hormones, *follicle-stimulating hormone (FSH)* and *luteinizing hormone (LH).*

FSH and LH

Called *gonadotropin hormones* and produced by the pituitary, FSH is critical during the first half of the menstrual cycle, called the *follicular phase,* and LH is critical during the second half, called the *luteal phase.*

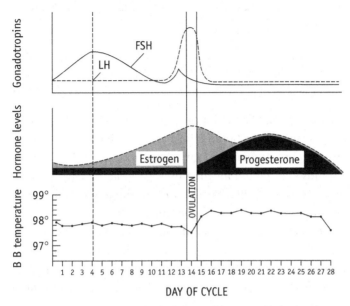

During a normal menstrual cycle, the balance of four reproductive hormones shifts, reflecting changes in the body's body temperature.

The first day of a woman's menstrual period signals Day 1 of a new menstrual cycle. On that day, the pituitary releases FSH, which signals the ovaries to increase production of the major female hormone, estrogen. Under the influence of estrogen, the uterine lining, or endometrium, enters a proliferative phase; that is, it grows and thickens in preparation for implantation by the fertilized egg.

As its name implies, FSH causes several follicles—which house the eggs—in the ovaries to develop and ripen. By Day 7, one of the follicles begins to grow rapidly. The others lag behind and are eventually absorbed by the body.

By Day 14 of an ideal 28-day cycle, LH begins to take over. There is a sudden, dramatic rise in LH levels, called the *LH surge,* which culminates in ovulation. During the surge, LH helps stimulate several important follicular functions. Like every cell in the human body, the egg cell has 46 chromosomes—strands of

Watch Out!

Don't wait until you think you're ovulating to have sex, because you may ovulate sooner than you think. And no sex means no sperm to fertilize the egg.

genetic material. The LH surge prepares the egg cell to expel half of its chromosomes. Sperm, the male reproductive cells, also each have 46 chromosomes to start. They, too, must shed half their chromosomes before meeting up with a mature egg. In this way, the fertilized egg will have a full complement of chromosomes—half from the egg and half from the sperm.

LH also helps ripen the follicle further, causing it to rupture and release a mature egg. The ovum, or egg, is expelled from the follicle on the ovary, grabbed by the fimbria at the end of the Fallopian tube, and journeys down the narrow Fallopian tube on the road to possible fertilization.

Progesterone

LH then signals the remnant of the newly ovulated follicle that has just released an egg to become a sort of endocrine gland, the *corpus luteum.* LH tells the corpus luteum to produce another major female sex hormone, progesterone. Like estrogen, progesterone targets the uterine tissue lining.

When it reaches the uterus, progesterone prompts the lining to undergo a change that enables it to support and nourish a newly fertilized egg. This preparation of the uterine lining takes approximately five days, the same time it takes for a fertilized egg to reach the cavity of the uterus.

Estrogen

Estrogen is the major female sex hormone and is responsible for sex characteristics such as skin texture, hair distribution, and body contour. During the first half of the menstrual cycle—that is, the half prior to ovulation—this ovarian hormone stimulates the endometrium (uterine wall) to become lushly supplied with blood. In the second half of the cycle following ovulation, progesterone is produced. This hormone, too, acts on the endometrium, increasing the growth of secretory cells, which are needed for a new life to grow in the uterus.

In other words, estrogen grows the uterine lining. Progesterone makes it soft and spongy to support the life of an embryo to latch onto the endometrium. Estrogen also increases the amount and changes the consistency of cervical mucus. At approximately Day 14 of the menstrual cycle, estrogen causes cervical mucus production to increase and the mucus to become thinner.

If pregnancy does not occur, the corpus luteum degenerates and progesterone production ceases after 14 days. Estrogen production tapers off during the second or luteal phase of the menstrual cycle. Deprived of hormonal support, the top layer of the endometrium begins to pull away from the uterine wall. No longer able to maintain this state of anticipation or preparation for a fertilized egg, the uterine lining crumbles and sloughs off. Rhythmic uterine contractions expel the built-up blood, the extra growth of the uterine lining, and the disintegrated egg. This is the menstrual discharge that flows through the cervix into the vagina over a three-to-five-day period, marking the end of one reproductive cycle and the beginning of another.

HCG

If pregnancy occurs and the fertilized egg starts implanting in the uterine wall, the early pregnancy begins to produce *human*

 Bright Idea

If you're in your late 30s or older, it may be a good idea to have a complete hormone evaluation now. It may save you precious time later.

chorionic gonadotropin (HCG). HCG is usually produced only when a fertilized egg reaches the implantation stage. Sometimes called the "pregnancy hormone," HCG is necessary to support a pregnancy. In fact, it's the HCG that "switches off" the menstrual cycle and ensures that no more eggs are produced during the pregnancy.

The male reproductive system

The male reproductive system—like the female reproductive system—has both external and internal parts. For the male, however, the major parts on the outside are the *testes, scrotum, epididymis,* and *penis*. On the inside are the *seminal vesicles, vas deferens,* and *prostate*. And, unlike the female's eggs that stay secure in the inner sanctum of the upper reproductive organs, the male's sperm journeys from parts in the external organs, into the internal organs, and finally out an external organ.

The testes or testicles

The testes are the main male sex glands. These sperm- and testosterone-producing factories are housed in a sac, called the scrotum, which lies below and slightly to either side of the penis. The testes contain hundreds of tightly coiled microscopic tubules called *seminiferous tubules*. It is here that sperm are produced, though they are not yet able to fertilize an egg. Testes hang in a sac away from the body and are two to four degrees cooler than the normal body temperature; the cooler temperature is necessary for sperm production.

Epididymis

After production in the testes, sperm, bathed in testicular fluid, leave the testicles and enter the epididymis. The epididymis is a 15-foot-long, tightly coiled cluster of microscopic tubes attached to a testicle. Here the sperm stay about two weeks, during which time they develop the ability to swim.

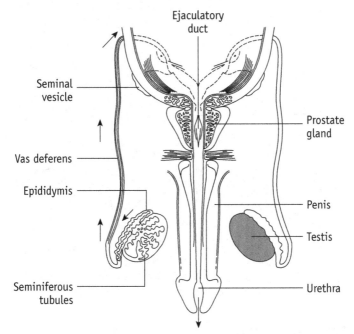

The male reproductive system. During ejaculation, sperm follow the direction indicated by the arrows in the diagram.

Vas deferens

Once mature, sperm are propelled by contractions to the end of the epididymis near an internal structure called the vas deferens. The vas deferens is also a tubal structure. It connects the epididymis with two other male sex glands, the seminal vesicles and the prostate. Both glands produce semen, which mixes with the sperm. Sperm and seminal fluid are stored in the vas deferens, awaiting their entrance to the urethra and out to the penis during orgasm and ejaculation.

Penis

It is through the urethra, which runs the length of the penis, that semen-containing sperm are ejaculated during orgasm.

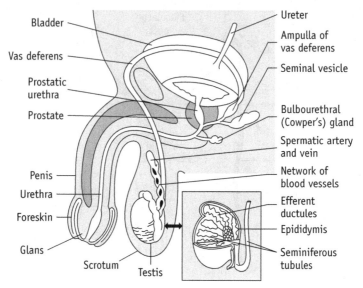

The male reproductive system, side view showing internal genitalia.

Male hormones

Male hormones are responsible for the all-important task of sperm production and release (ejaculation).

The male reproductive system falls under the influence of several hormones, generally called *androgens*. Just as estrogens are primary female sex hormones, androgens are the major male sex hormones. In truth, however, both sexes have both types of hormones. It's just that one plays a predominant role while the other plays a minor role.

Androgens play a significant role, starting with puberty when they become responsible for a young man's growth of pubic and facial hair, a lowering of his voice, the growth of his muscles, and a surge in his sex drive.

Androgens also play a major role in sperm production. The most important androgen for male reproduction is *testosterone*.

Testosterone

Produced in the testes, testosterone—as the primary male sex hormone—is responsible for the characteristics of the male body, including skin texture, hair distribution, voice quality, and sex drive. Along with FSH, testosterone helps stimulate *spermatogenesis*, the production of sperm. Three key hormones are necessary for the production of testosterone: *GnRH, FSH, and LH.* The latter two are known as *gonadatropins,* these hormones probably sound familiar to you. That's because they all play a major role in female reproduction and were described earlier in this chapter.

Gonadotropin-releasing hormone (GnRH)

GnRH starts the process of testosterone production. It is secreted by in the hypothalamus and then released to the pituitary gland, where it produces LH and FSH.

Luteneizing hormone (LH)

LH, which is secreted by the pituitary gland, stimulates the production of testosterone in the testes.

Follicle-stimulating hormone (FSH)

FSH is also secreted by the pituitary gland and is necessary for testosterone production. Along with testosterone, it stimulates the production of sperm in the testes. FSH also plays a key role in the maturation of sperm.

Sperm: Their production and release

As we've mentioned, hormones in the testes are also responsible for sperm production. Each minute of the day, approximately 50,000 new sperm are produced inside the tubules in the testicles. They start off as germ cells—precursors of sperm. During a process called meiosis, the germ cells go through a series of changes, or cellular and chromosomal divisions, on their way to becoming mature. One dramatic change is in their shape—from round cells to the tadpole-like shape of mature sperm. Once the

Watch Out!

If a man has had an infection, flu, or other serious illness in the past few months, it can temporarily render him infertile. The good news is that usually, new, healthy sperm will once again be produced. The bad news? It will take almost three months for sperm to replenish itself.

sperm cells have divided, they start to mature. Only when sperm mature completely are they capable of fertilizing an egg.

The whole process of sperm formation and maturation takes about 72 days. Sperm are stored in the epididydmis where they wait until a man ejaculates. It takes about 40 hours for the epididymis to become restocked with mature sperm after ejaculation.

The journey toward conception

Although only a single sperm is needed to fertilize an egg, about 300 million sperm are released with each ejaculation. Such large numbers are released to ensure that a high percentage of normally shaped, mobile sperm are able to swim fast enough up to meet with an egg as it moves down the Fallopian tube. The sperm actually travel in a relatively straight line up the vagina, through the cervix, into the uterine cavity, and finally into the Fallopian tube and hopefully into the welcoming arms of a mature ovum. This process can take anywhere from about 45 minutes to 12 hours. Sperm are actually carried through the Fallopian tubes by contraction of the tube muscles and the beating of the tubal cilia, as well as the movement of the sperm themselves. The chance of conception is diminished considerably if a man doesn't have millions of normally shaped, fast-moving sperm. The good news is that recent medical advances have helped men with low, or even very low, sperm counts to produce children. This is discussed in Chapter 9.

Despite this enormous, mobile army, only a few hundred or thousand sperm reach the Fallopian tube where the egg or eggs are. The other hundreds of thousands are lost, falling prey to a very hostile environment. Here are some of the problems sperm may encounter:

- Many sperm are killed by the natural vaginal environment.

- Cervical mucus may be too thick to allow the sperm to penetrate it and enter the uterus.

- Sperm cell movement may be so poor that too few can survive. In rare cases, the cervical mucus may contain antibodies that can incapacitate sperm. It's unclear, however, how significant these antibodies are in preventing pregnancy or causing infertility.

- Once out of the vagina, sperm movement may be hampered by structural damage in the uterus or tubes, making it mechanically difficult for sperm to reach an egg.

Of those sperm that reach the cervical canal, half enter the wrong Fallopian tube in search of an absent egg. Of those that enter the correct Fallopian tube, many are lost in the maze of the tube's folds. During this journey, the remaining sperm will undergo a process called *capacitation,* which gives them the capacity to penetrate and fertilize an egg.

Pregnancy is not an instantaneous event. It's a sequence of physiological milestones that take place over several days. From egg to embryo, here are the eight sometimes not-so-simple steps:

1. Ovulation is the first, but sometimes, most difficult step in the path to pregnancy. Mid-cycle each month, a mature egg, or ovum, is released from its follicle on the ovary surface.

 Bright Idea

Here's a good reason to have sex more often: Studies have shown that couples who have sex less than once a week are unlikely to conceive within the first six months of trying.

2. A single sperm penetrates the dense outer coat surrounding the ovum, called the *zona pellucida*. This coat makes the ovum impervious to other sperm and fertilization occurs. The single cell that results from this fertilization is called the zygote.

3. Beginning a few hours after fertilization, the zygote begins its long, dramatic growth—starting with a single cell, dividing, and redividing in a process called cleavage. First, two cells are formed, then four, then eight—the number of cells doubling with each division.

4. As the zygote continues to divide, it travels down the Fallopian tube into the uterus. Although the number of cells increases with each division, the size of the cells becomes smaller. If the overall size of the zygote increased, it would become too large to travel down the narrow passageways of the Fallopian tube into the uterus.

5. The fertilized egg enters the uterus—powered by the muscular contractions of the Fallopian tube and guided by the minute, fringelike projections on the tube's surface. The rapidly dividing zygote lies here for two or three days, growing and differentiating into cells that are destined to perform various functions.

6. On Day 7 after fertilization, the fertilized egg loses its protective coating. This new hollow sphere of cells floating freely in the uterine cavity is called a blastocyst. The blastocyst must now attach, or implant, itself in the uterine wall.

7. Now totaling about 100 cells, the blastocyst nestles against the uterine wall and prepares to attach itself. At this stage the blastocyst has two distinct portions—an inner cell mass and an outer wall of flattened cells called the trophoblast. This trophoblast becomes a hormone-producing organism, secreting human chorionic gonadotropin (HCG).

8. During implantation, the trophoblastic cells penetrate the uterine wall, embedding themselves into the endometrium. The blastocyst is firmly attached, or implanted, by Day 12 after fertilization.

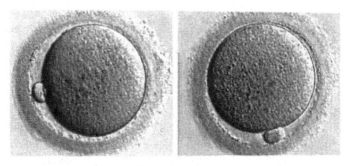

A mature unfertilized egg. (Photo courtesy of Lucinda Veeck Gosden, Weill Medical College of Cornell University)

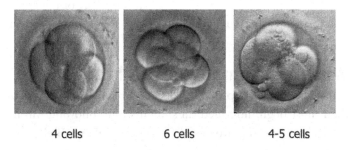

| 4 cells | 6 cells | 4-5 cells |

A fertilized egg that has divided into a four-cell embryo. (Photo courtesy of Lucinda Veeck Gosden, Weill Medical College of Cornell University)

A blastocyst occasionally becomes implanted inside the Fallopian tube or somewhere other than inside the uterine cavity. This is called an *ectopic pregnancy*. Such pregnancies are life-threatening and are usually terminated either surgically or with the use of medications.

The trophoblast is designed to become the nutritional organ of the embryo; the inner cell mass will become the embryo itself.

The point where they meet becomes the umbilical cord. During implantation, the trophoblast grows fingerlike projections, called *villi*, into the surrounding maternal tissue. They radiate out like porcupine quills and pierce the lush blood channels in the endometrium, which allows the villi to be microscopically bathed in nourishing blood. These villous lakes are the start of a new organ growing between the embryo and the mother. Called a *chorion*, it permits maternal circulation to sustain and nourish the embryo. Part of the chorion will form the placenta, which becomes a hormone-producing organ that supports the pregnancy.

> 66 The best time for fruitful intercourse is...when urge and appetite for coitus are present, when the body is neither in want nor too congested and heavy from drunkenness and indigestion, and after the body has been rubbed down and a little food been eaten... 99
>
> —Soranus, Roman physician, 2nd century AD

When everything goes right...

Although you now probably know more about reproduction than most beginning medical students, the following will help you understand the process of conception in a nutshell:

- The woman must ovulate a healthy, ripe, fertilizable egg.

- Fallopian tubes must be unobstructed in order to receive the egg.

- The couple must have sexual intercourse prior to or at the time of ovulation.

- The man must ejaculate millions of healthy, viable sperm deep into the woman's vagina.

- Many sperm must travel through the cervix into the uterus and finally into the open Fallopian tubes.

- The egg must be fertilized in the Fallopian tube and then travel back into the uterus.

- The fertilized egg must implant itself in a hormonally primed, normally shaped uterus, and grow into a healthy embryo.

You can see where there is a lot of room for error. This is why it takes many couples—fertile as well as infertile—so long to conceive, a subject that is discussed in the next chapter.

Misconceptions

Now that you know the facts about conception, it's time to sort the facts from fiction. There are many myths and misconceptions you're bound to encounter during your pursuit of pregnancy. While some may have elements of truth, most ultimately don't hold up to scientific scrutiny, or have yet to be proven or disproven.

Here are some popular myths about conception:

1. **The "missionary position" is best if you want to conceive.** The reality: Many people assume that if the female partner is on top during sexual intercourse, sperm will leak out of the vagina, reducing the chances for conception. Somehow, however, the sperm manage to make it to where they need to be, whether or not the couple engages in the missionary position. The force of the ejaculation, regardless of the man's position, is enough to propel sperm into the cervical mucus. And it's only the sperm that get into the cervical mucus that will pass through the cervix and enter the uterus. Whatever sperm don't reach the cervical mucus will probably be rendered useless in the vaginal environment anyway. So, use the position that's most comfortable for you. It's having sexual intercourse that's important.

2. **Having an orgasm increases a woman's chance of conceiving.** The reality: While having an orgasm increases a woman's pleasure, it's not necessary for conception; that

depends on whether or not a sperm fertilizes an egg. This can happen during pleasurable sex, unwanted sex, and even no sex, as in artificial insemination and in-vitro fertilization (IVF). Although some scientists theorize that the contractions of a female orgasm may facilitate the movement of the sperm toward the Fallopian tubes, healthy sperm—the kind that are most likely to fertilize an egg—will swim there on their own. And while an orgasm is usually necessary for a man to ejaculate sperm, occasionally small amounts of sperm are released prior to ejaculation.

3. **You should stay in bed for at least a half hour after intercourse if you want to conceive.** The reality: This is a corollary to the "missionary position" belief. Some women have been told that rushing out of bed will cause millions of sperm to flow out of the vagina. As we've mentioned, the sperm manage to get to their destination in spite of the spillage. Some doctors do, however, recommend that women do stay in bed awhile with their hips elevated on a pillow. While there doesn't appear to be any medical proof for this advice, there certainly is no harm in it. Trying to conceive can put enormous strains on a couple, so while by no means necessary, languishing in bed a bit in the afterglow of the moment is soothing. Enjoy the quiet time together.

4. **Sperm can only live for about a day.** The reality: Although many sperm live for only 24 hours, they can live for up to 72 hours in the woman's reproductive system. And in some cases, sperm have been known to have lived as long as five days!

5. **Ovulation always occurs on Day 14 of your cycle.** The reality: The day you ovulate depends on many factors, including the length of your cycle. Most women have a 28-day cycle and tend to ovulate on the 14th day. However, many

women have shorter or longer cycles and will ovulate accordingly. If a woman has a 25-day cycle, she's likely to ovulate on Day 11. If her cycle is 30 days, she'll probably ovulate on Day 16.

6. **You can conceive only one day each month—the day you ovulate.** The reality: A woman can conceive up to six days each month—five days prior to ovulation and on the day of ovulation. Conception after ovulation, however, is unlikely to occur. How to determine when you ovulate is discussed in detail in the next chapter.

7. **If you ovulate from one ovary one month, you'll ovulate from the other the next month.** The reality: Ovulation does not alternate between ovaries, but is a random event with each ovary having about a 50 percent chance of ovulating each month. Some women do, however, have a dominant ovary and will ovulate from that one more than the other.

8. **If you've been pregnant before, you'll have no trouble conceiving the second time around.** The reality: Having had a previous pregnancy—especially with your current partner—is a good sign, but it's not definitive proof of your current fertility status. A lot could have happened to you or your partner physiologically that could delay or interfere with conception. For one thing, you're both older and—as we mentioned in Chapter 1—that alone can make conceiving more difficult. And some women develop antibodies against their partner's sperm, making another pregnancy unlikely without treatment. (Anti-sperm antibodies are discussed in Chapter 4.) If you have a different partner, it's a whole different ballgame. Having been pregnant with a previous partner in no way ensures that a woman will easily conceive with her new partner. And if a male partner impregnated his previous partner, it doesn't guarantee that he's as fertile as he was in the past.

Last but not least is perhaps the most pervasive and frustrating myth of all:

9. **"Take a vacation and you'll get pregnant" or "Relax and you'll get pregnant."** The reality: Taking a vacation can help you relax, and when you're relaxed you're more likely to want to have sex. It also affords you the time to have sex, and having sex certainly increases your chances of conceiving. But the unfortunate implication behind this myth is that you're too stressed to conceive, and therefore need to relax more. This, however, has absolutely no scientific basis. Another similar myth—"Adopt and you'll get pregnant"—has also been disproven. We'll return to both of these myths in later chapters.

Just the facts

- An understanding of how the male and female reproductive systems work is an important part of preparing to conceive.

- The average young, healthy couple has only a 20 percent chance of conceiving each month.

- It takes approximately 72 days for sperm to be produced and matured.

- A woman can conceive up to six days each month.

- By learning the facts about getting pregnant, you can disregard the many myths and misconceptions.

Pursuing Pregnancy

PART II

GET THE SCOOP ON...
Why it takes so long ■ Monitoring your body for
ovulation ■ Sperm and male infertility ■ What to
do before consulting a specialist

Try, Try Again

By now you should have had your preconception exam, taken steps to correct any medical problem or problems you or your partner might have, and are concentrating on living a healthy lifestyle. You're probably raring to go, and if you're like most people, expect to conceive pretty quickly once you start trying. You undoubtedly spent much of your young adult life being very careful *not* to get pregnant or to father a child.

You might even, as many people do, plan to conceive at a certain time of the year so your child will be born at a convenient time or even under a favorable astrological sign. But if you're like the average couple, you might be in for a big disappointment. As you read in the previous chapter, a lot has to go right at the right time each month to achieve a pregnancy. There are, however, things you can to maximize your chances of conceiving as quickly as possible, taking into consideration your particular circumstances.

Realistic expectations

It's important to have a realistic sense of your chances of conceiving. As we mentioned in the previous chapter, you might be surprised to learn that the average, healthy, young couple has about only a 20 percent chance of conceiving each month. That's why it takes most couples from six months to a year to get pregnant. If the couple is older or has some health problems it's likely to take them even longer. But remember, we're talking about averages here. Of course there are countless couples that do conceive the minute they want to, but they're definitely in the minority.

Age

As we mentioned in Chapter 1 and will emphasize throughout the book, age is a key factor in fertility. While a healthy woman under age 30 has a 20 percent chance of conceiving each month, her chances drop to just 5 percent by age 40.

The older you are, the longer it will likely take you to conceive, and the greater the risk of having infertility, miscarriages, problem pregnancies, and babies born with birth defects. So, if you're in your mid 30s or older and haven't gotten pregnant after six months, and haven't already consulted a fertility specialist (reproductive endocrinologist), now's the time to do it. Consider that it may take you a few weeks or even several months to get an appointment, so the sooner you call the better. In Chapter 5 we give you helpful hints for finding the right specialists for you and your partner.

> ❝It never occurred to either of us that (my wife) would not get pregnant within a reasonable period of time. We thought it might even happen the first month we tried. After all, we had been using birth control for years.❞
>
> —Roy, 38

Good timing

The previous chapter outlined all the physiological elements necessary for conception to take place. If one of those elements is out of kilter, you probably won't get pregnant that month. Good timing is necessary for the sperm and egg to meet. There's one fairly simple—not to mention pleasurable—thing you can do to help ensure that your chances are maximized each month: Have sex often enough to ensure that you don't miss your most fertile days.

Recent research has found that the average woman is fertile for six days a month—the five days before ovulation and the day she ovulates. The two days before ovulation are usually the days a woman is most likely to conceive. But as we shall see, it's difficult to predict those two optimal days. So, to take advantage of the six-day "window of fertility," it's a good idea to "schedule" sex every other day around the time you think you might ovulate. That means usually starting on day 10 of the ideal 28-day menstrual cycle. This pattern helps ensure that enough sperm are present whenever the woman ovulates, since sperm usually are viable for 48 hours.

Of course, you might prefer to cover all your bases and have intercourse *every* day starting around day 10. It's ultimately up to you and your partner to decide how often to have sex as long as you have it during your fertile period. There is, however, some evidence that having sex several times a day or frequent masturbation can deplete the sperm pool. In fact, the concern about depleting a man's sperm supply is behind the fairly common advice that men should save up their sperm by abstaining from sex for several days prior to their partner's fertile period.

 Bright Idea

If your male partner travels a lot, he can have his sperm frozen. Then your doctor can inseminate you with your partner's sperm if you ovulate while he's away. This procedure, known as artificial insemination, is discussed in Chapter 7.

A recent large-scale study in Israel—which was presented to the European Society of Human Reproduction and Embryology in 2003—tested this theory in couples trying to conceive. The researchers discovered that even though the volume of semen and the number of sperm increased after several days of abstinence, abstaining from sex before ovulation was of *no* benefit to either fertile or infertile couples. In fact, abstinence was actually *counterproductive* when the male partner

> **❝**There had not been a time when we had unscheduled sex when I hadn't wondered beforehand whether it would be detrimental to my getting pregnant because we might use up the good sperm.**❞**
>
> —Sue, 36

had a low sperm count (subfertility); after one or two days of abstinence, the number of immotile and malformed sperm increased in these men. The longer they abstained from sex, the poorer their sperm quality. Their sperm, in effect, grew stale and were no longer able to fertilize an egg.

There are also some things you *shouldn't* do when having sex. If possible, don't use vaginal lubricants. If you do prefer to use lubricants, don't use any that contain spermicides—as their name implies, they kill sperm! In addition to reading the label, it's a good idea to ask your doctor or pharmacist about their contents. Even lubricants without spermicides can hamper sperm motility. Body oils and creams can trap sperm, too. If you must use a lubricant, choose only water-soluble ones. Of course, the best lubricant is the natural vaginal secretion.

 Moneysaver

If you want to use lubrication, look in your kitchen rather than the drug store. Egg whites and milk are good substitutes for commercial products. And they'll be easier on your pocketbook and your partner's sperm.

Ovulation: a woman's key to conception

Pinpointing ovulation can further ensure that you have sex at the right time. Unfortunately, the precise time of ovulation is typically only known retroactively; that is, after it's already occurred. Pregnancy is unlikely to occur even a day after ovulation. The trick, then, is to anticipate when ovulation is most likely to happen. Luckily, there are some easy, fairly accurate, noninvasive ways of determining whether or not you ovulate.

Monitoring your body

Certain body signals can indicate impending ovulation and even ovulation itself. One such sign is called *mittleschmertz*, a feeling that many women experience in their abdominal region around the time of ovulation. Some feel a twinge, some a sharp pain, and others mild discomfort in or around the ovaries.

One of the best signs of ovulation, however, and one most women experience, is a change in the quality and quantity of the cervical mucus during the menstrual cycle. By checking your cervical mucus you can tell whether you're approaching ovulation. A few days before you think you may ovulate, insert your finger into your vagina and get a small sample of mucus from around your cervix. Then try to stretch the mucus between your finger and thumb. If the mucus is thick, pasty, sticky, and/or opaque, you're unlikely to conceive because sperm can't live or swim in this hostile environment. But if the mucus is clear, thin, and stretchable, it's an indication that you're approaching ovulation. You're most fertile when you can stretch the mucus an inch or more without it breaking—a characteristic of cervical mucus called *spinnbarkheit*. Your partner's sperm will also be able survive and swim more easily to your awaiting egg in this friendly, moist environment. The reason women can become pregnant for up to six days *before* ovulation is because sperm can survive in this "nonhostile" cervical mucus for several days.

Lack of cervical mucus and having thick cervical mucus are not always signs that you aren't ovulating. Some women produce good cervical mucus at the time of ovulation, but it stays in the cervical canal, making it difficult to detect. And, infection or prior cervical surgery can have adverse effects on cervical mucus, causing it to thicken. But for most women, the changes in cervical mucus are very reliable predictors of ovulation.

Charting your temperature

Another way to find out if you ovulate is by keeping a basal body temperature (BBT) chart. This usually involves tracking your temperature each morning. The BBT is sometimes used to determine the LH surge (see Chapter 2), which is an indication of ovulation. To chart your BBT, you should take your temperature orally, rectally, or with an ear probe every morning before getting out of bed, or if you prefer, later on in the day as long as it's the same time each day. You should then plot the temperature changes on a chart, and mark which days you menstruate and have sexual intercourse.

> 66 When my doctor told me to keep track of my temperature every morning, I wasn't sure what she meant. She told me I could take it orally, rectally, or vaginally—even at night—as long as I was consistent. 99
>
> —Sally, 29

Over two or three months, the typical chart of an ovulating woman will show a pattern of a slight temperature rise (0.4 to 1.0 degrees F) at mid-cycle. The rise in temperature remains fairly level until about the time of menstruation, at which point the temperature drops. This is called a *biphasic* pattern and is a good indication that you ovulated. If no temperature elevation is apparent for several months—what's called a *monophasic* pattern—you're

probably not ovulating and should see a reproductive endocrinologist as soon as possible.

Some couples mistakenly think that they should have sex
when they see the temperature rise. Although the LH surge
usually occurs a day or two before ovulation, by the time the
temperature rise is apparent, you've probably already ovulated. If so, it's too late to conceive. Indeed, there have been
no documented cases of a pregnancy occurring the day after
ovulation.

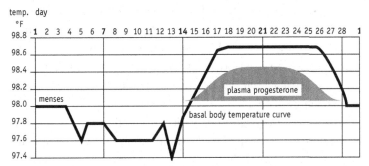

This is a BBT chart of a typical 28-day ovulatory cycle. The lowest point in
temperature may indicate ovulation. The rise in temperature is a result of
the progesterone, which is produced only after ovulation. When progesterone
levels drop so does the temperature, and the woman gets her period.

Unfortunately, BBT cannot determine ovulation ahead of
time, only after the fact. For that reason, many doctors don't recommend its use. However, it can give you some indication of your
ovulation patterns before seeing a doctor. It can also help you and
your doctor determine whether your cycles are abnormally long
or short. Another advantage is that it can be an indirect indication of an early pregnancy. If an egg does become fertilized, your
temperature will probably continue to stay elevated instead of
dropping as it does when you're about to get your period.

Moneysaver

Invest in a digital thermometer, which is nonbreakable and gives a more accurate reading than a glass thermometer.

Using ovulation prediction kits

Ovulation predication kits—or more accurately, tests—can be especially helpful in pinpointing ovulation and can be done most anywhere. By directly measuring LH levels, usually in the urine, these tests can detect the LH surge that precedes ovulation.

Ovulation prediction tests are performed daily for four or five days at mid-cycle—which is about eleven days after the first day of a woman's period. It's important to know the length of your menstrual cycle ahead of time when using these kits. If you've kept a BBT chart, you'll be ahead of the game.

There are many good ovulation prediction kits on the market. There are two kinds you can buy—one tests your urine and the other tests your saliva.

Urine tests

Most ovulation monitoring kits test LH in the urine. The LH surge is a good indication that ovulation will occur in about 24 hours, on average. Since the range is from 16 to 48 hours, the LH surge can help predict the two most fertile days of a woman's cycle.

In addition to LH in the urine, a good indication of impending ovulation is the presence of estradiol—a form of estrogen produced in and released by the ovary. Estradiol is responsible for the cervical mucus changes mentioned earlier that help the sperm to swim easily and survive long enough to reach an egg. While the LH measurement alone can predict when ovulation is about to occur, the additional monitoring of estrone-3-glucuronide (E3G)—a metabolite of estradiol—can tell you when your fertile time is actually beginning, thus widening your window of fertility.

Urine tests are easy to use: You either dip a test stick in a cup of urine or hold the stick under a stream of urine. You get the results—which are indicated by a color change in the test stick—in about 5 to 10 minutes. Most ovulation monitors are quite accurate in helping women determine their most fertile days as long as they follow the instructions very carefully. Although many tests claim to be 98 or 99 percent accurate, a more realistic range is 85 to 88 percent, and some are even less accurate. This method of fertility monitoring isn't worthwhile for women who have very long cycles (more than 42 days) or short cycles (less than 21 days).

The prices of urine tests can vary considerably, often depending on the sophistication of the monitoring device. A simple, single-use dip stick can cost as little as a dollar or two. More sophisticated monitors usually cost between $12 and $35, and you will need to buy a new one each month you are trying to conceive. Some high-tech computerized models can cost as much as $150 to $300, but these models are easier to use and interpret, and can be used for several months. If you're undecided about which test you should use, ask your OB/GYN for his or her opinion.

Saliva test

Several fertility kits using saliva have been introduced recently. As estrogen production increases near ovulation, a fern pattern often appears in dried saliva, which is appropriately referred to as *ferning*. While a saliva test may be easier to use, it may be harder to interpret than the urine test because it involves reading the results under a built-in microscope. Also, not all women's saliva will fern during their fertile period, or will do so only sporadically. In addition, eating, drinking, smoking, and

 Watch Out!

Not all home tests are accurate. Make sure that the one you are considering using is regulated by the U.S. Food and Drug Administration (FDA). You can find information about home tests on the FDA website at www.fda.gov.

Bright Idea

Consumer Reports rated the 11 top-selling ovulation prediction kits and also has information on their costs. You can get the article on their website at www.consumerreports.org.

brushing your teeth can throw off the test's accuracy. For these reasons, some experts claim the saliva tests are not as accurate as urine tests in predicting ovulation, although, not surprisingly, the manufacturers claim they are. Saliva and urine tests cost about the same, but the saliva kits contain enough test strips to last for several months.

Sperm: the key to male fertility

Just as the ovulation of a viable egg is the key to female fertility, ejaculation of healthy sperm is the key to male fertility. You might hear that it takes only one egg and one sperm to achieve a pregnancy, but that's only partially true. While it does, indeed, take one egg, millions of sperm are required to ensure that one sperm will be healthy and strong enough to fertilize that one egg.

There are approximately 100 to 300 million sperm in the average ejaculate; if there are fewer than 200 million sperm, the chances of conception are diminished. Every man produces many sperm that are malformed (poor morphology) or are incapable of traveling fast enough in a straight line (poor motility) to make the trip up to the uterus and finally the Fallopian tubes. The cervical mucus filters out most of the abnormal sperm. Many thousands of healthy sperm now need to make the long trip—a process that can take anywhere from 5 minutes to 24 hours.

When the remaining healthy sperm meet up with the egg in the Fallopian tube, they bombard the egg's protective coating, called the *cumulus*. Thousands of sperm die in the process. It takes about an hour for the egg to be stripped of its cumulus, at which time new sperm arrive and try to penetrate the egg's next protective membrane, the zona pellucida. Only those sperm that have been capacitated (see Chapter 2) can penetrate the membrane and fertilize the egg. One—and, it is hoped, only one—will succeed. If more than one sperm penetrates an egg, called *polyspermia*, fertilization is unlikely to occur. But if it does, the woman will undoubtedly not even know she had conceived because she's likely to have a very early miscarriage.

From this complex process of survival of the fittest, you can see why it's necessary for a man to have an adequate number of sperm per ejaculation, *and* why the majority of those sperm must have good morphology and motility.

These three key factors—sperm count, morphology, and motility—can be evaluated easily by semen analysis. Previously, men had to go to a doctor's office or lab to have a semen analysis, or their partner or someone else needed to bring the specimen in for them if they, for some reason, couldn't or didn't want to bring it in themselves. But home sperm tests have recently become available and men can now evaluate their own sperm in the privacy of their homes. The test costs about $40 and there are two tests per box.

While not as accurate as having a semen analysis done by a lab, home sperm tests can give some indication of the man's fertility status. The test involves the man producing a sperm sample at home and then staining the sample with a special dye. The color is then compared to a chart that indicates whether the sample contains more than 20 million sperm/mL (positive) or fewer than 20 million/mL (negative). If the test result is negative, it should be repeated in three to five days. If negative again, consult a urologist who specializes in male fertility or an andrologist as soon as possible to have a more complete evaluation.

 Moneysaver

Shop around for ovulation prediction kits and home sperm tests at discount pharmacies and on the Internet. When considering price, check to see if a test can be reused or is a one-shot deal.

Watch Out!

A home semen analysis requires that the man abstain from sex for three days before using the test. The best time to do the test, then, is at a time when the female partner cannot possibly become pregnant, such as during her menstrual period.

When everything seems to be going wrong

If you haven't gotten pregnant yet, don't panic. You may or may not have a fertility problem. Even if you do, infertility treatments have become so advanced that your chances for conceiving are better than ever. But before you start running off to a fertility specialist, there's a lot you can do on your own. And if you do decide to consult a fertility specialist, the following preliminary steps will save you time by providing useful information to your doctor on your first visit.

Take control of the situation

Whether or not you're certain you have a fertility problem, there are some basic steps you should take before you see a specialist:

1. If you haven't already done so, get a physical examination. As mentioned in Chapter 1, both partners should be in good physical condition before starting a family.

2. If you haven't gotten pregnant within six months, the male partner should go for a semen analysis. Although this will ultimately have to be done and even repeated several times, doing it early can save time and even needless testing and treatment. Many women have gone through years of expensive, invasive infertility treatments only later to discover that their partners have low sperm counts. (Keep in mind that even if a man has fathered a child in the past his semen can change over time; he should still go for a semen analysis.)

3. Start looking for a fertility specialist—a qualified reproductive endocrinologist for the female partner, and a urologist or andrologist for the male partner (see Chapter 5). We mentioned earlier that women in their late 30s or older should make an appointment with a fertility specialist after six months of trying and failing to conceive. Younger women are usually advised to wait for a full year without conceiving before consulting a specialist. But regardless of your age, if you're at all concerned that you might have a fertility problem, make an appointment with a specialist now. If you want to give it some more time, you should at least start your search for a specialist now just in case things don't work out. It will save you a lot of precious time—and frustration.

Educate yourself

By reading this book, you've taken a major step toward being in control of your fertility. But don't stop here. It's important for you to become an expert on fertility—and infertility if necessary. After all, you want to do everything you can to become pregnant, have a successful pregnancy, and a healthy baby. Educating yourself about the process is essential:

■ Read everything you can about fertility. Go to bookstores, public libraries, and medical libraries if you have access. Don't be intimidated by the medical books or terms. While you won't necessarily understand everything you read, they can be helpful, especially as you progress through diagnosis and treatment.

 Bright Idea

Share the results of all your home tests with your doctors. It can give them invaluable information and may even save you the time and cost of having to repeat certain tests.

- Use the Internet. It provides a wealth of information on, as well as the opportunity to talk to others about, your pursuit of pregnancy while maintaining your anonymity. We've listed many websites and other sources of information in Appendix C. But read everything with a critical eye, keeping in mind that not all information on the Internet is accurate.

- If you are concerned that you might have a fertility problem, contact the National Infertility Association, RESOLVE, which is the largest national organization for infertile couples. With 50 affiliates nationwide, RESOLVE provides information on all aspects of infertility, publishes newsletters, offers lists of qualified fertility specialists, and offers emotional support. You can find out if there is an affiliate in your area by logging on to RESOLVE's website at www.resolve.org. If there's no RESOLVE affiliate where you live, try to find another support group in your community.

Just the facts

- Age and poor timing of sex are two factors that can slow down conception.

- Observing changes in your cervical mucus is one of the best, easiest, and cheapest ways to pinpoint ovulation.

- A minimum of 200 million sperm per ejaculation is usually necessary for conception.

- Before going to a fertility specialist, the male partner should have a semen analysis and the female partner should have some idea of whether or not she ovulates, and when.

GET THE SCOOP ON...
The difference between infertility and sterility ▪
Hormonal and structural factors in men and
women ▪ Genetic and congenital causes ▪
When there's no apparent explanation

What Conceivably Can Go Wrong?

Chapter 4

If you haven't gotten pregnant yet you're probably feeling perplexed, frustrated, upset, and nervous. You might be wondering, are we infertile? Will we *ever* be able to have a baby? You may be tempted to run off to a fertility specialist right now. But before you do so, read this chapter; it will help you better understand infertility and its causes.

Our purpose is not to describe every fertility problem that a man or woman might have. Nor is it to tell you how these problems can be resolved. (Infertility treatment is discussed in detail in Parts IV and V.) Rather, our purpose here is to give you an overview of some of the major conditions that can interfere with conception. This chapter will also help familiarize you with the medical terms you might come across in your pursuit of pregnancy. This will be invaluable to you if you do decide to see a fertility specialist. You will be better equipped to discuss your medical problems with your doctor in a knowledgeable fashion, and therefore, fully participate in your treatment and quest for a baby.

73

Coming to terms

There's a lot of misunderstanding about the meaning of the terms *infertility* and *sterility*, and many people confuse the two. Sterility is defined as the absolute inability to reproduce. Some men and women are born with genetic disorders that render them sterile from birth, while others become sterile as an unfortunate side effect of a medical condition or treatment. These are cases of *involuntary sterility*, which is quite rare. On the other hand, men who have vasectomies and women who have their tubes tied so they cannot reproduce are examples of *voluntary sterility*, which is much more common.

Infertility—which is also quite common—is defined as the inability of a couple to achieve a successful pregnancy after one year of unprotected intercourse. A woman is infertile, therefore, if she has not become pregnant after a year of trying, and a man is infertile if he cannot father a child. Infertile men and women are sometimes referred to as *subfertile*.

Infertility affects more than six million American women and their partners. That's about 10 percent of Americans who are of reproductive age. But some estimates put the figure as high as 20 percent! You may be surprised to learn that infertility affects men and women with equal frequency. The good news is that most cases of infertility are treatable. Recent advances in drug therapy, microsurgery, and assisted reproductive technologies are making pregnancy possible for up to 75 percent of couples seeking treatment for infertility.

Whose problem is it, anyway?

In the not-so-distant past, many people—even some doctors—assumed that the cause of infertility was entirely due to the woman. Although that assumption is still occasionally made today, there is increasing recognition that something may be amiss with the male partner as well as the female. Indeed, in half the infertility cases, the man has a fertility problem.

Infertility can be caused by a number of factors attributable to the man, the woman, or both. The man has the exclusive problem 30 percent of the time, and the couple has a combined problem 20 percent of the time. The term *female factor* is used to describe conditions or disorders that contribute to infertility in women; *male factor* is used to describe those that cause infertility in men.

Individually, each factor may not impact greatly on your ability to conceive, but together they throw the

> 66 The minute I found out that there might be a problem, I started reading about infertility, and I had read some statistics about the age of the man being a factor, so I was concerned about my husband since he was 40. 99
>
> —Lee, 28

odds against you. For example, a woman who has a subtle cervical mucus problem might not have trouble conceiving if her partner has a normal sperm count. However, if her partner has a low sperm count her chances of conceiving are greatly reduced.

What's the problem?

Successful conception and pregnancy depends on many factors, as we described in Chapter 2. Because the female and male reproductive systems are quite complex, their numerous different organs, and intricate and delicate sets of hormones, are subject to a variety of problems. Some of these problems can interfere with a woman's ability to ovulate, conceive, or carry a pregnancy to term; other factors can adversely affect a man's ability to produce viable sperm and deliver the sperm into a woman's vagina. And to further complicate things, each partner can have multiple problems.

Fertility problems are often divided into three categories: hormonal, structural, and genetic factors. But nothing with regard to reproduction is that simple or straightforward. Many of these categories overlap, as you'll see from the following descriptions.

Hormonal abnormalities in women

As we explained in Chapter 2, the primary function of the ovary—ovulation—is tightly regulated by hormones. So anything that throws off a woman's hormones can cause ovulatory problems and miscarriages.

Ovulatory disorders

Also known as ovarian-factor infertility, ovulatory disorders are among the most common causes of infertility. Irregular or abnormal ovulation accounts for approximately 25 percent—although some estimates place it as high as 33 percent—of all female infertility cases. Amenorrhea (total absence of menstruation), continuous menstruation, and abnormal periods—such as heavy flow, cramps, or irregular cycles—can all be symptoms of ovulatory dysfunction.

As mentioned in Chapter 1, certain lifestyle factors—such as being under- or overweight, excessive drinking, or the use of certain drugs—can interfere with ovulation. They can cause progesterone defects, which are one of the most common ovulation problems and among the most common causes of anovulation. Other possible causes include any impairment in hypothalamic, pituitary, or ovarian function—such as hyper- and hypothyroidism or diabetes—which can lead to irregular or total absence of ovulation. Indeed, uncontrolled diabetes can cause both infertility and pregnancy loss.

Polycystic ovarian syndrome (PCOS or PCOD)

This is a hormonal abnormality that typically starts around puberty and causes ovulatory problems. It is also known as Stein-Leventhal Syndrome or hyperandrogenism. This abnormality—which affects about 5 percent of all women—causes the woman's ovaries to produce an excess of androgens, the male hormones. The ovaries then develop an excess of immature egg follicles or cysts and become enlarged. PCOS causes irregular or anovulatory menstrual cycles, and, as a result, infertility. Women with PCOS also commonly suffer from obesity, severe acne, and *hirsuitism*—abnormal hair growth on the face, chest, upper arms, legs, and back, which gives them a masculine look.

Hyperprolactinemia

An excess of the hormone prolactin is another hormonal imbalance that often leads to fertility problems in both women and men. Prolactin—which is secreted by the pituitary gland—increases during pregnancy and is responsible for milk production after childbirth. One of the symptoms is *galactorrhea,* the abnormal production of milk in women who aren't pregnant.

Hormonal abnormalities in men

Although they are the most common cause of infertility in women, hormonal abnormalities are a less frequent cause of male-factor infertility. That said, some men do have hormonal imbalances that interfere with sperm production. As we mentioned, men, like women, can suffer from hyperprolactinemia. In rare cases, men may even develop enlarged breasts and produce milk. Because an excess of prolactin can interfere with sperm production, men with this condition may suffer from *oligospermia* (low sperm count), *azoospermia* (total absence of sperm), or impotence.

Hypogonadism—also called testosterone deficiency—is another hormonal condition that can cause oligospermia, azoospermia, or impotence. Hypogonadism is the absence or reduction of the male sex hormone, testosterone, in the gonads. It's been estimated that 13 million men in the United States suffer from testosterone deficiency; however, many are beyond the age when they would likely want to father a child.

 Watch Out!

Calcium channel blockers—drugs used to treat hypertension—have been known to interfere with the ability of sperm to fertilize eggs. Men who are taking this type of high blood pressure medicine should speak to their doctors about switching to a different class of drugs.

The causes of hypogonadism include infections, trauma to the testicles, and medical treatments such as radiation, chemotherapy, or surgery. Mumps, hypothyroidism, hyperprolactinemia, and pituitary, testicular, or other tumors can all cause hypogonadism in adolescent or adult men. Some cases of hypogonadism are *congenital;* that is, they are present at birth.

Genetic and congenital abnormalities

Most cases of infertility are caused by diseases or other medical events that occur during childhood or adulthood. However, in a small number of cases, the cause of infertility is of *genetic* origin. Genetic disorders are those in which the chromosomes are involved and are usually inherited. For example, a child can inherit a defective gene from one or both parents that renders him or her infertile or even sterile. Cystic fibrosis is an example of one of the more common genetic diseases that can cause infertility in men.

While all genetic disorders are congenital, not all congenital disorders are inherited. Some occur spontaneously when a sperm fertilizes an egg, while others occur during fetal development. These include such disorders as Turner Syndrome and Kleinfelter Syndrome, two *chromosomal disorders* that we describe next.

Girls and boys are normally born with 46 chromosomes, half from the mother and half from the father. (Chromosomes are composed of DNA, which carries all of an individual's genetic information.) But sometimes a child is born missing a chromosome or with an extra chromosome.

Turner Syndrome

This fairly common chromosomal disorder affects about 1 in 2,500 newborn girls each year. Girls born with Turner Syndrome are missing an X chromosome. As a result, they do not have functioning ovaries and are therefore usually sterile.

Kleinfelter Syndrome

This is the most common chromosomal disorder that affects men. It occurs in 1 in 500 men—and usually renders a man sterile from birth. Men with this condition are born with an extra X chromosome (XXY) rather than one of each (XY). Boys born with this condition appear normal at birth. However, when they reach puberty, they suffer from hypogonadism. As a result, they fail to develop normal secondary sex characteristics—such as facial and pubic hair—and tend to have small penises and testicles.

Y-chromosome deletions

The Y chromosome is the male sex chromosome, and some men are born with segments missing from their Y chromosomes. These gaps—which are referred to as *Y-deletions*—are so tiny that they cannot be detected by conventional chromosomal analysis. Y-deletions—which are associated with extremely low sperm counts or even sterility—are being increasingly detected in infertile men.

Congenital disorders

Some male babies are born with structural abnormalities—such as undescended testicles (*cryptorchidism*)—that cause infertility. Other structural causes of male infertility are described later in this chapter.

In addition to causing infertility, some genetic or chromosomal abnormalities in the mother can cause repeated miscarriages. Indeed, between 50 and 60 percent of first-trimester miscarriages are the result of these abnormalities. Most miscarriages in the second trimester, however, are caused by structural problems.

Structural abnormalities in women

Structural abnormalities refer to anatomical problems that can occur in the various organs or body parts. They can be congenital (present at birth) or occur later in life. The most common structural abnormalities that cause female infertility occur in the cervix, the uterus, or the Fallopian tubes. These anomalies can be the result of sexually transmitted diseases (STDs), other infections, physical trauma, or genetic disorders. They can also be *idiopathic;* that is, of unknown origin. Whatever the cause, structural problems can prevent ovulation, interfere with implantation of the embryo, or cause miscarriages.

Cervical factors

The cervix is a vital component of the female reproductive system. It is the entrance through which sperm must first pass on their journey into the uterus and up the Fallopian tube to an awaiting egg. And, as we saw in Chapter 3, good-quality cervical mucus is essential for sperm to survive and pass through this first hurdle on the journey to conception. The cervix is also an infant's exit door to the outside world, staying tightly closed until the baby is ready to be born. Cervical abnormalities, however, can cause the cervix to open prematurely. This condition—known as *cervical incompetence*—is a major cause of miscarriages later in the pregnancy. Indeed, 20 to 25 percent of second-trimester miscarriages are believed to be the result of an incompetent cervix.

Cervical problems are often the result of STDs and other infections or *in utero* exposure to certain drugs such as diethylstilbestrol (DES), which we discussed in Chapter 1. DES is responsible for poor cervical mucus, malformation of the cervical canal, and cervical incompetence.

These and other cervical abnormalities can also be caused by genetic or other factors, but many of these problems are, in fact, *iatrogenic*—that is, they are caused by medical procedures or interventions used to treat diseases or problems rather than diseases themselves. Some of the procedures that can cause injury to the cervix are cryosurgery, cone biopsies, conization, cauterization, dilation and curettage (D&C), and therapeutic abortions.

Tubal factors

The Fallopian tubes provide a meeting place for the sperm and eggs—a place where fertilization, it is hoped, will take place. The Fallopian tubes also provide nourishment for the newly fertilized egg. The movement of the cilia in the tubes and contractions of the tubal wall help guide the fertilized egg into the uterus, its new home.

Watch Out!

If you've had any pelvic surgery or an STD, don't waste any more time or money on ovulation kits. Consider making an appointment now with a fertility specialist.

Damaged or malfunctioning Fallopian tubes account for 20 to 35 percent of infertility cases. These abnormalities can prevent eggs from ever reaching the approaching sperm. The tubes may be blocked or immobilized by scar tissue, which makes it impossible for them to move and to pick up eggs.

Any number of conditions or procedures could also narrow or totally block the Fallopian tubes, hamper their natural movement or that of their *fimbriae* (the finger-like end of the tubes), or impair their ability to secrete important fluids. As with some cervical problems, tubal obstruction, blockages, and immobilization are also frequently associated with treatment for other medical problems. For example, women who have had pelvic surgery for a ruptured appendix, ectopic pregnancy, fibroid removal, or an ovarian cyst are at risk for tubal adhesions. Likewise, women who have used an IUD or had two or more therapeutic abortions may be at risk for tubal problems. Other possible causes of tubal disease are scars and adhesions from STDs or other infections. Endometriosis, which is discussed in a moment, is another cause of tubal-factor infertility.

Uterine factors

The uterus is where the newly created embryo will implant, grow, and be housed for the next nine months. Indeed, the primary reproductive function of the uterus is to provide a home, nourishment, and protection for the developing fetus.

Uterine problems can cause infertility by preventing a fertilized egg from implanting in the walls of the uterus, or by providing a poor environment in which an early embryo can grow into a fetus. Structural problems of the uterus can cause recurrent miscarriages as well as infertility. Indeed, 10 to 15 percent of women with recurrent miscarriages have some sort of structural problem in their uterus, such as a misshapen uterus. In addition to providing a temporary home, nourishment, and protection for the developing fetus, the uterus is responsible for pushing the fetus through the cervix into the outside world.

Some women are born with structural deformities of the uterus, such as a *bicornuate* (double uterus) or a *septate* (divided uterus). And as with cervical and tubal-factor infertility, uterine-factor infertility can be the result of STDs and other infections, and scarring or infections from medical procedures, such as incomplete abortions or D&Cs. Other major causes of uterine-factor infertility include polyps, fibroids, and endometriosis.

Endometriosis

This is a condition in which the endometrial tissue from inside the uterus is found outside the uterus. This endometrial tissue is sometimes found on the ovaries, Fallopian tubes, and on the bladder and bowel. As many as 35 percent of women who undergo a complete diagnostic work-up for infertility are found to have endometriosis. Doctors have known for some time that endometriosis tends to run in families. But recently, investigators have actually found specific chromosomal abnormalities in women with endometriosis.

Although endometriosis can sometimes be symptomless, many women do experience the following:

- Painful menstrual cramps
- Diarrhea or painful bowel movements, especially during their period
- Painful sexual intercourse

 Bright Idea

Because endometriosis tends to run in families, tell your doctor if your mother or sisters had symptoms or were diagnosed with the disease.

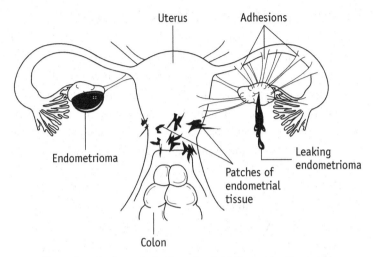

An illustration of endometriosis: the endometrial tissue migrating outside the uterus.

Polyps and fibroids

These are usually noncancerous growths that can distort or reduce the size and capacity of the uterine cavity. They can also interfere with the endometrium's blood supply as well as its ability to provide nourishment to a fetus. Fibroids are quite common. It is their location and size that determines whether or not they'll interfere with conception, embryo implantation, or carrying a baby to term. There are three types of fibroids:

- *Subserosal,* which grow on or protrude into the outer surface of the uterus, can compress the Fallopian tubes, interfering with their ability to pick up an ovulated egg.

- *Submucosal,* which grow inside the uterine cavity, can erode the endometrium, making it unable to prepare itself for embryo implantation.

- *Intramural,* which grow inside the uterus's muscle wall, may not hamper conception, but if they grow big enough to disturb blood supply, they can interfere with fetal growth.

Structural abnormalities in men

While structural problems are the second most common cause of infertility in women (after hormonal factors), they are the primary cause of male infertility. Structural anomalies typically occur in the testes or penis, and can block sperm production or delivery. They may be congenital or may develop later in life as a complication of illnesses such as STDs or other infections. Structural problems can also result from surgical procedures such as hernia repairs and surgery for prostate or testicular cancer.

The following are some of the more common structural abnormalities that can cause male infertility:

▪ **Varicoceles.** Varicoceles are not only the most common structural problem in men, they are the leading cause of male-factor infertility. They are also the most easily treatable. Varicoceles are a network of enlarged varicose veins in the scrotum, with more than 90 percent found in the left scrotom. They usually are associated with poor sperm morphology, but can also negatively affect sperm count and motility.

▪ **Undescended testicles.** This is a congenital condition in which the testes do not descend normally from the abdomen into the scrotum during fetal development. If the testes remain in the abdomen too long, sperm production is impaired.

▪ **Congenital absence of the vas deferens.** This is another structural abnormality present at birth. Men born with this condition are sterile because they are missing the duct— the vas deferens—through which ejaculation occurs.

▪ **Vasectomies.** A vasectomy is a voluntary version of the congenital absence of the vas deferens. In a vasectomy, the vas deferens is surgically closed off to prevent sperm from leaving the testes. Vasectomies can sometimes be successfully reversed.

▪ **Obstructions of the vas deferens and epididymis.** These
obstructions impair the sperm's ability to travel into and out
of the penis, and sperm need to travel from the testes to the
penis in order to enter the female reproductive tract. A
man can be born with these obstructions or acquire them as
a result of infection or surgery. Sometimes, however, their
cause is unknown (idiopathic).

▪ **Testicular torsion and trauma.** Testicular torsion is a condition in which the testis twists on the cord that attaches it to
the body. The sudden interruption of blood flow to and
from the testicle causes dramatic and painful swelling and
reduced sperm production. Testicular torsion may occur
after strenuous exercise or have no apparent cause.
Testicular trauma, or injury to the testicles, can also be
extremely painful and result in impaired sperm production.

Common Causes of Male Infertility	Percentage Among Infertile Men
Varicoceles	42 percent
Obstructions	14 percent
Other causes	21 percent
Idiopathic (unknown cause)	23 percent

Problems with sperm delivery

In addition to structural abnormalities, other problems can
interfere with ejaculation and the delivery of sperm into a
woman's vagina. The two most common are impotence and retrograde ejaculation.

Impotence (erectile dysfunction)

As we learned in Chapter 2, achieving and maintaining an
erection depends on a healthy supply of blood vessels to the
penis and healthy nerves to signal those blood vessels to open

and allow blood to flow into it. Many factors, from psychological stress to chronic diseases, can cause a man to be impotent. The problem may be a symptom of a minor, easily treatable problem—such as the side effect of an antidepressant or antihypertensive drug—or it may reflect a more serious condition, such as diabetes or atherosclerosis. Because male potency is such a key element in fertility, any man suffering from impotence should consult a urologist as soon as possible.

Retrograde ejaculation

Retrograde ejaculation is a condition in which semen goes into the bladder instead of into the urethra and out of the penis. Normally during ejaculation, the bladder sphincter closes so that semen can be expelled out the urethra. But some surgical complications, medications, or diseases—such as diabetes—can cause damage to the nerves that lead to the bladder sphincter. As a result, the bladder sphincter cannot close properly, and the semen takes the path of least resistance—backwards into the bladder rather than into the ejaculate.

Problems with sperm

As we explained in Chapter 3, a sufficient number of sperm—ideally at least 20 million—is necessary for conception to occur. The quality of the sperm is also important. Sperm quality is judged according to their motility (ability to move) and their morphology (shape). Without good motility, sperm cannot make that long swim up to an awaiting egg. If they are abnormally shaped, they may have difficulty swimming properly and penetrating an egg.

Deformed sperm come in many shapes and sizes. Those with more than one head or tail—or with too long or too short a head or tail—cannot fertilize an egg. Chapter 6 has more detailed information on evaluating sperm count, quality, and motility.

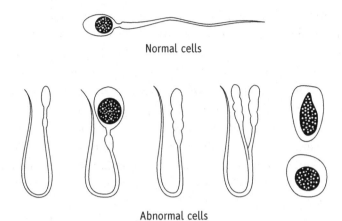

Normal cells

Abnormal cells

Normal and abnormal sperm cells. A large number of abnormally shaped sperm cause male infertility.

Unexplained infertility

Specific causes can be found in about 85 to 90 percent of infertile couples. However, in the remaining 10 to about 15 percent of couples with fertility problems, no cause is found. Because these couples don't have a specific diagnosis, they are said to have *unexplained infertility.* It's not that there isn't anything wrong with these couples, it's just that existing diagnostic methods cannot pick up every condition a couple may have. New research, however, is uncovering the cause in more and more cases of unexplained infertility. For example, up to 18 percent of men with unexplained oligospermia have been found to have an abnormality on their Y chromosomes.

Antisperm antibodies and other autoimmune disorders

It's been estimated that between 40 to 50 percent of cases of unexplained infertility are actually due to undetected autoimmune diseases. However, how significant a role the immune system plays in infertility is of considerable controversy among fertility specialists.

Some men do appear to have a rare autoimmune disorder called antisperm antibodies (ASA), in which they develop antibodies to their sperm; in effect, they become allergic to their own sperm. Normally, the immune system protects the body from "foreign intruders" such as viruses, bacteria, and other organisms. Sperm are usually protected from the immune system by a protective mechanism called the *blood-testes barrier*. Sometimes sperm cross this barrier after an injury to the testes, infection, or surgical procedure. The immune system responds by forming antibodies to attack what it considers foreign invaders—sperm.

An estimated 60 to 70 percent of men who have had vasectomies or vasectomy reversals, for example, develop ASA. If their sperm leak from the vasectomy site, the sperm mix with their blood and provoke an autoimmune reaction. The antibodies then attach themselves to the sperm and immobilize them or cause them to clump together (*agglutination*). This interferes with the sperm's ability to swim through a woman's cervical mucus and penetrate her egg. Once the immune system reacts to a substance as foreign—even a benign substance like sperm—it continues to attack the intruder each time it's exposed to it.

Women, too, occasionally develop antisperm antibodies and become allergic to sperm. Their bodies respond to their partner's sperm as foreign intruders and start attacking them. Women who have pelvic inflammatory disease (PID) also appear to be at increased risk.

 Bright Idea

After reading this chapter, write down the causes of infertility that you think may be relevant to you and your partner's situation to discuss with your doctor. Something in your medical or family history that may strike you as pertinent may not occur to your doctor.

Other even rarer autoimmune disorders can cause infertility. For example, some women produce antibodies that destroy their own ovarian tissue; as a result, they can't produce eggs and ovulate. Women with this type of autoimmune disorder are likely to have premature ovarian failure during their 20s or 30s, causing them to go through premature menopause.

The issue of antisperm antibodies in infertility is quite controversial. Some experts doubt their existence; others say that if they do exist, they don't play a significant role in infertility. Others theorize that antisperm antibodies may play a more important role than previously believed; that they not only kill sperm, they also interfere with the implantation and survival of an early embryo. *Implantation failure*—as this is called—is an area of current active investigation.

Stress

Unfortunately, for many couples, the cause of their infertility or recurrent miscarriages remains illusive—an extremely frustrating situation for both the couple and their physician. The good news is that in the majority of these cases, the couple will ultimately become pregnant either on their own or through treatment.

It's also unfortunate that unexplained infertility is too often blamed on stress. As we've mentioned, every infertile couple has heard the irritating line, "relax and you'll get pregnant." This advice implies that it's the woman's fault that she hasn't yet conceived—that she's probably too stressed or uptight to become pregnant. But if stress causes infertility, there would hardly be a need for birth control!

There is, in fact, no good scientific evidence that stress can actually *cause* infertility. What we do definitively know is that infertility is a major cause of stress. In fact, most of the so-called evidence about stress and infertility is anecdotal. We all know of cases where women try to conceive for years and years, take huge doses of fertility drugs, undergo countless surgical procedures, and nothing happens. Then they stop all treatment, and lo and behold, they become pregnant—presumably because they stopped trying so hard and finally "relaxed." But, statistically speaking, this outcome is the exception, not the rule. And when it does happen, the pregnancy may be a delayed consequence of all those fertility drugs and treatments. Or the couple may have just needed more time for all the elements to fall into place.

That's not to say that stress doesn't affect fertility in certain ways. The ability of a man to achieve and maintain an erection, as well as the frequency of intercourse, can be adversely affected by stress. Also, stress can throw off a woman's menstrual cycle. But that effect is usually temporary, and fertility drugs work very nicely to regulate a woman's cycle. We'll take a closer look at the role of stress in infertility in Chapter 15.

Now that you know what the various conditions are that might be interfering with your ability to conceive or father a child, you may feel ready to pursue the next step—finding a good fertility specialist who can both diagnose and treat your problem. Not only is this one of the most important steps you will take in your pursuit of pregnancy, it may also be one of the most challenging ones. The next chapter helps facilitate your search for the right fertility specialist for you and your partner.

Just the facts

- Fertility problems occur equally in men and women.

- Hormonal problems are the leading cause in infertility in women, while structural abnormalities are the primary cause in men.

- Some babies inherit or are born with disorders that render them sterile from birth.

- Specific causes of infertility cannot be found in up to 15 percent of infertile couples.

Doctors and Diagnoses

GET THE SCOOP ON...
Why people put off seeking treatment ▪ Finding
a good fertility doctor ▪ Making the most of
your visits ▪ Taking control of your treatment ▪
The doctor-patient relationship ▪ Knowing when
to switch doctors

PART III

Choosing the Right Doctor

Chapter 5

If you've read this far in this book, you're undoubtedly concerned that you have a fertility problem that needs to be addressed by a physician. Choosing the best possible fertility specialist is perhaps the most important thing you and your partner will do in your pursuit of pregnancy. Couples with fertility problems should consult qualified fertility specialists, and this chapter will help you do just that. But you or your partner may still be hesitant about taking such a step. If so, it may be helpful to explore some of the reasons why some couples wait month after frustrating month before picking up the phone and calling a specialist.

Putting off the consultation

One of the most common reasons people postpone seeking infertility treatment is denial. Most of us would have a hard time admitting to ourselves that we can't do what everyone else seems to do with ease—reproduce. It's also easy to be in denial when there are no physical symptoms present. Most people go to doctors because they have pain or discomfort, but this is rarely the case with infertility. Although infertility is a physical disorder, the majority of patients don't suffer from physical distress. Rather, theirs is an emotional pain that is the result of not being able to have something they desperately seek—a baby. Because there is usually no pressing need for physical symptom relief, people suffering from infertility can postpone going to the doctor indefinitely. But this form of denial can't last forever. When their emotional pain or frustration becomes too great, they usually do seek medical treatment.

When a person decides to consult a fertility doctor, it's an admission that something is probably wrong with his or her reproductive system. That person is then faced with the possibility of not only potentially painful and expensive diagnostic tests and treatment, but the more painful possibility of never being able to have a biological child. But remember, if you delay consulting a doctor, you'll be wasting precious time. And you won't be any closer to conceiving.

Many people also find the label "infertility" stigmatizing and embarrassing. Both men and women often see infertility as a reflection of their sexuality—a man may feel less of a man, and a woman less of a woman. Men tend to equate fertility with virility and infertility with impotence. While the ability to have and maintain an erection is an advantage when it comes to getting a woman pregnant, it's not a necessity. Many infertile couples conceive through artificial insemination with the husband's sperm, regardless of whether the husband is impotent or not (see Chapter 7).

Some men are so embarrassed by infertility—even when it's their partner who has the underlying physical problem—that

 Bright Idea

If you and your partner are at odds about going to a specialist, it may be helpful to consult a therapist or marriage counselor who can help you resolve your conflicts about this issue.

they're reluctant to consult a specialist. Some are afraid that if they consult a fertility doctor, they will have to discuss their sex lives with a total stranger, often another man, and they find that prospect threatening.

Women, too, may feel that it is too stigmatizing or embarrassing to see a fertility doctor and feel more comfortable seeing their regular OB/GYN. In fact, many women naturally gravitate to their regular OB/GYNs when they think they have a fertility problem. This may seem like the logical choice to you. After all, your OB/GYN knows you and has probably been handling your contraceptive needs and gynecological problems for many years. While this may be okay as a preliminary step, seeing your regular OB/GYN is ultimately not the best choice unless he or she is a qualified fertility—or infertility—specialist. Both these terms are commonly used and can be used interchangeably. Most fertility specialists who treat women are OB/GYNs, but most OB/GYNs are *not* fertility specialists. That is, they have not had the necessary advanced training in reproductive endocrinology necessary to effectively diagnose and treat many infertility problems.

> **❝**My OB/GYN was a very kind, sensitive, wonderful, dedicated person. But infertility was not his field of expertise and after a while I thought he was futzing around. And I wondered why he didn't say, you should go to a specialist.**❞**
>
> —Yvonne, 29

Looking for Dr. Right

Infertility is a couple's problem and its treatment requires specialized knowledge of both the male and female reproductive systems. This is especially true since in up to half the cases, male-factor infertility is a primary or secondary cause of a couple's inability to conceive.

A fertility specialist should be a licensed medical doctor who has extensive postgraduate training in reproductive medicine, and usually reproductive endocrinology and reproductive surgery as well. Usually fertility specialists are initially trained as OB/GYNs and urologists. Depending on your particular problem and needed treatment, you and your partner may see one or more of the following types of doctors. Make certain, however, that the person you see is *board qualified* or *board certified* in his or her area of reproductive endocrinology or another subspecialty of infertility.

- **Obstetrician/gynecologists (OB/GYNs).** These physicians are board certified in the medical and surgical specialties of obstetrics (the management of pregnancy and child-birth) and gynecology (the diagnosis and treatment of the female reproductive system). They may or may not be qualified reproductive endocrinologists (see below).

- **Reproductive endocrinologists (REs).** These are OB/GYNs who have completed a fellowship in reproductive endocrinology. This involves three years of intensive training in infertility, focusing on the role of hormones in reproduction. To become board certified, they must pass special examinations conducted by the American Board of Obstetrics and Gynecology. They are also trained in the assisted reproductive technologies (ARTs) such as IVF.

  While most OB/GYNs devote a large portion of their time to obstetrics, those OB/GYNs who become reproductive endocrinologists usually devote most or all of their practice to infertility.

- **Gynecologists (GYNs).** These doctors have usually been trained as OB/GYNs but have chosen to specialize in gynecology.

- **Reproductive surgeons.** These physicians have additional advanced training in microsurgery, and are usually trained in the assisted reproductive technologies such as in-vitro fertilization (IVF).

- **Urologists.** These physicians specialize in the diagnosis and treatment of the urinary tract in men and women, as

Watch Out!

Some doctors claim to be fertility specialists even though they don't have the necessary postgraduate or specialized training. Remember, just because doctors advertise themselves as fertility specialists, it doesn't mean they are. Specialists should be board certified in their area of specialization.

well as the male reproductive organs. Urologists are also qualified surgeons. They may or may not have had advanced training in the diagnosis and treatment of male infertility. Again, check their credentials.

■ **Andrologists.** Physicians, usually urologists, who specialize in the male reproductive system and male hormones. Many andrologists also specialize in infertility.

Now that you know what the different specialists do, how do you go about finding the right doctor for you? For one thing, keep in mind that there is no such thing as "the best doctor." There are many good, competent doctors, and your job is to find one who is well suited to your needs.

There are many ways to find a good fertility specialist, and you should probably not depend on one source. The first step is to collect names. The second step is to check their credentials to make certain they are, in fact, qualified fertility specialists. If several names come up repeatedly as good—or bad—doctors, it will help you narrow down your list. To collect a preliminary list of names, here's where to go:

■ **Support groups.** RESOLVE—the not-for-profit national support, education, and advocacy organization for infertile men and women—is a good place to start. Local affiliates keep an up-to-date list of fertility specialists that includes information about their qualifications. Log on to www.resolve.org to find a local affiliate. If there is none in your area, other fertility organizations can give you the inside scoop on local fertility doctors or clinics (see Appendix C).

- **Your personal physicians.** Your doctors—especially OB/GYNs, internists, and family physicians—can be excellent sources of referral. They can also give you feedback on the doctors you're already considering.
- **The American Society for Reproductive Medicine (ASRM).** Formerly called the American Fertility Society, ASRM is an organization of professionals interested in reproductive medicine. ASRM can provide you with the names of its members in your location; log on to www.asrm.org to learn more. Because professionals from many infertility-related fields can become ASRM members, you'll need to further check out their credentials and particular areas of expertise and interests.
- **Friends.** It's a good idea to ask friends who have experienced infertility for their recommendations. But keep in mind that just because a doctor helped your friend get pregnant doesn't mean he or she is the appropriate doctor for you and your particular problem. Physician friends can be especially helpful since not only might they know the names of some good fertility specialists, they can also check out a doctor's credentials *and* reputation.
- **Local hospitals.** You can call your local hospital or medical center to find out which doctors on staff specialize in infertility. Again, you should check out their credentials further.
- **Yellow Pages.** If you have no other choice, you may want to consult the Yellow Pages. But a name or an ad in the Yellow Pages is no guarantee that the doctor is indeed a competent fertility specialist.

Bright Idea

Go to as many infertility talks, meetings, or symposia as you can. You'll have a chance to meet local fertility specialists informally and possibly even ask them questions for free.

Watch Out!

Be wary of doctors who guarantee that they will help you get pregnant. No doctor can or should guarantee this.

Once you have the names of several good fertility specialists, check to see which physicians are covered by your insurance plan and then start calling for appointments. It's best to make appointments with several different doctors for consultations, since you won't immediately know if the doctor you've initially chosen to see is the right one for you. If you find one you like, you can cancel the other appointments if you give them enough notice. However, it may be a good idea to keep the appointments for second opinions or as alternatives if the first doctor doesn't work out.

As you can see, finding a good doctor takes some work. And it should. Your success in overcoming infertility depends heavily upon the doctor you choose, so you should be prepared to devote some time and care in choosing your specialist. Some people balk at the idea of questioning prospective physicians— they may feel intimidated or they just may not want to go through the effort. If that describes you or your partner, ask yourselves this question: Would you buy a new house or car without researching and carefully inspecting it? Your medical care should be even more important. You'll be investing a lot of money and time in your doctor. Your chances of fulfilling your hopes and dreams for a family depend, to a large extent, on this doctor. That's why it's important to choose this person very carefully.

There are basically three important things you need to look for in a fertility specialist: credentials, convenience, and compatibility. It may be helpful to think of them as the three Cs. Let's take a closer look at each.

Credentials

You should always ask about the doctor's postgraduate training. Some doctors say they're fertility specialists but lack the necessary training.

Fertility specialists should be *board certified* in reproductive endocrinology and infertility. A physician who is a board certified reproductive endocrinologist (RE) must have completed a residency in obstetrics and gynecology. He or she then has to take a three-year fellowship in reproductive endocrinology and pass both written and oral exams. Those who have done all of the above except taking or passing their oral exams are considered board eligible reproductive endocrinologists. Once they pass their oral exams, they become board certified.

There are about 940 board certified REs in the United States, 835 of whom are ASRM members. The others most likely are retired or no longer practicing. Most of these REs practice in large cities or medical centers.

There are several ways of checking a doctor's credentials:

▪ Contact a support group such as RESOLVE or the ASRM (see earlier contact information).

▪ Call your county medical society. Local county medical societies have directories of physicians that give information such as medical school attended, year of graduation, and board certification or eligibility in a specialty or subspecialty. You can usually find these directories in your local public library or on the Internet.

▪ Check with the appropriate medical board, such as the American Board of Obstetrics and Gynecology or the American Board of Urology.

 Moneysaver

If you decide to interview several fertility specialists before choosing one, you may be able to consider it as seeking a second opinion—and treat it as such for insurance purposes.

Bright Idea

Ask the doctor what percentage of his or her practice is devoted to infertility; fertility specialists should devote most, if not all, of their time to treating infertility patients. Also, if you see mostly pregnant patients in the office, chances are the doctor is primarily practicing obstetrics and may not have the necessary time or experience to treat infertility.

- Ask the doctor. You can ask the doctor directly about his or her qualifications, or check the diplomas on the wall. You can always double-check by calling the medical school or hospital where the doctor says he or she was trained or contacting the organizations mentioned above.

- Check the Internet. Some websites will do a search for specialists in your area as well as check credentials for you. There is usually a fee for this service.

Convenience

Infertility treatment is a major inconvenience in most people's lives. Therefore, it is helpful to find a doctor who is conveniently located, has convenient hours, and offers other amenities. Here's a list of convenience factors you might want to consider:

- **Convenient location.** Infertility testing and treatment can be very time consuming. For example, you may have to go in for blood tests, sonograms, or inseminations several days in a row. Getting away from work in the middle of the day for doctor appointments can be difficult, so the location of your doctor's practice is important. On the other hand, you don't want to sacrifice quality of care for a convenient location.

- **Flexible office hours.** If you aren't always able to get away from work for doctor appointments, a doctor with early morning hours or evening hours might be best for you. Weekend coverage and weekend hours can sometimes be important. Be sure to discuss scheduling issues with the doctor ahead of time.

■ **Phone hours.** Some doctors have special hours set aside for patients to call about test results or other important medical matters. You should feel free to call your doctor whether or not there are special phone hours, but be brief, out of consideration for both your doctor and the other patients who may need to reach him or her. Many doctors don't charge for short calls. However, if your phone calls become too time consuming, your doctor will most likely charge you an amount predetermined by your insurance policy. Sometimes phone calls are handled by your doctor's nurse or other assistants. This can be fine, especially if they're familiar with your case.

■ **Type of practice—solo or group.** A solo practice provides consistency of approach, continuity of care, and regular contact with the same physician. A group practice tends to have more flexible hours than solo practices, including weekend coverage. However, while you're always guaranteed to have a physician available at all times, you probably won't always get to see the doctor of your choice.

■ **Help with insurance.** Since infertility treatment can be incredibly expensive, a physician's willingness to help you with medical insurance issues can be crucial. In fact, some fertility specialists hire people just to help their patients— and themselves—with insurance matters. Your doctor should be willing to provide the insurer with the necessary information about your case, and his or her staff should be willing to help you fill out the appropriate forms. But

 Moneysaver

Some insurance policies cover e-mail communications with doctors, so be sure to call your insurance company to find out.

keep in mind that your health insurance policy is a contract between you and your insurer. Whether or not you get reimbursed is ultimately up to your insurance company, not your doctor.

■ **On-site lab and other equipment.** Ideally, your doctor will have the necessary equipment in or near his or her office so that you don't have to run all around town for various tests. Most reproductive endocrinologists have the necessary equipment to do routine and sometimes advanced tests and procedures. Some doctors may not have room for all the necessary equipment, but they should be able to refer you to convenient nearby facilities.

Compatibility

Compatibility with one's doctor, while very important, can be difficult to assess. And you certainly can't assess it until you actually go and see the doctor. You may instantly "click" with your doctor and then, after a few months, feel differently. Or you may not take to him or her right away, but as you become more comfortable with each other, you may develop a compatible doctor-patient relationship.

Compatibility is not the same thing as liking or loving. You just have to have a good working relationship, one in which you and your viewpoints are respected, and one in which you participate equally in the major decisions about your treatment.

Go with your gut feelings. If something about the doctor doesn't sit well with you, look elsewhere. You're going to be spending a lot of time with your doctor as well as the office staff. You should feel comfortable with them, feel free to ask them questions, and feel that you are being respected as a person and patient. And most important, you should feel that your medical needs are being met in an emotionally sensitive manner.

Making the most of your consultation

When you finally do get to the point of seeing a specialist, you want the consultation to be as useful and informative as possible. The following suggestions will help you get the most out of both an initial consultation and subsequent office visits:

■ Bring your partner. It's important both medically and emotionally to involve your significant other right from the beginning.

■ Perhaps the most important thing you can do is write down your questions ahead of time and bring them with you.

■ The second most important thing you can do is for both you and your partner to take notes and jot down any questions or concerns that occur to you during the consultation.

■ Make sure any important medical records and test results that may be of use to your new doctor have been sent to his or her office ahead of time. Call at least one week before your appointment to make sure your new doctor has received your medical records. If he or she hasn't, get them yourself and bring them to your first appointment. Also, don't forget to bring any fertility charts you've kept, including the results of home tests (see Chapter 3).

■ If you feel uncomfortable having your partner present during a physical exam or when your history is taken, you can request that he or she leave. Infertility treatment often involves revealing very personal information, especially about your past and current sexual activity. You might also feel uncomfortable discussing these issues with your doctor. But keep in mind that one of the cornerstones of the doctor-patient relationship is confidentiality—that is, the doctor cannot reveal what you say to others outside his or her practice.

Moneysaver

It's important to keep a complete set of all your medical records for your own purposes and to send to any doctors you might consult. Since many doctors charge by the page to copy medical records, if you have your own copies, you can make as many subsequent copies as you want—and save money.

Taking charge of your fertility treatment

Once you've settled on a good fertility specialist, you may be tempted to sit back and let the doctor do all the work. But infertility, like any important issue in your life, requires you to make important decisions. While many people prefer to have their doctor call all the shots (since the doctor is, after all, the expert), keep in mind that you're ultimately responsible for your own health care. This does not mean you become your own doctor. It *does* mean you become an active participant in your treatment. You and your physician form a partnership, based on mutual cooperation and respect. As an equal partner in that relationship, you have important responsibilities. For example, it's up to you to provide accurate information to your doctor and ask questions when you don't understand something.

Infertility treatment requires your full participation. You have to constantly evaluate and reevaluate the situation so you can make the best decisions for yourself. This can only be done with the help and support of your doctor and, ideally, your partner.

Becoming medically knowledgeable about infertility is perhaps the best way to work positively with your doctor toward your ultimate goal—achieving a successful pregnancy. Remember, knowledge is power. And most doctors will appreciate an involved, well-informed patient. Here are some tips:

- Keep a copy of all your medical records at home.
- If you have any questions or concerns about tests or treatments, call your doctor. Make sure all your questions get answered.

- Always weigh the pros and cons, the risks and benefits of every test, drug, and treatment your doctor recommends.

- Read everything you can on infertility. Become an expert on your and/or your partner's particular problem. Go to bookstores, medical libraries, public libraries, and the Internet.

- Join a RESOLVE or other support group, and go to infertility meetings, seminars, and symposia.

- Talk to as many people as you can who have had or currently have fertility problems.

- Trust your instincts. If you have doubts about your doctor, find another one (see "Switching doctors" on the following page).

The doctor-patient relationship

As we've said, your relationship with your fertility doctor is a partnership based on mutual cooperation and it should be a smooth one. After all, you both are working toward the same goal. But in every relationship there are times when things don't go so smoothly. If you have a difference of opinion with your doctor, discuss it with him and try to resolve the issue.

You might feel intimidated about discussing your differences. But keep in mind that you have nothing to lose and a lot to gain. Discussing these issues can help your doctor better understand you and your needs. But if you find that you and your doctor repeatedly have unresolved differences, you may want to consider finding a new doctor.

One problem that young couples sometimes face is not being taken seriously by their doctor. When a couple finally consults a doctor about infertility, they expect something to be

---

 Bright Idea

Make an appointment periodically just to talk to your doctor so you can both reevaluate your situation and discuss your options.

done about it. The woman is usually ready to begin her infertility work-up so that her problem can quickly be diagnosed and treated. But some OB/GYNs may not take the couple's concerns about their fertility seriously, and advise them to relax and give it more time. This is another reason why it's critical to see a fertility specialist, someone who understands how couples—regardless of their age—are concerned about their biological clocks ticking.

Many older couples face a similar problem. Despite the evidence that infertility increases after the age of 30, many nonspecialists treat their older patients in much the same way they treat their younger ones.

> 66 The doctor's whole attitude was very relaxed. He never gave me the feeling that it was a terribly urgent thing that I must immediately check out. And he kept saying, "Well, wait a few more months and see."...He said, "Maybe you should take a vacation." 99
>
> —Janet, 38

They follow the general rule that you wait one full year before initiating an infertility work-up or treatment. Most fertility specialists, however, believe that a woman over the age of 35—or even 30—who has not conceived in six months should start an infertility work-up. If you're convinced you have a fertility problem and your doctor isn't, find another doctor—someone at least willing to explore the possibility.

Switching doctors

Infertility patients are notorious for doctor shopping and doctor hopping. Patients often switch doctors if they feel their doctors can no longer help them. When conflicts cannot be resolved, or you believe your doctor can't help you conceive, it may be time to change doctors.

How can you tell if your doctor won't be able to help you conceive? If you feel that you aren't making progress—that you're no closer to a pregnancy or a clear understanding of why you're not getting pregnant after a reasonable period of time—it's time to move on to another doctor, or at least get a second opinion. Whether or not you stay with your doctor or even continue treatment varies from patient to patient. It depends on your age, diagnosis, prognosis, and emotional and financial limits. What it *shouldn't* depend on is false hope or unrealistic expectations about your doctor's abilities. No fertility specialist—no matter how famous or well qualified—can help every patient. Sometimes even the best doctor can miss some subtle aspect of a medical condition. That is why second opinions can be extremely helpful to both you and your doctor.

Countless patients have wasted considerable time and money by sticking with their OB/GYNs—or even fertility specialists—when they should have moved on to another doctor. On the other hand, skipping from doctor to doctor can be counterproductive. It may take a doctor many months or even years to help you achieve a pregnancy. What is important is that you feel that you are making progress, that another piece of the puzzle has been found, and that different treatment methods are tried.

Just the facts

- Some couples are hesitant to consult a fertility specialist because they feel stigmatized and embarrassed.

- It's important to shop around until you find a doctor who has the right credentials, a convenient location and hours, and with whom you feel compatible.

- Take charge of your fertility treatment by reading up on infertility, asking your doctor questions, and keeping your own medical records.

- Your relationship with your fertility doctor should be a partnership based on mutual cooperation and respect.

- If you feel your doctor has not given you the care you deserve, or if you feel you're making no progress in your infertility treatment, it may be time to switch doctors or at least seek a second opinion.

GET THE SCOOP ON...
The basic infertility work-up ▪ Specialized tests
for women ▪ Specialized tests for men ▪ Genetic
testing ▪ Gearing up for treatment

Chapter 6

Getting to the Root of the Problem

Once you've found a good fertility specialist, the next step is to find out what's wrong. Keep in mind that infertility is unlike other physical conditions. First and foremost, it's a couple's problem, so two patients are involved. Uncovering the cause or causes of a fertility problem—and finding a solution—must involve both partners. And, unlike most disorders, diagnosing the cause can easily take several months, or even more than a year.

The infertility work-up

The first step in diagnosing a fertility problem is the infertility work-up—a systematic process that takes some time, not to mention patience, to complete. But it doesn't have to be a long drawn-out affair; to save precious time, some components can and should be done simultaneously. A basic but thorough infertility work-up includes a history, physical examination, routine office and laboratory tests, and—if deemed necessary by your doctor—more specialized tests.

Moneysaver

Bring any earlier test results with you to the doctor's office—it may save you the cost of repeating tests. Keep in mind, however, that some tests might have to be repeated because your fertility status can change over time.

Any investigation into the cause of infertility should involve both partners from the very start. If the male partner does not yet have a urologist or andrologist, his partner's doctor can refer him to one. The couple should go to the initial appointments—and to as many of the subsequent ones as possible—together.

History

The first thing your doctor will do is obtain a complete history: medical, surgical, and sexual. This is often part of the initial interview.

Personal and family medical history

A complete medical history contains information not only about your personal health, but your family history as well. In addition to questions about your overall health, the doctor will ask you specific questions about your current and previous fertility status. Because sexually transmitted diseases (STDs) are a major cause of infertility, your doctor should seek clues of present or past infection.

- **Current infertility.** How long have you been trying to conceive? What contraceptives have you used? For how long? What infertility tests have you had? What treatments have you had?

- **Previous fertility.** If you're a woman, have you ever been pregnant? If so, did the pregnancy end in a live birth? If you're a man, have you ever fathered a child?

Your doctor will also question you about diseases or disorders that "run in the family," as well as your use of medications or drugs, and any lifestyle factors that may have an effect on your fertility.

- Do you have diabetes, hypertension, asthma, arthritis, ulcers, colitis, or thyroid disease? Have you had cancer? Were you treated with surgery, radiotherapy, or chemotherapy? Did your mother use DES (diethylstilbestrol) when she was pregnant with you? Does either partner have a family history of genetic disorders such as cystic fibrosis, sickle-cell anemia, Tay-Sachs disease, muscular dystrophy, or hemophilia? If you're a man, were your testicles normal at birth? Did you have mumps as an adult?

- What prescription and over-the-counter medicines do you take?

- Do you currently or have you ever smoked cigarettes? Used or abused alcohol? Taken illicit drugs? If so, how much do you use or have you used them?

- What type of work do you do? What hobbies do you have? Have you ever come in contact with chemicals, pesticides, or radiation?

- Have you ever had an STD? If you're a woman, have you ever had any, even vague, *genitourinary* (abdominal, bladder, or vaginal) symptoms?

The doctor may also ask you about other risk factors for pelvic inflammatory disease (PID), such as number of past sexual partners.

Surgical history

If you're a woman, have you ever had an appendectomy or other abdominal or pelvic surgery? If you're a man, have you ever had surgery to correct a varicocele, undescended testis (cryptorcidism), or hernia? Have you had any other groin, pelvis, or bladder operations? (Refer to Chapter 4 for more information about conditions and operations that might interfere with fertility.)

Sexual history

How frequently do you have intercourse? Do you have pain during sexual intercourse? What positions do you and your partner use? Do you achieve an orgasm? If you're a woman, do you douche, or use lubricants or feminine hygiene products? Does your partner's penis enter and penetrate your vagina? If you're a man, do you achieve and maintain an erection? Do you enter and penetrate your partner's vagina? Do you ejaculate into your partner's vagina?

Special questions about the woman's medical history

Besides current and previous fertility status, the doctor will ask the woman more in-depth questions about her gynecologic and obstetric history:

- **Gynecologic history.** When did you first start menstruating? Are your menstrual periods regular? How long, heavy, or painful are they? Do you experience *mittelschmerz*— mild pain on one side of your abdomen near the time of ovulation? Do you have vaginal discharge? What gynecologic or urologic problems have you had? Have you had a *tubal ligation* (sterilization, sometimes called having your "tubes tied")?

- **Obstetrical history.** Have you ever been pregnant? When? How long did it take to get pregnant? Did you carry to term? Were there any complications? Did you breastfeed? For how long? Did you ever have a stillbirth? Have you had an abortion, either spontaneous or induced? Were there any complications?

 Bright Idea

Some aspects of the initial interview may be embarrassing, particularly when they deal with sexual histories and practices. If a couple wishes, they should ask their doctor if these interviews can be conducted separately, and, of course, confidentially.

Special questions about the man's medical history

The doctor will also have specific questions for the male partner to answer, specifically pertaining to his urologic history. Such questions will include: Have you ever had undescended testes (cryptorchidism), a varicocele, testicular injury, testicular torsion, or been told you have Kleinfelter's Syndrome? Have you ever had any infection such as epididymitis, prostatitis, or sexually transmitted diseases? Have you had a vasectomy? Have you been exposed to direct excessive heat, radiation, or toxic chemicals? When did you enter puberty?

The physical examination

Next comes the physical exam. Your doctor will be looking more for factors that might be contributing to infertility than for the cause of infertility itself. These can range from malnutrition to obesity, from renal to thyroid disease. Very importantly, the doctor will look for signs of hormone imbalance.

The physical examination of the woman

A complete physical exam of the woman includes vaginal, pelvic, and rectal examinations. Your doctor will look for obvious structural defects, such as the size, shape, or position of your reproductive organs, which might be interfering with conception. The exam might also suggest fibroids, tumors, adhesions, or endometriosis, all risk factors for infertility. When inspecting the vaginal canal, the doctor will be looking for lesions and vaginal discharge, both of which might suggest an STD; and cervical tears, polyps, or infection, any of which might interfere with sperm survival. The presence of excessive hair (hirsuitism) on the face, back, and abdomen; acne; or obesity might be clues to a hormonal imbalance that can interfere with reproduction.

The doctor might perform a routine Pap test to rule out cervical cancer or other abnormalities and take a sample of cervical secretions for culture to rule out infection. In particular, the doctor should be looking for that silent, prevalent organism *Chlamydia trachomatis,* which is a leading cause of infertility. (See Chapter 1 for more information about this and other sexually transmitted diseases.)

The physical examination of the man

The doctor—usually a urologist or andrologist—will examine the testes, penis, scrotum, and prostate, looking for any signs of structural deformities or infection. Your doctor will also note the size and texture of the testes. In particular, the doctor will look for a varicocele, penile deformities, and undescended testes, as well as examine the status of the epididymis and vas deferens. The doctor might also take a sample of urethral secretions or prostate fluid to be cultured to rule out infection.

Your doctor will look for outward signs of a hormone imbalance, such as enlarged breasts. In particular, the doctor will note your secondary sex characteristics, those that are regulated by testosterone, such as facial and body hair, and voice depth.

Narrowing the possibilities

After your medical history has been taken, your doctor will have some clues as to where the problem(s) may lie. For example, a man might have had a vasectomy, or a woman might know ahead of time that she has endometriosis. But just because a cause is known ahead of time, it doesn't rule out other contributing factors that warrant further diagnostic testing. So how does the doctor narrow the range of reasons for your infertility?

This is where your medical history comes in. For example, a woman with a history of irregular, heavy menstrual periods would certainly undergo hormonal testing first. Because ovulatory and sperm problems are by far the most common causes of infertility, confirming ovulation and assessing sperm count and quality should be the first steps any doctor should take.

Your doctor will also want to explore other common causes of infertility, such as poor sperm and cervical mucus interaction and Fallopian tube or uterine problems. The diagnostic principle here is to start with the least difficult and invasive tests and go on to the more difficult or invasive ones as needed. Basically, your doctor will be trying to determine four facts:

- Is the woman ovulating?
- Does the man have sufficient, healthy sperm?
- Can the sperm and the egg meet?
- Can a fertilized egg implant itself successfully?

Your doctor will now order routine office and laboratory tests designed to look more closely for specific female and male infertility factors. These tests are quite simple and will seek answers to the first two questions above: Is the woman ovulating? Is the man producing enough healthy sperm?

Is the woman ovulating?

Because several hormones secreted in specific amounts and sequences regulate ovulation, testing for ovulation involves looking for signs that these hormones are present and measuring them at different times during the menstrual cycle. Keep in mind that these hormones are just markers, or indirect measures, for ovulation.

Your gynecologic history can provide clues to your ovulatory status. A history of irregular or absent menstrual periods points strongly to an ovulatory problem. As we saw in Chapter 3, some of the most common tests for ovulation can be done at home, including charting basal body temperature (BBT); evaluating cervical mucus; and measuring LH, estradiol, progesterone in the urine, and sperm survival and quality.

These tests—whether done at home or in the doctor's office—not only provide valuable information, they are also helpful in the scheduling and timing of intercourse and other tests and procedures.

If it appears that you are not ovulating at all—or doing so only sporadically—your doctor will order blood tests to measure hormone levels. These tests can also give the doctor invaluable information about other factors that might be interfering with your ability to conceive.

- A *FSH (follicle-stimulating hormone) test* helps distinguish ovarian failure from hypothalamic or pituitary problems. A basal measurement FSH on the first, second, or third day of the menstrual cycle is frequently done to see if a woman is experiencing premature menopause and to evaluate egg quality.

- An *LH (luteinizing hormone) test* shows if the hypothalamic/ pituitary and gonadal systems are working properly. It can help diagnose polycystic ovarian disease.

- An *estradiol (E2) test* assesses how well the ovaries are functioning and whether egg follicles are maturing properly.

- *Thyroid tests (TSH, T3 uptake, and T4)* detect hyper- or hypothryoidism, either of which can cause infertility.

- *Progesterone testing* shows whether ovulation has occurred and the corpus luteum is functioning normally. It's useful for determining that the uterine lining can receive a fertilized egg for implantation. Progesterone is another hormone that will give clues to a luteal phase defect.

- *Prolactin testing* shows the presence or absence of prolactin. Abnormally high levels can interfere with or disrupt ovulation and/or progesterone production.

Is the man producing enough healthy sperm?

The diagnostic work-up of the male partner should be done at the same time as the female partner. Luckily, the most important diagnostic test for male-factor infertility, the semen analysis, is a simple, noninvasive, and certainly not painful test, although some men may find it embarrassing.

Semen analyses evaluate the quantity and quality of sperm and seminal fluid. More than one analysis—usually three—may be done because semen quality varies and results can change over time. Semen analysis looks at several specific factors:

Bright Idea

Because not all technicians performing semen analysis are trained to interpret sperm morphology, make sure your doctor uses a lab with specially trained personnel.

- **Volume** shows whether the ejaculate has the right amount and mix of substances needed to keep sperm alive and well.

- **Sperm count,** sometimes called sperm concentration or sperm density, shows whether enough sperm are being delivered with the ejaculate to make conception possible. (Sperm production can be normal in the testis, but a blockage may cause sperm to be absent in the ejaculate.)

- **Sperm morphology** shows whether the sperm are shaped normally. There is another more sophisticated examination of sperm shape called the *strict sperm morphology determination*. In this test, specially stained sperm are examined under a microscope. Precise measurements of sperm heads and tails are taken. Doctors pay particular attention to the width, length, and contour of heads and the length of the tails.

- **Sperm motility,** which may actually be more important than their number or concentration, shows whether the sperm can swim, and whether they can swim fast and forward.

- **Sperm viscosity** shows whether semen—which is delivered into the vagina as a thickish, jelly-like substance called coagulum—will finally liquefy. If it doesn't, it may affect sperm function.

- **White blood cells (WBC),** if found in the semen, might point to an infection or inflammation. Sometimes WBC are difficult to distinguish from early sperm forms, so special stains may be added to help.

A semen sample is usually collected by masturbation after two or three days of sexual abstinence. If you're prohibited from masturbating for religious reasons, you might try using a condom with a pinhole in it during sexual intercourse. This allows some sperm to enter the vagina, and the rest to be collected from the condom for a semen analysis. Some men find it difficult to masturbate on demand, or at all. Because of this, many facilities have special private rooms, replete with erotic literature and videos, and some encourage the partner to participate, to help the process along. It's important that the sample be kept at body temperature, and that it be analyzed within about an hour after collection. If you need to bring a semen sample in for analysis, keep the container at body temperature by putting the container in a pocket close to your body.

Ask your doctor about the lab doing your semen analysis, particularly if the lab is right there in your doctor's office. If it doesn't specialize in infertility assessment and handle several dozen analyses a month, it may not have the expertise to make accurate evaluations. Some doctors are using computer-assisted systems. While they have their place, they shouldn't be relied on solely, either. They require a well-trained and experienced person to make assessments. And the equipment needs to be calibrated. It's easy for the computer to count every little speck as a sperm, leading the male partner to believe he has a higher sperm count than he really does. But it takes a skillful eye to evaluate other sperm characteristics, such as how well formed they are.

 Watch Out!

When in a car, don't leave semen samples on your dashboard or near the heater; they can get baked in the sun or fried from the heater. Avoid air-conditioning vents as well.

Table 6.1: Semen Analysis (Based on at Least Two Analyses)

Parameter	Normal Range
Volume	2 to 5 mL (may be as low as 1 mL)
pH	7.4
Sperm count	50 to 200 million per mL (20 million is the lowest count that will allow pregnancy to occur naturally, without special treatment)
Sperm motility	40 to 80 percent progressive motility one hour after ejaculation
Sperm morphology	30 to 50 percent (4 to 14 percent for *strict sperm morphology test*)
Liquefaction time	10 to 20 minutes after ejaculation
Content	No or only minimal white cells or epithelial cells

More specialized tests may be needed if the results of the semen analyses show a problem. If sperm count is low, a man's blood testosterone FSH and LH levels should be checked.

Can the sperm and egg meet?

The first test commonly used to answer this question is rather simple. It's also one that you and your partner start at home—the doctor views the results in the office. It's called the *postcoital test* (PCT), but is also known as the *Sims-Huhner test*. If the results of this test show a good number of moving sperm, other factors are likely to be interfering with fertilization.

The PCT has come under a lot of scrutiny lately, and its usefulness as a tool for predicting pregnancy has been challenged. One criticism is that there is little standardization in how the test is conducted and interpreted.

That said, the PCT can be useful in detecting cervical mucus problems that may be causing infertility. It also gives some idea of how the sperm react in the lower female reproductive tract, as well as whether enough sperm are being deposited in the vagina. In fact, for years it has been considered the gold standard for determining sperm survivability after intercourse. However, the PCT should never take the place of a complete semen analysis.

The PCT is performed just before ovulation, so BBT charting and urinary LH kits are helpful in scheduling this test. Ultrasound can also be useful to confirm if ovulation is imminent. You should engage in sexual intercourse the night before or on the morning of the test. Don't douche, use any lubricants, or use any vaginal medications, sprays, creams, or powders! The doctor will take a sample of the woman's cervical mucus—a painless procedure—and examine it under a microscope to see how many sperm are there and how well they're moving. There is some debate about exactly how long after intercourse the test should be done. Generally, about eight hours later is considered to be the best time, but the range can be from three to twenty-four hours.

If too few moving sperm are seen under microscopic examination, it could mean that sperm production or delivery into the vagina is impaired. If the sperm are not moving, it could signal a problem with the timing of the test or the cervical mucus itself. If the quality or quantity of the cervical mucus is poor, it may indicate a cervical abnormality or an infection.

Sometimes, your doctor will order this test a second time and set up your office visit earlier or later in the cycle than he or she did for the first test. For example, you may be asked to come into the office as soon as possible after sexual intercourse if the test wasn't well timed before.

Can the fertilized egg implant itself successfully?

For a pregnancy to occur, a blastocyst—which is formed about seven days after an egg is fertilized—needs to implant itself in the uterine lining (endometrium), where, if all goes well, it will grow into a healthy fetus.

Why some blastocyts implant and others do not is not well understood. However, recent research at the Center for Reproductive Medicine & Infertility at the Cornell Medical Center has found the age of the mother is the most important factor in implantation success. After age 36, women undergoing in-vitro fertilization (IVF) have a significantly lower implantation rate than younger women, and the rate continues to steadily decline with age.

Progesterone, which is produced by the corpus luteum, is another key factor; adequate levels are necessary to prepare the endometrium for implantation of the fertilized egg. Progesterone is also necessary for the survival of the newly fertilized egg and the prevention of early miscarriage. Progesterone can be measured in the blood or through an endometrial biopsy, which is described in the next section.

In addition to maternal age and progesterone levels, such factors as uterine fibroids or polyps or the abnormal development of the endometrium can interfere with implantation. If a problem is suspected, there are several diagnostic tests that identify the cause. These tests include endometrial biopsies, hysterosalpingograms (HSG), and vaginal ultrasounds or sonograms. Occasionally hysteroscopies are performed if implantation continues to be a problem.

Specialized tests for women

The following tests help evaluate the reproductive organs directly. These tests tend to be more invasive—and therefore more painful—than the previously mentioned diagnostic procedures. Some, such as a laparoscopy and a hysteroscopy, are surgical procedures. Therefore, they are usually the last steps in the diagnostic work-up and they may not necessary or appropriate for all infertile women.

Watch Out!

Be sure your doctor gives you a pregnancy test before you have an endometrial biopsy or any other invasive procedure. These procedures—and the medications you may need to take for the procedures—can potentially harm a fetus.

- An *endometrial biopsy* is used to evaluate both ovulation and luteal-phase defects, which can interfere with the ability of a fertilized egg to implant itself in the endometrium. Comparing the results of endometrial biopsy and blood hormone tests can show if ovulation and uterine preparation are normal.

  Performed quickly in the doctor's office, an endometrial biopsy is scheduled anywhere from the mid-luteal phase, or about Day 21 of a 28-day cycle, to just before a woman expects her menstrual period; that is, when progesterone-induced effects on the uterine lining are at their peak. A small piece of tissue is removed from the endometrium and examined under a microscope. A trained eye can tell if the tissue is responding properly to progesterone. While similar in some ways to having a Pap test, the endometrial biopsy is somewhat more invasive and painful. You might want to ask your doctor for a painkiller to take *before* the procedure.

- An *hysterosalpingogram* is a special X-ray using a contrast dye to evaluate the size and shape of the uterus and determine if the Fallopian tubes are open. It's performed after a menstrual period, but before ovulation. Injected through the cervix, the dye fills the uterus and should flow freely into the Fallopian tubes. Your doctor will be looking for uterine scar tissue, polyps, fibroids, and deformities— conditions that prevent sperm and egg from meeting or embryo implantation, or induce a miscarriage.

This test can be very uncomfortable for some, so you may want to ask for painkillers or anti-inflammatory drugs to ease the situation. Your doctor might also prescribe an antibiotic. You may have some discomfort as well as discharge for a few hours after the test as dye is expelled. The uterus stretching as it fills with dye is the cause of the discomfort. If the tubes are blocked, pressure might build up and may also cause some pain. But the pressure from the injected dye might even open up small blockages.

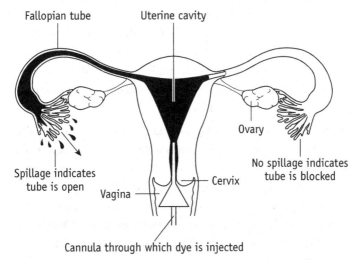

Illustration of an hysterosalpingogram. Reprinted with permission from the American Society for Reproductive Medicine (ASRM).

■ A *vaginal ultrasound* helps confirm ovulation. Because ultrasound works on the principle of sound waves bouncing off fluid-filled objects, if the follicle, which is a fluid-filled sac beneath the surface of the ovary, ripens, enlarges, and then collapses after an egg is released, the sonogram will detect it. Again, just because a deflated follicle is detected doesn't mean that it released an egg or had one in it to begin with. But a positive test result here plus positive results from LH surge and BBT charting raise the likelihood that you're ovulating. Occasionally, a series of sonograms—starting after the LH surge and continuing until a collapsed follicle is detected—may be taken to monitor ovulation. Another benefit of the vaginal ultrasound is that it can provide information about endometrial lining thickness, an important factor in implantation. This information is important if your doctor suspects a luteal-phase defect. Your doctor can also use the test to assess uterine and ovarian position and size and detect any cyst or pregnancy.

- *Transabdominal (pelvic) ultrasounds*, which are done externally rather than internally, are sometimes used instead of vaginal ultrasounds; however, they don't provide as much data. Vaginal ultrasounds also provide a cleaner image and are more easily tolerated by patients. Transabdominal ultrasounds require the women to drink large amounts of water to inflate their bladders.

- A *laparoscopy* is a surgical—usually outpatient—procedure done under general anesthesia. (See the illustration of a laparoscopy in Chapter 8.) It allows the doctor to look directly at the Fallopian tubes, ovaries, and the outside of the uterus through a telescopic instrument inserted through a small incision in or near the navel. Occasionally, other small cuts are made to allow a better look at the pelvic organs. Your doctor will check for endometriosis, adhesions, fibroids, and ovarian cysts. The doctor can also inject a solution through the cervix and uterus to see if the Fallopian tubes are open. You may have some pain, stiffness, and soreness for a day or two after the procedure.

 Watch Out!

Bring your partner or a friend with you when you have invasive tests. They can offer you emotional support as well as help get you home after the test if necessary. Some of these tests—and the medications that go with them—can impair your ability to function well for several hours.

Moneysaver

If you're having a laparoscopy or hysteroscopy, discuss in advance with your doctor the possibility of correcting any problem found at the same time as the diagnostic procedure. It will save the expense—and discomfort—of undergoing surgery a second time. But be certain the doctor performing the test is qualified to surgically correct any problems you might have.

■ An *hysteroscopy* is also a surgical procedure usually done on an outpatient basis. While the woman is under general or local anesthesia, a telescopic instrument is inserted through the dilated cervix into the lower end of the uterus. Gas or a clear fluid is injected into the uterus so that the uterine cavity expands and blood and mucus are cleared. Your doctor will be looking inside the uterus for fibroids, polyps, scarring, and congenital deformities.

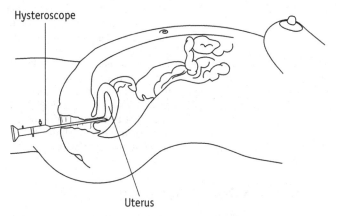

Hysteroscope

Uterus

Illustration of an hysteroscopy. Reprinted with permission from the American Society for Reproductive Medicine (ASRM).

Timing is everything, especially in infertility treatment. Here's a chart to help you see which tests are performed at the various points in the menstrual cycle. Remember, Day 1 is counted from the first day of real bleeding. (These estimates are based on a 28-day cycle.)

Watch Out!

If you're told that uterine fibroids are causing your infertility—but you don't have a distorted uterine cavity or tubal occlusion, or feel a lot of pelvic pressure—there might be other factors involved. Uterine fibroids are rarely the sole cause of infertility.

Table 6.2: The Timing of Some Basic Infertility Tests

Cycle Day(s)	Test	Why It's Done at This Time
Day 12 to Day 15	Postcoital exam	This test checks to see if sperm live well in the cervical mucus. It is scheduled during the point in the cycle when cervical mucus conditions are likely to be most favorable to sperm.
Day 19 to Day 24	Progesterone blood test	This test checks the levels of progesterone being produced. Progesterone production increases at the time of ovulation, so this test is scheduled during that part of the cycle when its levels in the blood are highest.
Day 19 to Day 28	Endometrial biopsy	This test permits the evaluation of the tissue that lines the uterus to if it can develop the structures see necessary to support an implanted fetus. The test is done after ovulation, when the tissue lining the uterus is best developed.

Specialized tests for men

In male-factor infertility, it's important that the man undergo an extensive urologic evaluation to ensure that any possible causes of infertility are not overlooked, and that the infertility is not an indication of some significant underlying health problem.

If routine laboratory test results are inconclusive or don't point to a specific problem, more sophisticated testing might be needed. Some evaluate sperm quality, some sperm production.

Others assess sperm transport. Here are some of the tests that might be ordered and why:

- An *acrosome reaction test* determines whether sperm heads can actually undergo the chemical changes needed to dissolve an egg's tough outer shell and penetrate it.

- A *testicular biopsy* can determine how well sperm are being produced. In this test, a very small piece of tissue taken from the *seminiferous tubules* and surrounding areas *(interstitial tissue)* is examined under a microscope for signs of abnormal sperm production.

- *Hormone tests* are sometimes as important in evaluating male-factor infertility as they are for female-factor infertility. Blood samples are taken and assessed for FSH and LH, which are both critical for sperm development and maintaining testosterone levels. Elevated prolactin levels may be associated with low testosterone levels and even impotence.

- A *vasography,* which is an X-ray of the vas deferens, is used to detect a blockage or leakage of sperm.

- *High-resolution scrotal ultrasonography* and *venography* are tests to find varicoceles in the testicles too small to be felt during physical examination.

- *Ultrasonography* is used to find damages or blockages in the male reproductive tract, including the prostate, seminal vesicles, and ejaculatory ducts.

- A *hypo-osmotic swelling test* is sometimes used to help predict whether sperm can fertilize an egg. Normal sperm tails will swell when put into a special sugar and salt solution. Poorly functioning sperm membranes don't seem to possess that characteristic. However, the significance is questioned by many fertility experts.

- A *sperm agglutination test* is a laboratory test in which sperm are looked at under the microscope to see if they clump together. Clumping prevents sperm from swimming through cervical mucus and attaching to an egg. Antisperm

Bright Idea

Several semen analyses should be done over the course of treatment. Because sperm quality can vary over time, and even a slight fever can change the results of an analysis, reevaluation can be very helpful.

antibodies or an infection can cause sperm agglutination. (See Chapter 2 for more information about antisperm antibodies.) As we noted earlier, the importance of antisperm antibodies and the need to test for them is controversial. Current data have raised questions about the usefulness of this test, so it's being used less and less frequently.

Other tests that were used in the past but are rarely used today are the *hamster penetration assay* or *sperm penetration assay (SPA)*.

Genetic testing

Genetic testing can be an important screening tool, not just for pregnant women, but for infertile couples as well. There are two types of genetic testing that can be extremely helpful in both the diagnosis and treatment of infertility: *pre-pregnancy genetic testing*, which involves testing the potential parents; and *pre-implantation genetic diagnosis*, which involves testing an embryo before it is implanted in an IVF setting.

Pre-pregnancy genetic testing can be a useful diagnostic tool for men who have extremely low sperm counts—and for couples who suffer from recurrent miscarriages—when no cause has previously been found. Pre-pregnancy genetic testing can also be used for carrier screening. This can help determine if potential parents are carriers of certain serious genetic diseases that run in families or certain racial groups—such as Tay-Sachs disease, cystic fibrosis, sickle cell anemia, and thalassemia—that can be passed on to their offspring. If it's discovered that both partners are, in fact, carriers, they may choose not to risk having their own biological children and decide to pursue third-party reproduction instead (see Chapter 11).

But there is another option that many infertile couples prefer: having further genetic testing after they undergo IVF or the other assisted reproductive technologies. This type of genetic testing—called pre-implantation genetic diagnosis or PGD—involves testing the embryo *before* it's implanted to rule out serious genetic disorders. Pre-implantation genetic diagnosis is discussed further in Chapter 9.

The third type of genetic testing that many couples undergo when they become pregnant is *prenatal genetic testing*. This involves testing the fetus *during* pregnancy through *amniocentesis* or *chorionic villus sampling* to rule out Down syndrome and other serious genetic diseases.

Diagnostic decisions

Now that you know what the various tests are, you and your partner can participate with your doctor in the decision as to what diagnostic tests, beyond the very simple ones, you should undertake. If possible, you'll want to avoid unnecessary, time-consuming, or expensive tests. Here are some questions you can ask your doctor that will help you make an educated decision about diagnostic testing:

- Is the test necessary?
- What will the test show?
- How much will it cost?
- Will my insurance cover it?
- Will it hurt? If so, what can I do to ease the pain?
- Should my partner or a friend accompany me?
- Does it require anesthesia or hospitalization?
- Will I need to miss work?
- How long will it take to get the results?
- If the test is negative, what's the next step?
- If the test is positive, will I need to take more tests?

Remember, it's up to you and your partner—hopefully with considerable input from your doctor—to decide what diagnostic tests you take and, ultimately, what treatments you accept. It's important to understand the implications of testing or not testing. Keep in mind that these decisions may impact on how rapidly and accurately a diagnosis is made and how successful treatment may be.

Getting ready for treatment

As we've emphasized, because infertility is a couple's problem, the road to fertility must be a joint effort. Before embarking on any type of treatment, you and your partner should consider separately and then discuss together what lies ahead. Ask yourselves: "What do I (we) want?" "What am I (we) prepared to do?" Of course, circumstances—whether physical, emotional, or even financial—change. So what you decide today doesn't have to be written in stone. You can, and probably will, change your mind. But having some idea of what you're willing to undergo will help you set up a plan of action and a timetable. This puts you in control and will help relieve anxiety.

Just the facts

- A basic infertility work-up involves a history, physical exam, and diagnostic office and laboratory tests.

- Specialized tests for women involve x-ray, ultrasounds, and occasionally minor surgery.

- Specialized tests for men involve blood or other lab tests, and occasionally a biopsy.

- Genetic testing is indicated for men who have extremely low sperm counts—and couples who have recurrent miscarriages—when no cause has previously been found.

- After discussing your options with your doctor, it's up to you and your partner to decide what diagnostic tests and treatments you will undergo.

Traditional Treatments

GET THE SCOOP ON...
When are fertility drugs an option? ▪ The latest
fertility drugs ▪ Multiple births and other side
effects ▪ Monitoring drug treatment ▪ Fertility
drugs for men ▪ Artificial insemination

PART IV

Fertility Drugs and Other Nonsurgical Treatments

Chapter 7

O nce you've found a qualified doctor who you and your partner are comfortable with and you've gone through a thorough diagnostic evaluation, you're probably anxious to get going on treatment. Infertility treatment typically begins with noninvasive, nonsurgical measures—such as fertility drugs—unless there is an obvious need for surgery.

Indications for fertility drugs

Fertility drugs are a mainstay of infertility treatment. Certainly, you'll be given fertility drugs if you have obvious ovulatory dysfunction—the major cause of female infertility. Infertility due to hormonal problems can be treated successfully with *ovulation induction*— as treatment with fertility drugs is called—in as many as 75 percent of all cases. This figure is similar to the rate of conception in the normal population.

Moneysaver

Shop around in drug stores and on the Internet for the best deals on your fertility or other prescription drugs. And call around periodically. Prices can change frequently.

You may be surprised to learn that the fertility drugs—and other hormones that are typically used to treat female infertility—are also used to treat some types of male-factor infertility. Also, in cases of male-factor infertility, the female partner is sometimes given fertility drugs to ensure *that* she ovulates and to pinpoint the time *when* she ovulates. With these assurances, procedures such as *therapeutic insemination,* or TI, more commonly known as artificial insemination, can be carried out at the woman's most fertile time. These procedures will be discussed in more detail later in this chapter.

If you're an older woman, or the cause of your infertility is not identified, fertility drugs are often prescribed to help boost the quality of your ovulations. And sometimes when both partners' fertility is not up to par—if the woman's ovulations are not regular and the male partner's sperm count is a bit low—fertility drugs may be just the thing to compensate for these subtle fertility shortcomings.

Finally, fertility drugs are an integral part of assisted reproductive technologies (ARTs). Here they're used to increase the number of eggs produced and to schedule these high-tech procedures. (See Chapters 9 and 10 for more information on ARTs.)

It's likely, then, that at some point in your infertility treatment, fertility drugs may be an option for you. So it makes sense for anyone facing infertility treatment to understand these drugs and what they can do for you. Of course, fertility drugs are not the only noninvasive infertility treatment available. In this chapter, we'll look at several other options—such as artificial insemination—as well.

Back to basics

Before we get started on the treatments themselves, however, a quick review of key points in the hormonal orchestration needed for ovulation, fertilization, and implantation is in order. (For a more detailed description of the female reproductive system, including hormonal control, see Chapter 2.)

Here are the steps involved in the natural, untreated menstrual cycle:

1. The hypothalamus releases gonadotropin-releasing hormone (GnRH) in a series of discrete, pulsed bursts that increase in the later part of the menstrual cycle.

2. In response to the GnRH signal, the pituitary gland releases follicle-stimulating hormone (FSH) and luteinizing hormone (LH). It's primarily FSH that stimulates follicles to mature. (Anywhere from two to fifteen eggs and their follicles emerge from a resting state in the ovaries during each cycle. But only one or two become dominant and eventually release their eggs.)

3. As they mature, follicles release their own set of hormones, primarily estradiol, a type of estrogen.

4. In response to estrogen, the pituitary gland releases less and less FSH. If all goes correctly, only enough hormones, in particular FSH, are produced to keep the best follicles maturing.

5. At mid-cycle, the follicle fully matures or ripens. LH levels increase, or surge, to stimulate the follicle to ovulate; that is, release its egg.

6. The empty follicle after ovulation becomes the corpus luteum, a hormone-producing structure, and begins releasing progesterone, which helps the endometrium become receptive to implantation of a fertilized egg.

Ovulatory disorders and fertility drugs

As we've mentioned, ovulatory dysfunction is by far the most common cause of female-factor infertility, accounting for one quarter to one third of all infertility cases. Ovulatory dysfunction is the failure of the ovaries to produce or release an egg regularly, usually because of a hormonal imbalance. The aim of ovulation induction using fertility drugs is to bring these hormones back into line so that an egg is regularly available for fertilization each cycle.

What fertility drugs treat

Fertility drugs help treat a variety of ovulatory disorders, including:

- Failure to ovulate (anovulation)
- Infrequent ovulation (oligo-ovulation)
- Erratically occurring periods
- Luteal-phase defects, both short and long
- Absence of menstruation (amenorrhea)
- Progesterone deficiencies

First, the aim of fertility drugs for these problems and for the procedures we'll discuss later in this chapter is to stimulate the production of a limited number of eggs—one or two of them. This is sometimes called *controlled ovarian hyperstimulation.* Obviously, having eggs available is critical for pregnancy to occur.

Second, fertility drugs help to regulate the ovulatory cycle. This allows you to time sexual intercourse and schedule an artificial insemination if indicated.

Third, fertility drugs play a vital role in ARTs as well. In ARTs, fertility drugs are used to increase the number of viable eggs per cycle—sometimes to more than a dozen—with the hope of improving the chances of fertilization and implantation. (See Chapter 9 for a full discussion of ARTs.)

Finally, hormones are often given to prepare the uterus for embryo implantation, for ART procedures, and particularly when using third-party reproductive procedures involving donor embryos. (See Chapter 11 for more on third-party reproduction.)

Important considerations

There are some particulars to remember when you're considering taking fertility drugs. Keep in mind that ovulation induction is a custom-tailored therapy. That's one reason why you need to be under the care of a specialist—usually a reproductive endocrinologist—who understands how to use these drugs appropriately. Several factors determine what fertility drug or drugs you're given and how much of them you should take.

First, your doctor will determine which hormone or hormones are malfunctioning. Depending on your hormonal profile, you may be prescribed one or more fertility drugs. And, depending on your clinical picture, treatment can take several directions. One strategy may be to replace a missing hormone. Another is to prescribe one hormone that will stimulate the release of the missing one. Other strategies include giving low doses of a drug for a prolonged period and giving high doses for a short time.

Second, it's important to remember that not every treatment cycle ends with a viable and available egg. Sometimes the hormonal juggling takes time to refine. It could be several months before a good-quality ovulation occurs. Remember, too, that a treatment cycle might have to be abandoned if your ovaries look ready to release too many eggs because it would increase the risk of having a multiple birth. Of course, if you're planning an ART procedure, the goal of ovulation induction is to have many good-quality eggs available for retrieval and fertilization. But this is not the aim of ovulation induction when sexual intercourse or therapeutic insemination is the mechanism for fertilization.

And last but not least, age matters. As we've discussed, as a woman ages, her ovaries become more resistant to hormonal stimulation, either by infertility treatment or by the body itself, producing fewer follicles and eventually causing abnormally elevated serum FSH levels. Also, ovarian production of estrogen

Watch Out!

While the notion of a multiple birth might seem appealing, a singleton birth—that is, one baby per pregnancy— is healthier for both mother and baby (see Chapter 10).

and progesterone declines, sometimes causing irregular menstrual cycles or even making the uterus less able to accept a pregnancy. Finally, fertilized oocytes are less likely to develop successfully into live births.

It's been known for years that a woman's chances of getting pregnant, carrying a pregnancy to term, and delivering a healthy, normal baby diminish steadily as she ages. Today, doctors are realizing that this reduced reproductive ability is due largely to poor egg quality.

Older women given traditional fertility drug regimens don't always get good results. But new combinations are becoming available to help improve egg production in women over 40. Older women who have no other infertility problems and who are given injectable fertility drugs have a chance of ovulating normally. Unfortunately, older women are at increased risk of having a miscarriage.

Other considerations to keep in mind:

- Fertility drugs can throw your emotions off balance. These drugs can exaggerate the mood swings many women experience during their menstrual cycles. These premenstrual syndrome (PMS)-like symptoms can sometimes wreak havoc with your emotional state, which may already be shaky because of the anticipation and disappointments associated with any fertility treatment.

- Fertility drugs require careful monitoring. The oral ones such as clomiphene citrate (Clomid) and letrozole (Femara) require minimal monitoring. But the injectable ones containing FSH (either alone or in conjunction with LH) need intense monitoring. Your doctor must be able to gauge your response to therapy and calculate how much of a drug or drugs you need at a particular time. This part of the hormonal balancing act is guided by the results of tests you'll take throughout your treatment cycle.

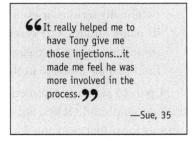

❝It really helped me to have Tony give me those injections...it made me feel he was more involved in the process. **❞**

—Sue, 35

▪ Fertility drugs often require daily injections for several days. To save you the cost and time involved in going to the doctor's office, the injections are usually given at home by your partner or a trusted friend. Your doctor will teach that person how to inject you as easily and as painlessly as possible.

Why monitoring is necessary

It's critical that you be monitored carefully for the effects these drugs are having on your ovarian system. Monitoring is done for several reasons:

▪ To assess your response to the fertility drugs and to make adjustments as needed.

▪ To be certain that too many eggs are not being produced in any one cycle. Because fertility drugs can cause more than one egg to be produced, the likelihood of a multiple birth increases. With a multiple pregnancy comes inherent risks: multiple births, premature delivery, low-birth-weight babies, and miscarriage. Certainly, these are issues for you, your partner, and your doctor to discuss. The majority of pregnancies—more than 75 percent—following ovulation induction are singletons, while about 20 percent are twins. Far fewer are triplets or more.

- To determine when ovulation occurs. This allows doctors to maximize the chance of fertilization, whether done through sexual intercourse, therapeutic insemination, or assisted reproductive technology (ART).

- To avoid ovarian hyperstimulation syndrome (OHSS), a potentially serious or even life-threatening condition. As its name implies, OHSS results when the ovaries are over-stimulated to produce eggs. The ovaries may enlarge and fluid may accumulate in the abdomen.

Up to 10 percent of women undergoing ovulation induction may develop mild OHSS, but fewer than 1 percent get a more serious form that occasionally requires hospitalization. In fact, the risk of OHSS is rare with some fertility drugs, such as clomiphene citrate and letrozole. Women with *polycystic ovarian disease (PCOD)*, sometimes called *Stein-Leventhal Syndrome* or *hyperandrogenism* (see Chapter 4), are at particular risk for OHSS. They tend to develop many small follicles rather than a few large ones, which increases the chances of OHSS.

The early warning signs of OHSS include pelvic pain, nausea, vomiting, weight gain, and reduced urine output. In more serious cases, fluid can accumulate in the lungs, causing difficulty breathing. In extreme but rare cases, an ovary can rupture. OHSS can also lead to blood clots, damaging the liver, kidneys, lungs, and brain. Rarely, OHSS can lead to death, even if the drug is carefully administered and properly monitored

OHSS onset can be sudden and usually occurs about one week after ovulation. If you're on FSH-containing regimens, you'll need to be monitored for at least two weeks after ovulation and, if pregnant, through early pregnancy.

The good news is that although fertility drugs do carry some risks, with today's improved drug regimens and advanced monitoring techniques, by and large the use of fertility drugs is very safe when prescribed and monitored by qualified doctors.

How ovulation induction is monitored

When you're taking fertility drugs you'll be undergoing tests periodically throughout your treatment cycle. The most critical tests are:

- Ultrasound, which is used to measure the number of follicles, their growth, and their diameter.

- Blood tests, which measure hormone levels throughout your treatment cycle. Your doctor will use the test results to determine any dosage adjustments needed.

In addition to these important tests, your doctor will examine you for signs of possible side effects of the medication. (There's more information on the risks of fertility drugs later in this chapter.) Your doctor may also perform a postcoital test to evaluate cervical mucus quality. The postcoital test is used if you're taking hormones that have anti-estrogen properties, which can thicken your cervical mucus, making it less amenable to sperm movement.

Your doctor may also have you chart your basal body temperature (BBT) and use ovulation kits along with ultrasounds to help assess the way you're responding to oral drugs.

Now that you've got a pretty good idea what fertility drugs are supposed to do, how your doctor will monitor your response to them, and what pitfalls are involved, we'll give you some specific questions to ask your doctor before you start treatment.

Just as we said in Chapter 4 concerning diagnostic tests, you should feel free to ask questions. Always ask, "What does this drug do?" "What are its side effects?" "How long do I have to be on it?" "When can I expect to see results?" "What are its risks?" "What monitoring will I need while taking this drug?"

 Bright Idea

If your partner travels a lot, recruit a back-up person to give you your injections.

Be sure to also ask your doctor if you need to restrict any activities while taking the drugs. And get written instructions for the medicines you are prescribed. This includes information about storing, handling, and, particularly, administering the drugs. Many of these drugs must be mixed and given by injection. The more you know about these drugs, the better prepared you'll be for some of the physical and emotional ups and downs that they can cause, as well as the ups and downs of success or failure during each treatment cycle.

A guide to fertility drugs

Now that you know about fertility drugs in general, knowing more about specific drugs is also important. To make this section easier to read, we've provided a detailed list of the common fertility drugs, using their generic or chemical names, followed by their brand names. For example, clomiphene citrate, a widely prescribed fertility drug, is a generic name. It's available under the brand names Clomid or Serophene.

Keep in mind most fertility drugs are actually the hormones themselves so they really don't have bona fide generic names. Human menopausal gonadotropin (hMG) is the hormone name and that's what's given. The table that appears later in this chapter should help guide you through the alphabet soup of hormones and fertility drugs.

Listed after the generic and brand names are their routes of administration; that is, how the drugs are given. You take most of these drugs by injection. In general, the older drug formulations are given intramuscularly (IM)—by injection deep into the muscle tissue. You probably can't give these injections to yourself, so you'll need to enlist the help of your partner or someone else.

Many of the newer drug formulations, particularly those developed through genetic engineering, are injected subcutaneously (SC)—under the skin using a small, thin needle. These are much easier to give to yourself. Some fertility drugs are taken orally. And, occasionally, a drug may be given in a nasal spray.

Moneysaver

If you're traveling while taking fertility drugs that need refrigeration, get a hotel room with a small refrigerator. It's cheaper than having to throw away spoiled medicine. You can also ask to have your medicine refrigerated during airplane flights.

Next comes a description of what doctors call the drug's mechanism of action—in other words, how it works. We'll then describe the drug's uses and tell you what to expect. As we said earlier, injectable fertility drugs require careful monitoring throughout your treatment cycle. We've already discussed some of the tests (for example, lab assessments, ultrasound exams, physical exams, and postcoital tests) you'll likely undergo and why. We'll just list the tests that are likely to be performed. You can refer to the appropriate section on drug monitoring for the rationale behind these tests.

Finally, we'll list some of the side effects and risks. (The list is not complete, but covers what appear to be the most common side effects and risks.) We're not going to go into dosages, because that depends on your hormone levels at any particular time. The dosage will likely be changed several times during your treatment. Suffice it to say that you should always ask how much of a drug you should be taking and ask again whenever the dosage is changed.

We're also not going to give you specifics on how long to be on any particular drug(s); that's a determination only you and your doctor can make. We'll just leave you with the caveat that you should not be taking any of these drugs for more than several months. Also, keep in mind that the side effects for most of these drugs are dose-dependent. This means the more of the drug you take, the more likely and worse the side effects. As when taking any drug, if you do have serious side effects, call your doctor immediately.

Clomiphene citrate

This is one of the most useful drugs available to treat female-factor infertility. It's certainly one of the oldest and least expensive.

Brand names: Clomid, Serophene

Route of administration: Oral

How it works: Clomiphene citrate is an anti-estrogen; that is, it blocks estrogen receptors in the hypothalamus, causing it to think you have an estrogen deficiency. As a result the hypothalamus signals the pituitary gland to secrete more FSH and LH. The rising FSH levels stimulate follicle development. As the follicle develops, it secretes estrogen on its own. After therapy is stopped, the hypothalamus senses the high estrogen levels and signals the pituitary to begin the LH surge and egg release. If you don't get your periods, you'll first be given a progesterone-like drug to produce menses.

Uses: To stimulate ovulation if you have infrequent periods, long cycles, or luteal-phase defect. (Sometimes, luteal-phase defect can be a side effect of clomiphene citrate therapy.) If you don't have any periods, you usually shouldn't be taking clomiphene citrate until pregnancy is ruled out.

What to expect: Clomiphene citrate is typically taken daily for five consecutive days, starting several days after your menstrual period begins. Exactly when to begin treatment depends on your particular hormone profile. If you haven't gotten your period in a while, your doctor might prescribe oral *progesterone* (Prometrium) or oral *medroxyprogesterone* (Provera) to trigger menstruation. If clomiphene works, you should ovulate about a week after your last pill.

Tests you'll take: Your doctor will probably order a postcoital test to be certain the drug's not thickening your cervical mucus. If it is, your doctor may prescribe estrogen or prednisone following clomiphene citrate therapy to help normalize cervical mucus consistency. If that doesn't work, *intrauterine insemination* (a procedure we'll discuss in more detail later in this chapter) or other hormones (LH or FSH) are options.

You may have to chart your BBT and use ovulation predictor kits. You might undergo a pelvic exam to see how you're

Watch Out!

Clomiphene citrate can have adverse effects on cervical mucus, so it's important to monitor your own cervical mucus and tell your doctor if it becomes opaque and sticky around ovulation.

responding to the drug. To make certain you aren't developing any ovarian cysts, you might undergo a pelvic exam or ultrasound test before another treatment cycle is begun. Unless you have a complex case or an ART is planned, extensive blood tests and ultrasound monitoring—as used for the injectable drugs mentioned later in this list—are rarely used if the ovulation tests are positive.

The majority of pregnancies occur in the first three cycles of clomiphene citrate use in women who ovulate regularly on this drug. The number falls dramatically after the first six cycles.

Risks: There's less of a risk of multiple births with clomiphene citrate than with other fertility drugs. The chance for twins is about 10 percent or less; the likelihood of more than two babies is 1 percent. Overstimulation of the ovaries may cause ovarian cysts, which is the reason a pelvic exam should be performed before each new cycle is begun. Severe hyperstimulation (OHSS) is rare with this drug.

Side effects: Hot flashes, mood swings, depression, nausea, and breast tenderness. If you develop severe headaches or vision problems, call your doctor immediately.

Letrozole

Letrozole, a new anti-estrogen drug used to treat breast cancer, is also being used to help induce ovulation. Unlike many other traditional anticancer drugs, it does not kill cells.

Brand name: Femara

Route of administration: Oral

How it works: Letrozole is an aromatase inhibitor, meaning it lowers estrogen production in the ovaries and behaves very much like clomiphene. However, it appears to clear from the body quickly, so it is less likely to adversely affect cervical mucus.

Uses: Letrozole has been found to be very successful in treating women who cannot tolerate clomiphene. It's also being used to treat endometriosis.

What to expect: Same as clomiphene

Tests you'll take: Same as clomiphene

Risks: Same as clomiphene

Side effects: Same as clomiphene

Human chorionic gonadotropin (hCG)

Produced in early pregnancy, the hormone hCG is derived from the urine of pregnant women.

Brand names: Profasi, Pregnyl, Ovidrel (produced through genetic engineering)

Route of administration: Intramuscular injection (IM) or subcutaneous injection (SC)

How it works: hCG is typically used in conjunction with clomiphene, letrozole, hMG, and FSH to facilitate ovulation. Chemically similar to LH, it produces an LH-type surge, which causes a mature follicle to release an egg.

Uses: Many women undergoing ovulation induction will not release eggs spontaneously. Although hCG does what LH does, it has a longer duration of action than LH and is cheaper and easier to use.

What to expect: Ovulation usually occurs about 36 hours after an hCG injection.

Tests you'll take: Ultrasound and blood monitoring. If you're just undergoing standard ovulation induction—not superovulation induction in preparation for an ART—hCG will not be given if too many follicles seem to be developing.

Risks: Multiple births, OHSS

Side effects: Lower abdominal tenderness, redness or tenderness at injection site, hot flashes, cramping

Human menopausal gonadotropin (hMG)

A combination of FSH and LH, hMG is derived from the urine of postmenopausal women. It is among the most potent fertility drugs available.

Brand names: Repronex, Menopur. (Pergonal is no longer being produced.)

Route of administration: Intramuscular injection (IM) or subcutaneous injection (SC)

How it works: Stimulates ovaries *(gonads)* directly to produce several eggs in one cycle

Uses: This family of drugs are the most potent fertility drugs available. If clomiphene citrate hasn't worked, particularly if you need more FSH, you may be given hMG. It will raise FSH levels substantially and keep them elevated for longer periods than clomiphene citrate. These drugs are also useful for women who do not menstruate. And, like clomiphene citrate, it's sometimes given if you're planning an ART procedure.

What to expect: Injections are usually given daily for seven to twelve days, starting between Day 2 and Day 5 of the menstrual period. Once one or two large follicles are seen and estrogen levels are appropriate, an injection of hCG is given to stimulate their release. (Occasionally, women taking hMG will release eggs on their own.) If too many developing follicles are detected, the hCG injection is withheld.

Unlike clomiphene citrate, these drugs have no anti-estrogen effects, so it won't adversely affect cervical mucus quality. In fact, it may have the opposite effect—it may make it easier for sperm to reach the cervix.

Tests you'll take: Ultrasound and blood monitoring

Risks: Because hMG is so potent, the risk of a multiple birth is higher than for clomiphene citrate. Ectopic pregnancy, spontaneous abortions, and premature deliveries may be increased in a woman taking hMG. There is also a risk of OHSS.

Side effects: Breast tenderness; pain, rash, swelling or rash at the injection site; abdominal bloating or pain; mood swings

Follicle-stimulating hormone (FSH)

FSH, which used to be derived from the urine of post-menopausal women, is now made synthetically.

Brand names: Follistim, Gonal-F, Bravelle

Route of administration: Subcutaneous injection (SC)

How it works: FSH stimulates follicle growth directly.

Uses: FSH is usually given when clomiphene hasn't worked. Because these drugs contain FSH with very little LH, they're also helpful when used in women with polycystic ovarian syndrome (PCOS), a common ovulatory disorder we discussed in Chapter 4. In PCOS the LH levels are high, but FSH levels are low or normal.

What to expect: FSH is usually given daily for about a week or so early in the cycle. Ovulation usually occurs within one to two weeks of treatment. Like women undergoing treatment with hMG, women taking FSH are monitored with ultrasound and blood estrogen tests and receive an injection of hCG to stimulate follicle release.

Tests you'll take: Ultrasound and blood monitoring

Risks: Similar to those for hMG

Side effects: Similar to those for hMG

Lutropin alfa (LH)

Lutropin alfa is the world's first pure form of LH. Previously derived from urine, it is now made by genetic engineering (recombinant human LH).

Brand name: Luveris

Route of administration: Subcutaneous injection (SC)

How it works: LH is responsible for egg maturation and ovulation.

Uses: It is licensed to be used for people who have severe pituitary suppression (LH and FSH deficiency). It must be given with FSH.

What to expect: Similar to hMG

Tests you'll take: Similar to those for hMG

Risks: Similar to those for hMG

Side effects: Similar to those for hMG

Bright Idea

To lessen the pain, swelling, or irritation associated with a hormone injection, alternate injection sites. Discuss it with your doctor first; if he or she agrees, you may be able to give it once in one buttock, next time in the front of the thigh, next in the other buttock, and then in the other thigh.

Bromocriptine

Bromocriptine decreases prolactin, the hormone responsible for milk production in women after childbirth.

Brand name: Parlodel

Route of administration: Oral or, in special cases, vaginally

How it works: Reduces pituitary gland secretion of prolactin

Uses: Bromocriptine is used for women with high prolactin levels, which inhibits FSH and LH release.

What to expect: Bromocriptine is used several times daily until prolactin levels return to normal and normal prolactin levels are maintained. Treatment is quite successful, although some women do need to take clomiphene or hMG as well.

Tests you'll take: Prolactin levels and scans of the pituitary may be ordered.

Risks: Bromocriptine does not increase the risk of a multiple birth.

Side effects: Nausea, vomiting, nasal congestion, headache, dizziness, fainting, decreased blood pressure. (Many of these side effects can be alleviated by using the vaginal suppository form of the drug. Side effects usually stop within seven to ten days.)

GnRH agonists

GnRH agonists influence the release of both estrogen and testosterone in the body.

Brand names: Lupron (leuprolide acetate), Synarel (nafarelin acetate), Zoladex (goserelin acetate)

Route of administration: Lupron, intramuscular injection (IM) or subcutaneous injection (SC); Synarel, nasal spray; Zoladex, skin implants

How it works: GnRH agonists cause LH and FSH release from the pituitary, eventually exhausting its supply, resulting in FSH and LH suppression.

Uses: GnRH agonists allow precise ovulation induction by suppressing normal ovarian function. GnRH agonists have been particularly helpful for women planning ART procedures. They have reduced the number of cancelled ART treatment cycles because of poor response to fertility drugs or premature ovulation. GnRH agonists are also sometimes given to women with polycystic ovarian disease (PCOD), endometriosis, or uterine fibroids.

What to expect: GnRH agonists require daily injections. Minor side effects (see below) may occur initially, but diminish over time.

Tests you'll take: Ultrasound and blood tests

Risks: Multiple births, OHSS when used in conjunction with ART

Side effects: When used alone, very similar to those seen in menopausal women, including hot flashes, headaches, mood swings, insomnia, vaginal dryness leading to painful intercourse, reduced breast size, and bone loss. When used with hMG and similar drugs, risks and side effects are similar to those for hMG.

GnRH antagonists

GnRh antagonists work in the opposite way as GnRH agonists. GnRh antagonists control the suppression of LH and FSH immediately, which induces ovulation.

Brand names: Cetrotide (centrorelix), Antagon (granirelix)

Route of administration: Subcutaneous injection (SC)

How it works: GrRH antagonists work by blocking the effects of GnRH and preventing an LH surge and preventing LH and FSH release.

Uses: GnRH antagonists are very useful for the timing of inseminations and other procedures.

What to expect: These drugs temporarily shut down the ovaries, thus preventing premature ovulation. hCG must be given to induce ovulation at the correct time.

Tests you'll take: Ultrasound and blood monitoring

Watch Out!

Fertility drugs should not be taken indefinitely, because they are very potent hormones. If a drug doesn't work within three to six cycles, you and your doctor should consider reevaluating the drug regimen and, of course, the subsequent treatment.

Risks: Similar to GnRH agonists

Side effects: Similar to GnRH agonists

Metformin

Metforim is normally used to regulate blood sugar levels in the treatment of type 2 diabetes. While currently approved only for the treatment of diabetes, it appears to be very successful in treating polycystic ovarian syndrome (PCOS).

Brand name: Glucophage

Route of administration: Oral

How it works: Metformin removes the inhibitory processes that prevent ovulation in PCOS patients. Metformin doesn't stimulate ovulation like other fertility drugs; rather, it permits ovulation to happen by reducing insulin levels. It also helps ovulation induction drugs function more efficiently in patients with PCOS.

Uses: Used for the treatment of PCOS

What to expect: Metformin is usually taken two or three times a day with meals. Gastrointestinal symptoms are fairly common but diminish over time.

Tests you'll take: Discuss with your doctor.

Risks: A rare but serious life-threatening condition, lactic acidosis, can occur, especially in women who abuse alcohol, have kidney or liver disease, are dehydrated, or have hypoxia (low levels of oxygen in the blood).

Side effects: Nausea, vomiting, loss of appetite, diarrhea, bloating

Fertility drugs for men

Although hormone deficiencies are relatively rare causes of male infertility, hormone replacement therapy is helping men with specific hormonal abnormalities (see Chapter 4). The following drugs are primarily used to treat female infertility but are also occasionally used to treat men. They are all described in the earlier section on fertility drugs for women:

- **hCG (Profasi and Pregnyl)** is usually given to stimulate the testes to produce testosterone and increase sperm production.

- **Clomiphene citrate (Clomid)** is used to stimulate sperm production.

- **hMG (Repronex)** is sometimes used to treat men with FSH and LH imbalances.

- **Bromocriptine** is used when it's certain that a man has hyperprolactinemia.

Whether these drugs work or not depends on the cause of the infertility and the drug used. Men with hypogonadism are frequently successfully treated with the administration of gonadotropins. Not only do they have normal sperm counts within a year, but their sperm have good morphology and motility.

Hormonal treatment with such drugs as Clomid is occasionally prescribed for men with idiopathic infertility—that is, the cause of their low sperm count is unknown. While these drugs might increase sperm count, studies show that sperm motility rarely improves, and the results for pregnancy rates are mixed.

> **“** My doctor put me on Clomid and I felt weird taking the same fertility drug my wife was taking! I was also afraid I'd grow large breasts, but I didn't. **”**
>
> —David, 38

These drugs are considered safe for men to take. However, some men who take Clomid have reported visual, gastrointestinal, and neurological disturbances and changes in libido and weight.

Watch Out!

Up to 25 percent of the drugs sold on the Internet have been found to contain no active substances. If you do buy online, buy only from websites with the Verified Internet Pharmacy Practice Sites seal, which identifies licensed websites.

Other drugs

There are other drugs besides hormones, such as antibiotics, that have been found to be helpful for male-factor infertility. Infections, for example, can interfere with sperm production and transport. The prostate, seminal vesicles, epididymis, urethra, and even the testes themselves can be infected. Once an infection is diagnosed, and usually confirmed by a culture, an appropriately effective antibiotic is prescribed.

In Chapter 4, we mentioned that both erectile dysfunction (impotence) and retrograde ejaculation are important causes of male-factor infertility. In retrograde ejaculation, the semen is released backward into the bladder during ejaculation. This problem can sometimes be overcome by removing sperm from a urine sample and using it to inseminate the partner. Some men can even be helped by taking common over-the-counter medicines, such as those that contain the decongestant pseudoephedrine. This type of drug affects nerve signals and may help the bladder neck close during ejaculation, thus restoring normal ejaculation.

Impotence—whether caused by psychological factors or medical conditions—can often be helped with drugs such as Viagra, Cialis, and Levitra.

Other treatments

Men suffering from neurological defects or injuries sometimes have difficulty ejaculating through sexual intercourse or masturbation. There are new *ejaculation stimulation* techniques to collect semen. Two primary ejaculatory stimulation methods are used:

- Vibratory stimulation, in which the penis is massaged with an electrically powered vibrating device.

■ Electroejaculation stimulation (EES), in which a probe is inserted into the rectum and a low-level electrical current is supplied to excite the nerves and induce an ejaculation. (If the patient has rectal sensation, anesthesia is used.)

The semen from these techniques is then processed and used for either in-vitro fertilization (IVF) or therapeutic insemination.

Artificial insemination

One of the most common, oldest, simplest, and successful treatments available to overcome several male and female infertility problems is *artificial insemination* (AI) with the husband's or a donor's sperm.

Some problems of the male reproductive system can make it difficult for men to deposit sperm directly into their partner's vagina. While these problems can sometimes be treated by surgery, some can also be treated by using artificial insemination, which allows the sperm to be deposited directly into the vagina.

AI is sometimes referred to as *therapeutic insemination* (TI). To confuse matters further, when the woman is artificially inseminated with her husband's sperm, the procedure is called AIH, the "H" standing for "husband." When sperm from a donor is used, the procedure used to be called AID, with the "D" standing for "donor." Donor sperm is discussed in greater detail in Chapters 11 and 12.

Whether using the sperm from the husband or a donor, the goal is to place a large number of sperm close to the point of fertilization. Sometimes the procedure is done several times during ovulation to optimize the chance of fertilization.

Once it's been determined that the woman doesn't have problems that would seriously impede fertilization, such as damaged Fallopian tubes or implantation problems, AI is quite useful. What's critical is that she be ovulating at that time. In fact, AI is often performed in conjunction with ovulation induction.

AIH is useful in men with retrograde ejaculation, premature or delayed ejaculation, or structural defects that prevent sperm from being deposited in the vagina. It's also helpful in bypassing the cervix when the woman's cervical mucus is poor or she produces antisperm antibodies. AIH is often used in couples with unexplained infertility. There are two AI techniques: *intracervical insemination* (ICI) and *intrauterine insemination* (IUI).

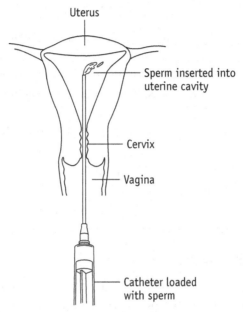

Intrauterine insemination. Washed sperm are injected through a catheter into the uterus.

■ In ICI, the male produces a semen specimen, typically through masturbation. If donor sperm are used, a frozen specimen collected at least six months earlier is thawed and used. The specimen is placed in the cervix using a syringe or cannula. Sometimes a cervical cap is used for a few hours to help keep the sperm from flowing out of the vagina.

■ In IUI, the sperm are separated out of the seminal fluid. This is necessary because seminal fluid contains substances that can irritate the uterus. Besides, separation selects the most motile sperm. The sperm are then concentrated in a small volume of medium.

Bright Idea

If you're planning on AIH, make sure your partner tells the doctor if he's had a fever or illness within the last three months; this can adversely affect sperm. If so, AIH—for that cycle—may be less likely to work.

Rather than placing the washed sperm near the cervix, the sperm are loaded into a fine catheter that's inserted through the cervix into the uterus. The sperm are released high inside the uterus, even closer to the Fallopian tubes than possible with ICI. The procedure is usually painless. In recent years, IUI has replaced ICI as the technique of choice.

If TIs don't work as a treatment for a male-factor problem, surgery is another option for many men, especially those with structural problems. Surgery is also an option for many women with structural problems, as discussed in the following chapter.

Just the facts

- Ovulation can be induced by fertility drugs in up to 75 percent of women with ovulatory problems.
- There are several promising new fertility drugs on the market, including letrozole (Femara) and lutropin alpa (Luveris).
- Fertility drugs for women can effectively treat some men with certain hormonal conditions.
- Multiple births are a potentially serious side effect of some fertility drugs.
- Women who take fertility drugs should be carefully monitored with blood tests and ultrasounds to avoid hyperstimulation of the ovaries and other serious problems.
- Artificial insemination can be a very effective treatment for some couples with either male- or female-factor infertility.

GET THE SCOOP ON...
The latest surgical innovations ▪ Surgical options
for women ▪ Surgical options for men ▪
Traditional surgery vs. the ARTs ▪ Considerations
before undergoing surgery

Surgical Solutions

Chapter 8

A s we saw in the last chapter, drug treatment can be highly effective for many infertile couples. However, for those who have structural or other nonhormonal problems, surgery may be their best bet.

Until quite recently, surgery often wasn't very successful in treating many cases of infertility. Surgeons had neither the tools nor the techniques that they do today. Recent therapeutic advances have overcome many of the obstacles surgeons have faced in the past, and now offer many couples a real chance of restoring their fertility.

Surgical innovations

Several new surgical innovations have contributed to the development of recent technical advances in the treatment of infertility. These include the following:

▪ **Microsurgery.** The use of high-power magnification has made the ability to reconstruct small structures on both the male and female reproductive organs more feasible and successful.

157

- **Laser surgery.** Lasers can be used to remove diseased or damaged tissues with virtually no bleeding and trauma and improve surgical outcomes.

- **Small precision surgical instruments.** These instruments allow surgeons to see, reach, and work within the confined spaces of the pelvis and other parts of the body.

- **Endoscopic equipment.** These narrow fiberoptic, telescope-like instruments allow doctors to look directly inside the body to examine damaged and diseased organs. They also have tremendous treatment implications and applications.

Initially designed to be used for diagnostic purposes, endoscopic equipment is now being used therapeutically during surgery. Doctors now can not only inspect your internal organs up close, but also correct many problems they see as soon as they're found, obviating the need for a second or more invasive (open) surgery.

> 66 After two years of taking fertility drugs, my doctor suggested a second laparoscopy. The surgeon found adhesions on my tubes and cysts on my ovaries and a large cyst at the end of my tubes...and he removed the cysts and adhesions. So I had my surgery—a little more than expected! 99
>
> Sarah, 30

The two endoscopic instruments commonly used in minimally invasive infertility surgery are *laparoscopes* and *hysteroscopes,* which we discussed in Chapter 6. When these instruments are used to diagnose or evaluate a problem, the procedure is called a *diagnostic laparoscopy* or *diagnostic hysteroscopy.* However, these instruments are now widely being used to correct—as well as diagnose—many uterine, tubal, and ovarian disorders, including uterine fibroids and endometriosis. When used to fix a problem, the procedure is called an *operative laparoscopy* or an *operative hysteroscopy.*

The following are descriptions of how these instruments are used operatively, rather than diagnostically:

- Laparoscopes are inserted through a small incision at or near your belly button. Your doctor will inspect your uterus, Fallopian tubes, and ovaries. If a correctable problem is discovered, operative instruments, such as laser equipment, surgical knives, and sutures, can be inserted through other small abdominal incisions. (See the illustration later in this chapter.)

- Hysteroscopes pass through the vagina and cervix and allow doctors to view your uterus. Again, if a correctable problem is uncovered, operative instruments can be passed through the hysteroscope. For example, if a minor blockage is seen at the area where the Fallopian tube joins the uterus, a flexible tube or wire is slid through the hysteroscope and used to push or scrape out the blockage. Hysteroscopic surgery can also be used to remove some types of fibroids and septum defects.

Operative laparoscopies have largely replaced open abdominal surgeries for many types of infertility problems, particularly tubal repair. Hysteroscopies eliminate the need to cut through major organs and can be done on an outpatient basis under local anesthesia. By contrast, more traditional surgeries require general anesthesia and are highly invasive. The surgeon must make a large incision in your abdomen just to reach organs needing repair.

Surgical solutions for women

Thanks to operative laparoscopes, hysteroscopes, and other innovations, surgery for infertility tends to be far less invasive and traumatic than in the past. This means less pain and discomfort, faster recuperation, and often, much better results for women being treated surgically for tubal, ovarian, pelvic, or uterine infertility.

Bright Idea

If possible, allow yourself the luxury of taking additional time off from work after a surgical procedure. You'll feel a lot better when you go back to the office.

Unblocking tubes

Fallopian tubes can become obstructed by scars and adhesions from such conditions as STDs, endometriosis, or even from a previous tubal surgery. Unblocking these tubal obstructions is one of the most common indications for surgical treatment of female-factor infertility.

The minimally invasive surgical procedures previously mentioned are very effective in removing the scars and adhesions that block the tubes. However, for more extensive tubal repairs, a laparotomy—a major open surgical procedure that requires general anesthesia—is usually necessary. In a laparotomy, the surgeon cuts through the abdomen to get to the Fallopian tubes. Working with microsurgical instruments, the surgeon then cuts out the damaged portion of the tubes and sews the remaining sections back together again.

The location of the obstruction dictates the particular type of laparotomy surgery you'll need. Here are three of the most common surgical options:

- *Salpingostomy* is a procedure in which a cut is made in the fimbrial end of the Fallopian tube and blockages or damaged tissues are removed.

- *Fimbrostomy* is a procedure that corrects any damage to the actual fimbria.

- *Tubal reimplantation* removes the Fallopian tube from the uterus and reconnects it to the uterine wall.

Reversing tubal ligations

Tubal obstructions are not the only reasons women need tubal surgery. About 10 percent of women who've "had their tubes tied"—that is, undergone *tubal ligation (tubal sterilization)*—later change their minds. Tubes can't simply be "untied" because they are actually cut, not tied. Reversing female sterilization requires a laparotomy, and is successful in opening the tubes in up to 90 percent of cases. However, only between 60 and 75 percent of women who have their tubal ligations reversed succeed in getting pregnant. Several factors help to determine success in reversing the sterilization and getting pregnant afterward.

- **How the original tubal ligation was done.** If rings or clips were used to block off the Fallopian tubes, you've probably had less tubal damage than if the sterilization was done by actually destroying your tubes with *electrocautery*. If your tubes were cut in their midsection, there is a good chance the tubal ligation can be reversed. While this may allow you to become pregnant, it doesn't guarantee that you will.

- **How much of the tubes remain after the reversal.** The more Fallopian tube left, the better the chances for pregnancy.

- **How experienced the surgeon is.** The reversal of a tubal sterilization is an exacting surgery using microsurgical techniques. You need to find a qualified surgeon who specializes in this type of microsurgery; the more experience the surgeon has had in doing this surgery, the higher the chance of success. This is obviously not only true for sterilization reversals, but for all the other surgical procedures as well.

 Watch Out!

If you've had tubal disease and you think you may be pregnant, see your doctor immediately. Even if you've had a tubal repair, your chances of having an ectopic pregnancy are increased, and you will need to undergo tests to determine where the early pregnancy is located.

Tubal surgery vs. assisted reproduction (ARTs)

As with any invasive procedure, it's important that you talk to your doctor ahead of time about the relative risks and benefits of having surgery. There are alternatives you might want to consider, especially in-vitro fertilization (IVF) and other assisted reproductive technologies (ARTs), which are discussed in Chapters 9 and 10. There are pros and cons for treating tubal disease with either surgery or ART, as shown in the following table.

Table 8.1: Comparison of Surgery to ARTs as Treatment for Tubal Disease

	Surgery	ART
Fertility drugs	No	Yes
Invasive	More	Less
Recuperation	Lengthy	Minimal
Success	Variable	Variable
Future success	Allows continued attempts at pregnancy	Permits attempts only through treatment cycles
Cost	Less	More
Insurance coverage	Usually	Variable

Treating endometriosis and pelvic adhesions

Endometriosis, as we explained in Chapter 4, is a condition in which endometrial tissue from inside the uterus is found outside the uterus. The tissue can build up, bind, and block reproductive structures and interfere with conception and pregnancy. Endometrial tissue can grow in and around the Fallopian tubes, causing tubal obstructions; or end up in the uterus or other sites in the abdominal cavity, causing pelvic adhesions.

When the tissue lodges in the ovary it can cause ovarian cysts, called endometriomas.

Although frequently treated with hormonal drugs such as Lupron, generically called leuprolide (see Chapter 7), endometriosis is sometimes severe enough to require surgery, either alone or in addition to drug therapy. If the doctor finds endometriosis during a diagnostic laparoscopy—which is really the only definitive way to tell if you do have it—the endometriosis tissue can be vaporized, using lasers or electric current.

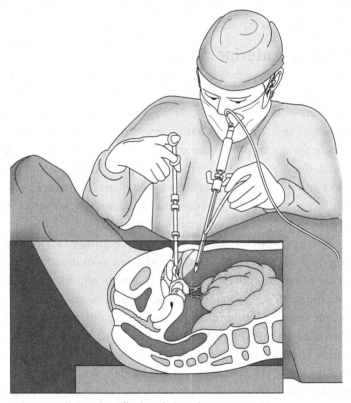

A surgeon is removing adhesions during a laparascopy.

In the past, laparatomies or other invasive surgical techniques were the standard for treatment of endometriosis. But the abdominal surgery itself could lead to scarring. Today, the current surgical management of tubal or pelvic endometriosis—as

Bright Idea

Most women don't need to have their uterus removed to treat uterine fibroids. If your doctor recommends a hysterectomy, consider getting a second opinion.

well as pelvic adhesions—involves laparoscopic surgery. Not only does this less-invasive technique require small incisions, but lasers and/or electric current are used to vaporize the adhesions.

Removing uterine fibroids

Uterine fibroids, sometimes called uterine myomas—are among the more common uterine disorders that can contribute to infertility—affecting about 20 to 25 percent of American women. These abnormal, but noncancerous, masses of smooth muscle tissue can prevent an embryo from implanting or growing in the womb. *Submucosal* fibroids grow inside the uterine cavity and pose the biggest threat to pregnancy. Uterine fibroids can be removed during an operative hysteroscopy, an operative laparoscopy, or by a laparotomy myomectomy.

There is, however, a new non-surgical treatment for fibroids called *Uterine Artery Embolization* (UAE)—or occasionally, *Uterine Fibroid Embolization* (UFE). UAE, which is normally done in a hospital under IV sedation rather than general anesthesia, involves having a small incision made in your groin through which the doctor passes a catheter through each of the two arteries that lead to your uterus. The doctor then injects tiny sand-like particles into the arteries where it blocks the blood flow to the fibroid. There is not enough blood flow to nourish the fibroids, and after about three to six months, many will decrease in size or disappear entirely. In general, after six months, about 70 percent of patients have a 70 percent reduction in fibroids.

Because UAE doesn't involve surgery or general anesthesia, it appears to be safer than a laparotomy myomectomy—the usual surgical treatment for fibroids. And recovery time is considerably shorter—about one week compared with one or two months for surgery. However, as with any medical procedure, there are some risks as well as side effects; some women have infections or severe cramps afterward. In rare cases, the procedure can cause an injury to the uterus, which may require a hysterectomy. There have also been a few reported cases of women going through early menopause after the procedure. There have been many reported cases of successful pregnancies after UAE, but the effects on fertility are not yet known since there are fewer than 1,000 recorded cases of women attempting pregnancy after this procedure. Still, because UAE appears to be a highly successful, minimally invasive treatment for fibroids, you may want to discuss this option with your doctor.

Surgical solutions for men

Many of the traditional surgical techniques for female-factor infertility we've just described are being replaced by the ARTs. However, surgery for male-factor infertility is on the rise. In fact, some of the newer sperm-retrieval procedures to help overcome male-factor infertility have their roots in the micromanipulation techniques that were refined for use in the ARTs.

Two of the more commonly used microsurgical techniques for male-factor infertility are *vasovasotomy* and *vasoepididymostomy*. These techniques are commonly used to reverse vasectomies and to correct obstructive azoospermia, both of which are described next.

Vasectomy reversals

Vasectomy has long been a safe, effective, popular contraceptive method for men, which up until fairly recently was not reversible. However, for a variety of reasons, many men decide to have their vasectomies reversed. Over the last two decades, vasectomy reversal—sometimes called a *microsurgical repair of vasal obstruction*—has been refined, and success rates are improving.

One key consideration affecting the chances of successful reversal is the length of time since the vasectomy was done. The best results—obviously measured in terms of the ability to produce a pregnancy—are achieved if the sterilization was performed within the last ten years. But it's not unheard of for vasectomies performed decades ago to be reversed successfully. And if the vasectomy was done less than three years ago, you could be looking at a pregnancy rate of about 75 percent.

Depending on your particular situation, a vasovasotomy or a vasoepididymostomy might be performed. The assisted reproduction technologies are also an option and are discussed in the next chapter.

Vasovasotomy is the most common vasectomy-reversal surgery currently being performed and it's simpler to do—not to mention say—than a vasoepididymostomy. Its goal is to remove the sections of the vas deferens that were destroyed during the original sterilization procedure, and are now blocking sperm transport, and to reconnect the clean open ends. (For a reminder of the physical details of the male reproductive system, refer to Chapter 2.)

In this exacting surgery, small incisions are made in each side of the scrotum. Depending on exactly where along the vas the original vasectomy was done, the incision may have to be extended higher, and the surgeon might need to bring the testes and epididymis out of the scrotum to work on them.

The damaged vas deferens portions are cut out. Before reconnecting the two clean ends, your surgeon will make a few critical observations and determinations. First, your doctor will want to verify that sperm are present. To do this, some fluid is removed from the vas deferens and examined under a microscope.

 Bright Idea

If you're planning a vasectomy reversal, ask to have your sperm removed and frozen for later use. If the reversal doesn't work, at least you may have enough sperm to produce a pregnancy by IVF later without going through the pain and expense of further surgery.

Moneysaver

Vasectomy reversals are much less expensive than ART procedures, so you might try a vasectomy reversal first, especially if time or age are not factors. But it can take up to a year to have a normal sperm count after the surgery, if it happens at all.

If sperm or parts of sperm are found in the fluid, the operation can proceed normally. This involves stitching back together both the inner and outer layers of the tube-like vas. The idea is that sperm will once again travel freely through the vas deferens and out the urethra during ejaculation.

If no sperm are present in the vas fluid, your surgeon will probably opt to perform a vasoepididymostomy—a more complicated procedure. This happens in about one third of vasovasotomy cases.

Vasoepididymostomy is performed if an obstruction has formed in the epididymal tubule. An obstruction sometimes develops if testicular fluid builds up after a vasectomy. It can also occur after an infection or injury. Sometimes it's due to a congenital defect.

Vasoepididymostomy is designed to bypass the obstructed area in the epididymal tubules. Instead of sewing the two ends of the vas back together after the removal of the damaged portion, one end is stitched directly to the epididymal tubules, below the point of the obstruction. The other end of the vas is left behind. This allows sperm to flow from the epididymis directly into the vas deferens, bypassing the blockage.

Both of these surgeries, which can last for a couple of hours, may be done as outpatient procedures with local or general anesthesia. You may be told to stay in bed for a day or so and not to resume strenuous physical or sexual activity for two to six weeks. You'll be given mild analgesics and maybe an antibiotic. After about six to eight weeks, you'll undergo monthly semen analyses to check on results.

Your doctor may be able to get some idea during surgery about how successful the procedures will be. Pregnancy rates following vasectomy seem to correlate with the quality of the sperm seen in the vas deferens fluid during surgery. The more motile the sperm, the better the outcome.

Most pregnancies occur within two years after a successful vasectomy reversal. If your semen analysis after the reversal is good but no pregnancy has occurred, your doctor may want you to be tested for antisperm antibodies. Nearly three quarters of men who have had a vasectomy are believed to develop antisperm antibodies. But because vasectomy reversals tend to turn out so well, antisperm antibody testing isn't routinely done. It tends to be a poor predictor of whether pregnancy can be achieved after surgery. Still, some doctors believe it can be a useful test.

And, of course, your partner needs to continue to be evaluated. She may have developed a fertility-related problem in the meantime.

Correcting obstructive azoospermia

Vasovasotomies and vasoepididymostomies are also performed on men with obstructive azoospermia, a condition in which no sperm are found in the ejaculate because of a blockage. The blockage might be something present from birth or acquired later in life. In either case, you'll undergo a few more diagnostic tests before having one of the microsurgical procedures mentioned earlier. Careful reading of the test results can help pinpoint the exact location of a blockage. Besides a physical exam and semen analysis, your FSH blood and seminal fructose levels should be tested. You'll probably also have a testicular biopsy to show if indeed you're producing sperm.

The FSH tests are especially important: If your FSH levels are very high, you're probably not producing any sperm. An attempt at reversal would therefore be pointless. If your semen has fructose in it, on the other hand, there is usually an obstruction in the vas that explains the azoospermia.

Fixing varicoceles

Varicoceles, or varicose veins surrounding the testicles, are quite common, particularly in men who suffer from infertility. While about 10 to 15 percent of all men have varicoceles, the rate is much higher for men who are infertile. Indeed, about 30 to 40 percent of men who go to the doctor for an infertility evaluation have this condition.

> **❝**It blew my mind that I not only have a fertility problem, but I'd need surgery to be able to have my own kid! Luckily, the varicocelectomy worked—I had a normal sperm count four months later. **❞**
>
> —Bob, 35

Varicocelectomy is a relatively simple and commonly performed surgery to correct this cause of male-factor infertility. It is performed as an outpatient procedure with local, regional, or general anesthesia. The surgeon makes a small incision in the groin and ties off the enlarged veins.

Semen quality seems to improve in some men undergoing this procedure. Unfortunately, it's hard to predict who'll be helped and who won't. A review of nearly 3,000 cases in one of the largest male infertility centers in the country showed that semen quality improved in about two thirds of the men having surgery, and about 40 percent successfully impregnated their partners.

Opening blocked ejaculatory ducts

A procedure called *transurethral resection of the ejaculatory duct* (TURED), is performed to open a blockage, which may be the result of infection or a congenital abnormality, in the complex systems of ducts leading from the testes to the urethra. Depending on where along the sperm transport route the blockage is, either microsurgery or endoscopic surgical repair is possible. TURED is usually highly successful in correcting this type of male infertility problem. The procedure takes only about 30 minutes and it's done with an instrument that passes through the urethra in the penis.

New sperm-retrieval techniques

Today, men who have too few sperm (oligospermia) or no sperm at all (azoospermia) in their ejaculate—including those who have had unsuccessful vasectomy reversals—are being helped through highly advanced microsurgical techniques. These procedures allow for direct sperm retrieval from men who, just a few years ago, had virtually no chance of fathering a child. There are two types of azoospermia:

▪ *Obstructive azoospermia.* In this condition, the testes produce sperm but their transport to the penis is somehow blocked.

▪ *Nonobstructive azoospermia.* In this case, it's not blockage that's the problem. It's that the testes are producing too few, if any, sperm.

Recently, several techniques have been developed to help men with obstructive and nonobstructive azoospermia. These procedures are used in combination with a technique called *intracytoplasmic sperm injection (ICSI)*, either performed immediately or at a later time with frozen sperm. (See Chapter 9 for more information about ICSI.) The new procedures include:

▪ *Microsurgical epididymal sperm aspiration (MESA).* This microsurgical technique is used to retrieve sperm in men with obstructive azoospermia. This occurs in men who have been born without the vas deferens or who have blocked vas deferens. Sperm are removed directly from the epididymis.

In this procedure, an incision is made in the scrotum and—using a micropipette or a cannula—either a small incision or a puncture is made into the individual tubules of the epididymis. If moving sperm are found in the tubule, the fluid is collected and used immediately for ICSI. (You can have some sperm frozen for later use as well.)

This technique is particularly helpful for men who have had a vasectomy that cannot be reversed or certain congenital abnormalities, or who suffer from a neurological disorder or injury that prevents ejaculation.

Bright Idea

If you have nonobstructive azoospermia but don't know its cause, consider having genetic screening to help identify any genetic abnormalities that might be responsible for the condition. If you have obstructive azoospermia—and were born without vas deferens—you should be tested for cystic fibrosis gene mutations.

- *Percutaneous epididymal sperm aspiration (PESA)* is a simpler, less invasive procedure than MESA and is also used to retrieve sperm from men with obstructive azoospermia. PESA involves passing a needle through the scrotum to repeatedly puncture the epididymis to aspirate sperm. Sperm collected this way are also used immediately in an ICSI procedure.

- *Testicular sperm extraction (TESE)* is a procedure in which sperm are extracted using a biopsy needle directly from the testicular tissue through a small incision made in the scrotum. A piece of testicular tissue is removed and examined in the lab to see if sperm are there. If they are, the sperm can be used immediately in an ICSI procedure or frozen for later use.

- *Percutaneous testicular sperm aspiration (TESA)* involves puncturing the testes repeatedly with a needle, aspirating the sperm, and using them immediately in an ICSI procedure. This procedure is usually reserved for men with obstructive azoospermia, although it has been used in nonobstructive cases as well.

To have or not to have surgery

As you can see, you often have several options in the surgical treatment of male and female infertility. Some involve deciding between traditional and minimally invasive surgeries. Others involve choosing between any surgery and ART.

Watch Out!

Keep in mind that some of the ARTs involve invasive procedures that require some form of anesthesia. All invasive procedures carry risks as well as benefits.

Before undergoing any surgical correction of an infertility problem, you need to have a frank discussion with your infertility specialist and/or surgeon. You should examine the pros and cons of any procedure and discuss all the options that are available, both at your infertility center and at others.

Remember that all of these microsurgical procedures require surgical expertise. So, if you need to undergo microsurgery for your infertility, it's important that you find a surgeon with a good track record for the specific procedure you need. Ask, "How often do you do this procedure?" "What's your success rate with this type of procedure?" "What's the success rate nationally or at other centers?"

In particular, a highly experienced surgeon is needed because, for many types of surgeries, and particularly for tubal repairs, one attempt at correction is usually all that can and should be tried. Repeated microsurgical corrections are not very successful.

With any surgery, there are certain questions that you should ask, such as "How long will the surgery take?" and "How long will I be in the hospital?" If the surgery is done as an outpatient procedure, find out how long you're actually going to be at the facility so you can make appropriate arrangements for transportation.

There are other important questions to ask that will make your recovery easier. Here's a helpful list to take with you when you're discussing a surgical option with your doctor:

- How much will it cost?
- How much pain should I expect?

- What painkillers can I take? (Get a prescription for any painkillers or antibiotics you might need *before* you leave the facility at which your surgery is done. In fact, some facilities have onsite pharmacies that will fill a small prescription to tide you over until you can get a full prescription filled.)
- What kind of follow-up care will I need?
- How long will I be laid up?
- When can I resume nonstrenuous activities? Strenuous ones?
- When can I go back to work?
- When can we attempt pregnancy again?

Finally, ask what follow-up tests, if any, you might need. And, of course, find out when you can expect to see results from the surgery.

While you're having your preliminary discussions about surgery with your regular physician, remember, if in doubt, it's a good idea to get a second opinion before undergoing infertility surgery. Most surgeons won't mind. Be certain to ask about the pros and cons of traditional surgery for your particular condition and situation compared with the ARTs.

Ironically, the surgical advances for infertility have, in some cases, made the traditional surgical techniques obsolete or less desirable. Many couples, particularly older ones, are now opting to skip conventional surgical procedures and going directly to high-tech ARTs to overcome their fertility problems. Rather than trying to permanently restore their fertility, they're choosing to temporarily bypass damaged and poorly functioning reproductive organs to achieve conception. These procedures, which are discussed in the following two chapters, are giving older couples—as well as many other couples with structural and other disorders—a better chance at conceiving and having a healthy baby than would traditional surgeries.

Just the facts

- Laser and microsurgery can correct many formerly untreatable forms of infertility.

- Tubal ligations and vasectomies are now being reversed surgically with encouragingly high rates of success.

- Men with varicoceles and oligospermia can be successfully treated by surgery and go on to father children.

- Traditional surgery can often permanently correct a problem that is interfering with conception, while IVF requires repeated cycles to treat the same condition. Traditional surgery is also more likely to be covered by insurance.

- There are important considerations to take into account before undergoing surgery, such as the skill of the surgeon, the risks involved, and the cost of the procedure.

The Assisted Reproductive Technologies

GET THE SCOOP ON...
Who can benefit from the ARTs? ▪ What's involved
in the procedures ▪ The ARTs from A to Z ▪ The
newest techniques ▪ Cryopreservation ▪ The debate
over stem cell research ▪ The cloning controversy

PART V

The Current and Future State of the ARTs

Chapter 9

In his 1989 book *Life Before Birth*, Dr. Robert Edwards, who, along with Patrick Steptoe, was responsible for the world's first "test-tube" baby, describes the moment: "On 25 July 1978, Louise Brown was born. She was a lovely baby...and her parents' joy was our joy...I waited for my turn to hold Louise in my arms and to marvel...at her tiny wrinkled perfection."

It's been over 25 years since Louise Brown was conceived and born in England through in-vitro fertilization (IVF). The news shocked the world, and dire predictions were made of deformed offspring resulting from this new, experimental technique. Since then, IVF and the other assisted reproductive technologies (ARTs) that have sprung from IVF have not only become commonplace, they have helped tens of thousands of infertile couples realize their dreams who otherwise would have had little or no hope of having their own biological child.

Who do the ARTs help?

Initially, IVF was developed for—and considered—a last resort to help women who had blocked, injured, or absent Fallopian tubes. While ARTs are still being used largely to treat tubal-factor infertility, their uses are expanding. Today they are also being used earlier in the treatment of infertility, and not necessarily as a last resort. Couples with unexplained infertility, men with low or no sperm counts, and older women are among the groups now realizing success through ARTs. The following table shows the most common conditions for which the ARTs are used in the United States. Keep in mind that these were primary diagnoses only and that couples probably had more than one factor contributing to their infertility.

Table 9.1: Diagnoses of Couples Who Had ART Cycles with Their Own Fresh Eggs

Cause	Percentage of Patients	Success Rate (Live-Birth Rate)
Tubal factor	14%	31%
Ovulatory dysfunction	6%	33%
Diminished ovarian reserve	6%	14%
Endometriosis	7%	32%
Uterine factor	1%	23%
Multiple female factors	13%	23%
Male factor	19%	34%
Multiple factors (male plus female)	19%	26%
Unexplained infertility	11%	30%
Other causes	6%	26%

Source: Centers for Disease Control, 2002

The ARTs are not appropriate for everyone in these categories. To be a candidate for IVF or the other ARTs, the maximum age for a woman using her own eggs is, ideally, 42. The American Society for Reproductive Medicine (ASRM) recommends that all women who wish to undergo an ART procedure, regardless of their age, should:

- Not have undergone premature menopause.
- Have at least one accessible ovary.
- Have a normal uterus.

In general, you and your doctor should take into account these other medical issues when considering whether the ARTs are appropriate for you:

- The length of time you've been trying to conceive with conventional treatments.
- Your chances of success with the more conventional treatments compared with the ARTs.

We'll be looking later at what else to consider before you and your doctor decide on a specific ART procedure. In the next chapter, we'll give you some tips on how to choose an ART program, but before we do that, it will help for you to know what's involved in ART procedures. We'll give you a handle on the subtle differences between the procedures that have evolved from the original IVF technology, and the newly developed sperm and egg micromanipulation techniques.

Some ARTs are best suited for specific female- or male-factor infertility. Some work well when both partners have problems, and it's not unusual to find that after one ART method fails, another is tried. Keep in mind when looking for an ART

 Moneysaver

There are many less expensive hormonal and surgical treatments you may consider before going to the ARTs. They may also be less invasive and time consuming.

program that what you think you need today may not be what you know you'll need tomorrow. Understanding the scope of the options available will make you better prepared to choose an ART program that's right for you.

What's involved?

IVF was not only the first, but is still the most widely used ART. IVF is a technique in which your eggs are removed from your ovary and mixed with your partner's (or donor's) sperm in a Petri dish (not a test tube). If the egg becomes fertilized and develops into an embryo, it can be transferred to your uterus where—if all goes well—it will implant and you will become pregnant and have a healthy baby.

There are several key steps involved that all the ARTs, including IVF, GIFT (gamete intrafallopian transfer), ZIFT (zygote intrafallopian transfer), and TET (tubal embryo transfer), have in common. The newer micromanipulation techniques are really adjuncts to these procedures, so the overall steps in all these treatments are the same. They are:

1. Ovulation induction
2. Egg retrieval
3. Fertilization
4. Embryo transfer
5. Implantation

Ovulation induction is used to stimulate the ovaries to produce several mature eggs in one cycle. The chance for pregnancy is greater if more than one egg is available for fertilization and transfer to the woman's uterus. (See Chapter 7 for more information about the role of fertility drugs in the treatment of infertility.)

As we saw in Chapter 7, a critical component in ovulation induction is timing. You'll be returning to the facility several times for blood tests and ultrasound monitoring to pinpoint when follicles are maturing and to watch for ovarian hyperstimulation syndrome.

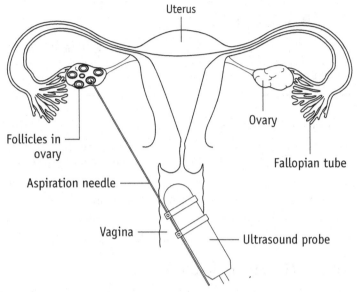

Egg retrieval with an ultrasound-guided needle. In egg retrieval, ripe eggs from the follicles of an ovary are aspirated through a needle that is inserted through the vagina, guided by an ultrasound probe.

Then you'll be given other hormones to induce follicle maturation and an egg retrieval session will be scheduled. If all goes according to plan, eggs are retrieved just prior to their actual release, fertilized, and the resulting embryos are then transferred to your uterus. You may also be given progesterone to help make the uterine environment more receptive to implantation. As we've mentioned several times, successful ovulation induction is tantamount to a hormonal balancing act and is as much an art as a science. That's one reason why not all ovulation induction cycles end in retrievals. Even if eggs are retrieved they may not fertilize, or the embryos may not survive. Despite the common use of GnRH agonists (see Chapter 7), which help prevent premature ovulation and inadvertent loss of follicles before retrieval, about 15 percent of cycles are cancelled before retrieval, and more than 23 percent before transfer.

Watch Out!

Although natural IVF cycles save you the expense and risks of ovulation induction, their success rates per cycle are much lower than for ovulation-induced IVF procedures.

Occasionally, an approach called *natural cycle IVF,* in which no fertility drugs are given, is used. It has several advantages as well as drawbacks. It's cheaper and requires less monitoring than ovulation induction, and, of course, it carries none of the risks of fertility drugs, like ovarian hyperstimulation. On the other hand, you probably will produce only one egg and that may not fertilize. The result is a variable pregnancy rate.

The ARTs from A to Z

In addition to classic IVF, there are several other variations of this procedure that are done on the female partner, including GIFT, ZIFT, and TET. Other ART techniques—such as assisted hatching—involve microsurgical procedures (described in a moment) on the egg or embryo in addition to one of these IVF-type procedures.

These techniques differ in the way eggs are retrieved, where fertilization takes place, what is transferred, and where it is transferred. For example, IVF waits until a fertilized egg has divided several times before transfer into the uterus; in GIFT, the eggs and sperm are placed into the Fallopian tubes for fertilization to occur. IVF relies on transvaginal retrieval and transfer, while GIFT uses a laparoscopic approach.

These and other differences allow your doctor to choose the treatment that's best for you. Some factors that you and your doctor will consider when choosing one of the IVF procedures are the status of your Fallopian tubes, whether you know your eggs can be fertilized, and whether you have mild or severe endometriosis. If your Fallopian tubes are blocked, for example, GIFT is not for you. Nor may GIFT be right for you if your partner's sperm quality is poor. But if you have mild endometriosis or unexplained infertility, GIFT may be a good choice. Today, IVF is done almost exclusively, primarily because IVF does not usually require laparoscopic surgery, and its pregnancy rate is equal to or higher than GIFT, ZIFT, or TET.

Now that you know the key steps in the IVF procedures as well as their overall differences, it's time to take a more detailed look at each technique.

In-vitro fertilization (IVF)

In IVF, a woman is given fertility drugs to produce several eggs, which are retrieved from the ovaries in one of two ways—by transvaginal ultrasound aspiration or occasionally, laparoscopy.

In *transvaginal ultrasound aspiration*, which is usually performed with local anesthesia or under mild sedation, an ultrasound probe inserted through the vagina uses high-frequency sound waves to identify mature follicles. If such follicles are found, a special narrow needle is guided through the vagina to the ovaries to suck up—or aspirate—the follicle's contents. During *laparoscopic aspiration*, which is performed under general anesthesia, the doctor inserts a narrow, telescopic device through a small incision in or below the woman's navel. If mature eggs are seen, the doctor guides a needle through the abdominal wall to retrieve them.

Regardless of the aspiration technique employed, each retrieved egg is mixed with the man's sperm, which have been separated from their seminal fluid through a process called *sperm washing*. The mixing is done in a lab dish containing a special culture medium. The mixture is then placed in an incubator set to the same temperature as a woman's body. If fertilization occurs and the cultured embryo starts dividing, a transfer is scheduled, usually in three to five days when the embryo reaches about an eight-cell stage or beyond.

Embryo transfer is done as an outpatient procedure without anesthesia (although sometimes the woman is given a mild sedative). The embryos and some of the culture media are

Moneysaver

Avoiding having triplets or quads can potentially save you tens of thousands of dollars in medical costs as well as the costs of rearing three or more babies at once, which is estimated to be five to seven times greater than raising singletons.

loaded into a special catheter, which is inserted through the cervix into the uterus. There they are gently deposited and, it is hoped, one successfully implants itself on the uterine wall.

To increase the chances of success, more than one embryo is transferred at a time—most commonly two, or sometimes three or more. Extra embryos can be cryopreserved for transfer during another cycle if pregnancy doesn't occur after the initial transfer. The ASRM recommends that you and your doctor agree in advance on how many embryos you want transferred, and that you sign an informed consent. Because of the desire to maximize the chances of a pregnancy during a particular cycle, some couples choose to have more than a few embryos transferred. This raises the risk of a multiple pregnancy, which many couples may hope for so they will be assured of having several children. While twins represent an acceptable risk, triplets do not. There are serious downsides to having multiple pregnancies and births, which are discussed in Chapter 10.

Gamete intrafallopian transfer (GIFT)

In GIFT, eggs can be retrieved as in IVF by transvaginal aspiration or laparoscopically. Then the retrieved eggs and sperm are mixed together. In GIFT, however, they're placed directly into one or both Fallopian tubes, rather than in a Petri dish full of culture medium. This is usually done laparoscopically. It's hoped that fertilization will occur while the mixed sperm and eggs are in the tubes. (Sometimes doctors wait a few minutes to give sperm time to attach to an egg's outer shell before transferring the mixture.)

Some couples find GIFT a more natural, and therefore more philosophically appealing, method for conception, since fertilization takes place within the woman's body. In the past, GIFT has worked better than IVF for some couples. But since pregnancy rates with IVF have steadily increased over the years (in most programs they equal or are better than GIFT), GIFT is being used less and less often. Another consideration is that GIFT, as well as ZIFT, requires laparoscopy, while IVF typically does not.

GIFT is only an option for women with normal Fallopian tubes. Women with mild endometriosis are also candidates for GIFT. Because it's impossible to determine fertilization unless a pregnancy occurs, GIFT is not used unless it's known that the sperm can fertilize an egg.

Zygote intrafallopian transfer (ZIFT)

ZIFT is sometimes known as PROST (pronuclear stage transfer) and can best be understood as an IVF-GIFT hybrid. It's not widely used, if at all, today. As in IVF, eggs are retrieved transvaginally and mixed with sperm in the lab. If fertilization occurs, resulting zygotes, which are fertilized but undivided eggs, are transferred via laparoscopy, as in GIFT, into the Fallopian tubes within about 24 hours. As we said earlier with GIFT, IVF success is obviating the need to use ZIFT and it eliminates the need for a laparoscopy.

If the quality of the woman's eggs is in doubt, ZIFT is sometimes advised over GIFT because fertilization can be detected. If GIFT fails, ZIFT might be tried next.

 Bright Idea

If you've had an ectopic pregnancy, choose IVF rather than GIFT, ZIFT, or TET because IVF does not involve the Fallopian tubes. These other procedures may put you at increased risk of having another ectopic pregnancy.

Tubal embryo transfer (TET)

This is another IVF-GIFT combination technique. Like ZIFT, it's not widely used today. As in IVF, more developed (four- to eight-cell stage) fertilized eggs are transferred. But, as in GIFT, embryos are transferred into the Fallopian tubes.

Intracytoplasmic sperm injection (ICSI)

Before ART, the only options available for men with low sperm counts were artificial insemination, adoption, or child-free living. However, in the last decade, micromanipulation and sperm aspiration techniques (see Chapter 8) have made it possible for men with very low sperm counts or those unable to provide semen specimens to father children. Unlike previous approaches to male-factor infertility that focused on increasing the quantity or quality of sperm, micromanipulation focuses on an individual sperm. In essence, as long as there is one good, viable sperm, which is all that nature needs or allows anyway, fertilization can occur.

In ICSI, the woman undergoes ovulation induction and egg retrieval. The man provides a semen sample from which one sperm is drawn into a microscopic needle and injected directly into a single egg. This is done repeatedly until all the mature eggs are injected or all the functional sperm are used up. If fertilization occurs, resulting embryos are transferred, as in an IVF procedure, into the woman's uterus.

ICSI is being used to help men who were born without the vas deferens, the conduit that transports sperm from the testis, or men who have obstructions that can't be repaired, and those with severely decreased sperm counts to father children. It has greatly reduced the use of therapeutic or artificial insemination with donor sperm.

Although pioneered only in the early 1990s, ICSI is now one of the most successful of the micromanipulation methods and is being performed by most IVF centers in this country. The success rates with ICSI are comparable to the success rates of standard

IVF *without* severe male-factor infertility. This is an amazing accomplishment since without ICSI, the success rates for couples undergoing IVF with severe male-factor infertility are very low.

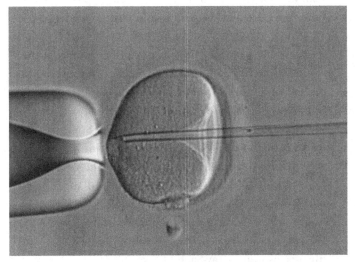

Intracytoplasmic sperm injection (ICSI) in which a sperm is injected directly into an egg to facilitate fertilization. Reprinted with permission from the American Society for Reproductive Medicine (ASRM).

Preimplantation genetic diagnosis (PGD)

PGD—a recently developed technique that is being used to test early embryos for various genetic and chromosomal disorders prior to their transfer. In this way, many serious disorders affecting babies can be ruled out *before* pregnancy.

In PGD, the woman undergoes IVF and after her embryos are formed, they are then cultured for a few days. Around day three, the embryos, consisting of five to eight cells, are biopsied using a technique that does not appear to damage the embryo. *Embryo biopsy* involves carefully drilling a hole in the outside layer of the embryo—the zona pellucida. One cell is then removed and analyzed for defects, and the results are usually available the following day.

PGD can help couples increase their chances of having healthy babies in the following ways:

- **Finding chromosomal and genetic disorders before pregnancy.** Prior to PGD, if there was a risk of passing on hereditary diseases, women would have to undergo prenatal genetic diagnosis (amniocentesis or *chorion villus sampling*, or CVS) in the early months of pregnancy. If the results showed the child was in danger of inheriting the disease or genes for certain devastating diseases, the only options would be undergoing an elective abortion or having a baby with a life-threatening disease. Some of these diseases, such as Tay-Sachs, cause infants or babies to die a very painful death. With PGD, however, the results are known even *before* an embryo is transferred and a pregnancy occurs. Researchers are hoping that PGD can be used to detect a variety of genetic disorders, such as Duchenne muscular dystrophy, hemophilia, and cystic fibrosis, as well as Tay-Sachs.

- **Picking good-quality embryos.** Doctors believe that one reason some embryos don't implant is that they contain a type of chromosomal abnormality called *chromosome aneuploidy*, or extra chromosome. In fact, some studies have shown that about half the embryos from what doctors call "difficult IVF patients" may have this genetic defect. PGD can be used to detect this chromosomal abnormality prior to embryo transfer. This would spare an infertile couple repeated unsuccessful treatment cycles because embryos with these defects could be identified and not transferred; only those embryos without identified defects would be transferred.

Studies have shown that PGD is very successful in detecting certain genetic and chromosomal disorders, and follow-up studies have found that PGD appears to be a safe procedure as well.

Bright Idea

If you have had PGD and become pregnant—and you're over 35—you should still consider having an amniocentesis or CVS. PGD is not a guarantee that the fetus is totally free from all genetic or chromosomal diseases.

Assisted hatching

This is a micromanipulation technique in which a small hole is made in the outer covering (zona pellucida) of a three-day-old embryo, as is done in PGD. This process makes it easier for the embryo to hatch and implant in the uterine lining. Usually embryos hatch out of the zona pellucida when the embryos are five or six days old. However, in older women, the zona pellucida often becomes harder or tougher, making it more difficult for the embryo to hatch.

Assisted hatching is being used to help improve implantation rates following IVF and has, until recently, been used for women over the age of 37. The use of assisted hatching is gradually expanding and many programs now use it for all women undergoing IVF. It's also being used when cell division is slow, and on embryos with thick outer shells, which can occur with frozen embryos.

Promising new techniques

Although thousands of babies have been born from ART procedures, success rates, while constantly improving, still range from about 20 to 50 percent, depending on the technique and severity of the couple's problem. Researchers are now learning more about why some couples undergoing ART procedures never produce a fertilized egg, have an embryo implant, or maintain an ongoing pregnancy. In the process, they're refining older techniques and developing new ones.

Immature ooycte (egg) maturation

Researchers are working on ways to help immature eggs mature in the lab (*in vitro*) instead of in the body. Rather than relying on fertility drugs to boost the number of mature eggs available for retrieval, immature eggs can be collected and grown in a special culture medium. In essence, the drugs would be given to the woman's eggs rather than to her.

The maturation of eggs in vitro would help women with polycystic ovarian disease (PCOD); fertility drugs can cause them to develop an excessive number of large follicles and lead to ovarian hyperstimulation syndrome (OHSS), a potentially life-threatening condition (see Chapter 7). So, rather than risk OHSS, these women can have their immature eggs collected without using fertility drugs. This technique can also be used in women whose stimulation cycles have to be cancelled because of the possibility of OHSS. Immature egg maturation will also be helpful to women who don't respond well to—or have serious side effects from—fertility drugs, and those who prefer not to take them because of cost or other reasons. Since the maturation of immature eggs is done with few or no fertility drugs—and therefore requires less monitoring—it will be considerably less expensive than standard IVF.

This is a major area of research around the world, and there have been a few successful pregnancies so far. Once perfected, this technique can have a profound effect on infertility treatment by assisted reproduction; the use of fertility drugs to stimulate IVF cycles may become the exception rather than the rule.

Fluorescent in situ hybridization (FISH)

A highly specialized PGD technique under study, FISH uses synthetic DNA segments that have special fluorescent markers attached to them. The bright color can signal a chromosomal abnormality, such as extra chromosomes or other genetic abnormalities. A number of genetic diseases, including Tay-Sachs disease, Huntington's disease, Duschenne dystrophy, and cystic fibrosis, have been tested using FISH analysis.

Blastocyst culture of embryos

Researchers are trying to imitate nature's own timing. During natural conception embryos don't implant until about five days after fertilization. At that point they're at the *blastocyst* or greater than eight-cell stage. In IVF, embryos are typically transferred about three days after fertilization, when they are in the five- to eight-cell stage. Researchers are looking into whether culturing embryos longer before transferring them into the uterus would improve implantation rates. Culturing embryos longer might also give doctors a longer time to see if the embryos are developing normally and then transfer only the apparently normal ones. This might allow fewer embryos to be transferred to achieve a successful pregnancy and birth, reducing the risk of multiple births.

Cryopreservation today and tomorrow

Cryopreservation is the freezing of cells, tissue, or organs at very low temperatures to keep them alive. Cells contain water, and normally when frozen they expand and ice crystals form, which can permanently damage their cellular structures. Cryopreservation uses special fluids called cryoprotectants that act very much like car antifreeze to prevent expansion and crystal formation. Unfortunately, this type of cryopreservation works well for some tissues—such as sperm and embryos—and not for others, such as eggs.

Frozen eggs

Freezing, successfully thawing human eggs, and producing pregnancies has proven very difficult, at least until recently. Researchers are now experimenting with both slower and faster freezing times, and faster thawing times. They're also developing new coolants that prevent the formation of ice crystals that harm the cells. So far, investigators have been quite successful with mouse eggs and embryos; less so with human ones. So far, about 100 babies have been born from frozen eggs. Scientists hope that the improved freezing and thawing methods being investigated will improve the pregnancy rates using frozen eggs and frozen embryos as well.

Women who are at risk of losing ovarian function because of cancer treatment, radiation therapy, or other medical treatments can freeze their eggs ahead of time (see Chapter 1). The possibility of freezing ovarian tissue—another option for women undergoing these treatments—is also under investigation. Some women, for a variety of reasons, delay childbearing. Having their eggs frozen while they're still young will allow them to use their own eggs, rather than donor eggs, when they are older and no longer ovulating. Women who are opposed to the use of frozen embryos on religious, ethical, or other grounds—as well as women without a male partner or donor—can freeze their eggs and have them fertilized at some later point in time.

Frozen embryos

Unlike eggs, embryos have been successfully frozen, thawed, and transplanted for the last two decades, resulting in thousands of babies. Women who go through IVF often have extra embryos that they can choose to have frozen for future use. They can then use their frozen embryos rather than going though another egg retrieval. As a result, they can avoid the inconvenience, risks, and high costs of going through ovarian stimulation with fertility drugs, as well as the egg retrieval. However, they will need to go through the second half of the IVF cycle—which involves taking hormones to prepare the uterus for implantation—and then going through an embryo transfer, as in IVF.

Watch Out!

Only about 30 percent of couples undergoing a fresh IVF cycle will have extra embryos for freezing.

Unfortunately, the success rate with frozen embryos is not as high as with fresh embryos. According to a 2002 survey by the Society for Assisted Reproductive Technology (SART) on the ARTs, the live-birth rate per transfer from fresh embryos per transfer was 35 percent, while for frozen embryos it was 25 percent. Still, frozen embryos are an important option for many infertile couples, and a 25 percent success rate is considerably higher than it was just five years ago.

It's up to each couple to decide whether or not they want to freeze any extra embryos they may produce. Most frozen embryos are stored by the ART clinics themselves, and only a small percentage (less than 2 percent) are at private for-profit storage facilities. The average cost for storing embryos varies from a few hundred dollars per year to up to $1,500 a year. Several countries, including England and Australia, have passed laws that limit the number of years embryos can be stored—often five years. In the United States, however, there are no such laws or guidelines; it's up to each individual program. If you do have frozen embryos, you must at some point decide that you no longer need them or want to keep them in storage. You will then have three options:

1. You can donate them to another infertile couple.

2. You can discard them.

3. You can donate them to stem cell or other research.

According to the SART survey, nearly 400,000 frozen embryos have been stored in the United States since the 1970s. Only the infertile couples themselves can determine not only whether they want to freeze extra embryos, but what they want done with them afterwards. The survey found that 88 percent (350,000) of the embryos were going to be used by the couples who created them, 2 percent (9,000) were slated to be discarded, and another 2 percent were being donated to other infertile couples. Almost 3 percent (11,000) were designated for research. The remaining embryos (4.5 percent) were being held in storage for various other reasons such as the patient could not be located, she died, become divorced, or abandoned her embryos.

Some couples reject the idea of donating their embryos to other infertile couples because they are not comfortable with the concept of another couple giving birth to and raising a child that is genetically theirs (and, if they have other children together, a full sibling to those children). This is similar to giving up a child for adoption except that the adoptive mother, rather than the genetic mother, is the one who becomes pregnant and gives birth. (Embryo donation and other forms of third-party reproduction are discussed in more detail in Part VI.) The federal government is currently developing legislation to delineate screening tests for infectious and genetic diseases that couples will have to undergo before they can donate their embryos.

According to the SART, only 3 percent of frozen embryos (11,000) have been donated to stem cell or other research. Because many embryos don't survive the thawing-out process and others have defects, only about 2,000 of those embryos will ultimately be usable for research purposes.

Embryonic stem cell research

If you undergo IVF, the issue of donating embryos for stem cell research is worth exploring since you may have to make that decision at some point. According to RESOLVE, almost 50 percent of

---

 Moneysaver

Donating excess embryos to other infertile couples not only helps others, but saves you the cost of years of storage.

Bright Idea

Because it's up to each individual program to decide how long they will store eggs, be sure to ask ahead of time how long the program stores embryos. If you are in your 20s or 30s, you may want to find a program that stores embryos for at least 10 years.

infertile couples would prefer that their unused embryos do some good. Furthermore, they believe it's extremely important to be able to use stem cells for research purposes to save lives.

Indeed, stem cells hold the promise of curing many serious and debilitating conditions such as Alzheimer's disease, Parkinson's disease, diabetes, and even cancer. And embryonic stem cells hold the most promise. Unfortunately, the issue of embryonic stem cell research is shrouded in controversy and confusion. Understanding what stem cells are—and what they do—can help clarify these issues.

What are stem cells?

Stem cells are undifferentiated cells that can, in culture, divide indefinitely and become specialized cells. In simpler terms, they are like a starter kit for creating replacement parts for the body. **Adult stem cells**—which can be extracted from umbilical cords, bone marrow, skin, muscle, fat, and testes—are *multipotent;* that is, they can only develop into the organ or tissue from which they are derived. For example, stem cells from bone marrow can only be used to replace bone marrow cells.

Embryonic stem cells, on the other hand, are *pluripotent* cells, meaning they can be stimulated to develop into virtually any type of body cell, and replace damaged cells in a sick individual. They continually renew themselves, potentially becoming an ongoing repair system for the body for such serious conditions as Parkinson's and Alzheimer's diseases, spinal cord injury, strokes, burns, heart disease, cancer, diabetes, osteoarthritis, rheumatoid arthritis, and birth defects. Most embryonic stem cells are extracted from three- to five-day blastocysts that were created and donated by couples undergoing IVF. They can also be derived from cloned embryos, which are discussed in a moment.

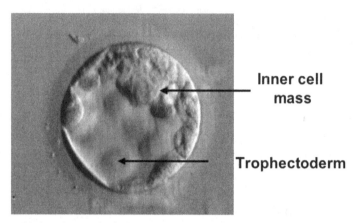

Inner cell mass

Trophectoderm

This is a photograph of a human blastocyst (five-day-old embryo). It is from such a blastocyst that embryonic stem cells are derived. Photo courtesy of Lucinda Veeck Gosden, Weill Medical College of Cornell University.

Stem cells and infertility treatment

Infertile couples who donate embryos for stem cell research may not only be helping people with deadly and disabling diseases, but may also be helping future generations of infertile couples. According to world-renowned embryologist Alan Trounson of Monash University in Australia, embryonic stem cells may—within the next 10 years—be used to create eggs and sperm for infertile couples, thus making infertility a thing of the past. For example, embryonic stem cells may help those who completely lack sperm or egg cells from either congenital disorders or as a result of cancer or other diseases. By receiving

 Watch Out!

Some ART programs require that couples donate their unwanted embryos to other infertile couples rather than to science or have them discarded. Make sure you ask in advance if a program has any requirements or restrictions about extra embryos.

embryonic stem cells, they potentially can develop sperm or egg cells and have their own children. Using embryonic stem cells may also be helpful for women who go through premature menopause and no longer produce eggs.

Scientists have recently had success in transplanting frozen sperm stem cells into sterile mice, which were then able to produce offspring. Adult sperm stem cells can potentially help human males, too. Freezing sperm is not always an option for infertile men; in some cases, the man's sperm is of such poor quality, it can't withstand freezing and thawing. If a man with poor-quality sperm has to undergo cancer treatments, for example, he potentially can have sperm cells extracted from his testes before treatment, and transplanted back afterwards so he starts producing healthy sperm. This technique may also be useful for young boys who have not yet started producing sperm, but who have to undergo chemotherapy or other treatments that

> ❝ Had we had the option available to us when we completed our treatment, we would have gladly donated our embryos for scientific research...we would have felt blessed to have donated them to help advance science and potentially save millions of lives. ❞
>
> —Barb Collura, IVF mother and Director, Chapter and Constituent Services for RESOLVE, ASRM press conference, May 23, 2005

might render them sterile in the future. In the same way, adult stem cells from ovaries may be able to be produced and used by infertile women. Keep in mind that this research is still in the experimental stage and is not yet a clinical reality.

Why are stem cells controversial?

So, if stem cells can be so helpful to millions of sick and dying individuals—not to mention infertile couples—why all the controversy? Actually, the controversy is over embryonic stem cells, not adult stem cells. Some religious and other groups—and some political leaders, including President George W. Bush—strongly oppose this practice because they believe that experimenting with human embryos is destroying human life.

Still, the overwhelming majority of Americans are in favor of using embryonic stem cells for research purposes. Some proponents point out that blastocysts—which are smaller than a pinprick—do not have brains, central nervous systems, hearts, lungs, or any body parts. Even some pro-lifers see no harm in extracting stem cells from these very early embryos. As pro-life Senator Orrin Hatch (R-UT) was reported to say on *Meet the Press,* "I just cannot equate a child living in the womb, with moving toes and fingers and a beating heart, with a frozen embryo sitting in a lab somewhere." More importantly, proponents believe that these embryos—many of which may either be destroyed or eventually die in storage—have the potential to cure previously incurable diseases and to save millions of lives. The bottom line is that it's ultimately up to each couple to decide what happens to their extra embryos.

Cloning

While the issue of stem cell research is extremely contentious, it doesn't come close to the controversy that cloning has inspired. Cloning, while intriguing to some, has terrified many. Fear abounds that cloning could be used for ill rather than good. Certainly, the popular Ira Levin book and movie from the mid 1970s, *The Boys From Brazil,* in which little Hitlers were cloned, reinforced this fear.

What is cloning?

Cloning is the duplication of biological material. There are actually two types of cloning:

1. **Reproductive cloning,** which would be used to produce an offspring that is genetically identical to its parent.

2. **Therapeutic cloning,** which can produce embryonic stems cells for research.

Bright Idea

For more detailed information about stem cells and cloning, check out www.genome.gov, www.asrm.org, or http://stemcells.nih.gov/info/basics/basics5.asp.

Reproductive cloning is what disturbs people the most. In 1998, to the dismay of many, Scottish researchers successfully cloned a sheep named Dolly, who gave birth to triplet lamb clones. To date, only animals have been cloned, and they tend to die in utero or soon after birth. Some that survive may have severe birth defects.

In spring 2005, Korean scientists announced they had successfully cloned 11 human embryos. Rather than fertilizing eggs with sperm, they used the nucleus from the skin cells from patients aged 2 to 56 who had either diabetes, an inborn disease of the immune system, or a spinal cord injury. Many people were once again alarmed, concerned that any kind of cloning—even this type of therapeutic cloning—will lead us down the slippery slope to reproductive cloning of humans.

How is cloning done?

Cloning is typically done through a technique called *somatic cell nuclear transfer* (SCNT). In SCNT, embryos are produced from eggs that are *not* fertilized by sperm, as in normal reproduction. Rather, the nucleus of a donor egg—which contains the DNA of the egg donor—is removed and replaced with the nucleus of a *somatic* (body) cell from the animal or person to be duplicated. This cell—which can come from any part of their body—contains the DNA of that animal or person. The altered egg is then stimulated to divide into an embryo. In reproductive cloning, the blastocyst (early embryo) would be implanted in a woman's uterus where, theoretically, it would develop into a fetus and baby that is genetically identical to the donor of the somatic cell (the woman who gives birth, unless a surrogate uterus is used)—in other words, a clone. This is the outcome that most people agree is morally unacceptable.

In the case of therapeutic cloning—the method used by the Korean scientists—the nucleus of the donor egg is replaced with the nucleus of a cell from a patient. (Skin cells were used in the Korean study.) The egg then divides and forms an embryo. Five or six days later, the stem cells are extracted from the blastocyst. The blastocyst, which contains only the DNA of the patient, not the egg donor, is therefore the patient's exact genetic match (clone). As a result, the stem cells that are extracted can be transplanted into the patient without being rejected by his or her immune system.

This accomplishment was hailed by many as a huge scientific leap in the advancement of stem cell research. Many scientists believe that getting embryonic stem cells through cloning rather than obtaining them from frozen embryos is the best method to use. For one thing, frozen embryos that are stored for long periods of time may not be usable. The most important medical reason, however, is that the cloned embryonic stem cells won't be rejected by the recipient's body since they are a perfect genetic match.

Others, however, have greeted the Korean cloning success with caution, concern, or condemnation. They fear it won't be long before one of these cloned embryos is transplanted into a woman's uterus to produce the first human clone. Indeed, polls show that most Americans are opposed to any cloning research that involves humans, regardless of the purpose, be it for research, reproduction, or rehabilitation. So, while most Americans are in favor of embryonic stem cell research when the stem cells are derived from embryos donated by infertile couples, they draw the line at stem cells derived from cloned embryos. Some even believe that cloning embryos should be legally banned.

On the other hand, many others—scientists and laypeople alike—strongly believe that *any* stem cell research, including therapeutic cloning, is vitally important and should be legal, encouraged, and funded. They do, however, tend to agree with the majority of Americans in condemning reproductive cloning. RESOLVE's position paper on the stem cell and cloning debate states that they, along with the Coalition for the Advancement of Medical Research, are in favor of therapeutic cloning but "oppose any effort that would allow reproductive cloning, a technique we believe, at this time, is unsafe, irresponsible, and unethical."

Improving embryo evaluation

Fortunately, not all embryo research is as emotionally and politically charged as stem cell research and cloning. Scientists are exploring other ways, besides PGD, to evaluate embryos before they're transferred. This would allow doctors to identify and transfer the embryo—or embryos—with the best chance of producing an ongoing pregnancy.

What these researchers learn about embryos may also help the thousands of couples who suffer from spontaneous miscarriages. It's estimated that about 60 percent of spontaneous miscarriages are caused by chromosomal abnormalities in the embryos.

Better embryo evaluation would have other benefits as well. For example, if more first IVF attempts were successful, fewer embryos would need to be produced and later frozen. Freezing better-quality embryos might mean that transfers with frozen embryos would be more successful. Perhaps most importantly, better embryo evaluation would mean that more pregnancies would be achieved with only one embryo transferred. This would dramatically reduce one of the most troubling aspects of the ARTs—mutiple births, especially triplets or more. ASRM guidelines recommend that in normal circumstances, only two embryos be transferred in young women with good-quality embryos. Because of the clinical and economic toll that multiple births place on the mother, the children, and society, some other countries have similar or even more restrictive guidelines and regulations. This critical issue is discussed in more detail in the next chapter.

There are many other serious issues related to the ARTs that require couples to make important, informed decisions. First and foremost is deciding whether or not to pursue the ARTs, and if so, how to find a good program. These and other key issues are addressed in the next chapter.

Just the facts

- Over the past 25 years, IVF and other ARTs such as GIFT and ZIFT have helped hundreds of thousands of severely infertile couples have their own children.

- Improvement in cryopreservation technique is helping boost pregnancy rates using frozen eggs as well as frozen embryos.

- Micromanipulation techniques in conjunction with the ARTs are helping severely infertile men and women have their own children.

- New ART techniques such as assisted hatching and ICSI are showing promising results.

- Stem cells can come either from embryos or adult body tissue. Embryo stem cells can potentially be more useful for curing disabling and deadly diseases than adult stem cells.

- There are two kinds of human cloning: reproductive cloning, the cloning of science fiction, which probably has never been done despite some unsubstantiated claims; and therapeutic cloning, the cloning of embryos to obtain stem cells, which was first done in 2005.

GET THE SCOOP ON...
Emotional, medical, and other considerations ▪
How to choose an ART program ▪ Assessing a
program's success rate ▪ Age, race, and other
factors that determine success

Considering the ARTs

Chapter 10

N
ow that you know what the ARTs are, there
are some things you and your partner should
think about before looking for a specific program. Making the decision to undergo ART is a
momentous—not to say expensive—one. And it's
not an easy one to make. It's difficult, for example,
to enter into an expensive treatment that has a much
greater chance of failure than success. But if this
might be your only chance of pregnancy, you need to
think long and hard about the emotional and physical, as well as the financial, toll of these treatments.
There are no guarantees in the ARTs; no guarantee
that viable eggs will be retrieved or fertilized, and no
guarantee that a fertilized egg will divide properly, or
that an embryo will implant and result in a pregnancy.
That said, the success rates for ARTs have improved
considerably over the past two decades, and now are
equal to or even better than the odds for an average,
fertile couple to conceive in any given month.

But before we look at success rates and choosing
a program, it's important to understand what the
risks are to both the mother, the couple, and their

Watch Out!

The average length of time a woman needs to devote to a typical ART cycle is two weeks but can be as long as six weeks.

offspring, as well as some of the key issues that must be addressed. Fortunately, the ARTs have proven to be very safe procedures. But—as with any medical treatment—there are always some risks, however slight, that you need to be aware of. And there are other issues, besides medical ones, that warrant consideration. These include emotional, interpersonal, financial, and ethical issues.

Emotional considerations

Pursuing the ARTs can be an emotional roller coaster for many couples. They must deal with the possibility that these methods are, in fact, the last resort in their attempt to have their own biological children. Then there is the waiting at nearly every step in these methods: Waiting to see if follicles will develop. Waiting to see if eggs can be retrieved. Waiting to see if they become fertilized. Waiting to see if the resulting embryos develop properly. Waiting to see if there are embryos to be transferred. Waiting to see if they implant. Waiting to see if the pregnancy continues. And, perhaps, even waiting for a coveted place in the ART program of your choice.

> 66 IVF is our last chance. It's also a big gamble for us financially. It's like shooting dice and winner takes all. If we lose, we lose both money and our dream for a child. 99
>
> —John, 30

It's no wonder that most couples going through the ARTs feel anxious, fearful, and, unfortunately for so many, disappointed, even devastated and angry.

These feelings are often exacerbated by the side effects of fertility drugs that play a large role in any ART therapy. These drugs can throw your emotions into turmoil. The emotional issues are not unlike that of most infertility treatment and are discussed in detail in Part V. The financial costs are, however, considerably higher, and may be out of reach for many couples—especially those whose health insurance policies don't cover the ARTs. Chapter 17 addresses the financial aspects of infertility treatment, including ART.

Medical considerations

The medical risks are usually short term and associated with the drug therapy and the egg retrieval typically involved in the ARTs. Long-term risk considerations include multiple births, birth defects, chromosomal abnormalities, and cancer.

The drug therapy

The major risk of fertility drugs is ovarian hyperstimulation syndrome (OHSS). As we mentioned in Chapter 7, up to 10 percent of women undergoing ovulation induction may develop mild OHSS, but less than 1 percent get a more serious form that occasionally requires hospitalization. The good news is that mild hyperstimulation is associated with a slightly increased chance of pregnancy. The most severe form, which occurs in fewer than one in a thousand cases, can usually be treated without hospitalization. (See Chapter 7 for more information about the risks and side effects of hormonal therapy.) Uncommon side effects include blood clots where the shots are given, and local swelling, redness, pain, and very rarely, death.

The egg retrieval procedure

As with almost any type of invasive medical procedure, there are the side effects from, and risks related to, local or general anesthesia or sedation. These can range from the more common side effects such as prolonged nausea and wooziness to the less common but serious ones, such as anaphylactic shock. In rare cases, death can occur. As in any invasive procedure, there is also the risk of infection, bleeding that can sometimes be severe, or organ damage. Informed consent is required when undergoing ART.

Watch Out!

When you go for a procedure—no matter how minor, or how little anesthesia or sedation you're given—bring someone with you. You probably won't be able to drive home afterward, and may not be very steady on your feet. A companion can help you get home as well as give you emotional support.

Multiple births

Multiple births can be a mixed blessing. After years of infertility, having two or more children at once certainly is cause for celebration for most couples. But multiple pregnancies can also cause serious problems for both the mother and her babies.

Women with multiple pregnancies are at increased risk of miscarriages and pregnancy complications such as preeclampsia (pregnancy-induced hypertension), gestational diabetes, and placental abnormalities. They are also at increased risk for premature labor and may have to be confined to bed rest or even hospitalized for weeks or sometimes months before delivery. Pre-term births occur in more than half of twin pregnancies and from 90 to 100 percent of pregnancies with triplets or quadruplets. Caesarian (C) sections are often necessary for twin births and virtually always required for the birth of three or more babies. Sadly, those women carrying large numbers of fetuses may also have to make the extremely difficult decision to undergo a fetal reduction to increase the survival probability and health of the remaining fetuses.

The babies that result from multiple pregnancies—especially triplets or more—are at increased risk for myriad problems, including prematurity, low birth weight, and even neonatal death. Indeed, compared with singletons, a twin is 7 times more likely and a triplet 20 times more likely to die within a month after birth. Being born prematurely puts a baby at risk for such serious conditions as respiratory distress syndrome, cerebral palsy, blindness, and lifetime disabilities.

In addition, the cost of having multiples adds considerably to a couple's total treatment costs. A study published in 1996 in the journal *Obstetrics and Gynecology* estimated that the cost of having children from in-vitro fertilization (IVF) was approximately the same for both twins and singletons: $39,000. However, the cost of having triplets or quadruplets was an astounding $340,000. These costs, which included the cost of IVF, maternal hospitalizations, and neonatal intensive care, are likely to be considerably higher today.

> ❝The objective of infertility treatment should be the birth of a single, healthy child.❞
>
> —The American Society for Reproductive Medicine (ASRM), 2001

The cost of raising multiples can be enormous as well, especially if there are health problems that lead to long-term disability. Even raising healthy multiples takes much patience, energy, and money.

The strain of raising multiples combined with the drain on a couple's finances can wreck havoc on the best of relationships. The good news is that there are ways to minimize the risk of multiple births. These include careful blood and ultrasound monitoring of the woman during ovulation induction (see Chapter 7) and limiting the number of embryos that are transferred, which we discuss later in this chapter.

Birth defects and other problems in offspring

There has been some concern that children born of IVF and the other ARTs such as intracytoplasmic sperm injection (ICSI) would be born with birth defects. According to a recent study, children born through ART procedures are at somewhat greater risk of having lower birth weight than babies born through natural conception. And another recent study found that there was a very small increase in the risk of birth defects among IVF babies compared with other babies. The study, however, did not prove that ART was the cause of these problems.

The researchers suggested that other factors not tested for may have been responsible. Other studies, however, suggest no increase in abnormalities. Indeed, a study in Belgium—which was reported at the European Society of Human Reproduction and Embryology in June 2005—found that 151 children born through IVF and ICSI had *higher* IQs at the age of eight compared with a control group of children of the same age whose mothers had not undergone IVF. The researchers, however, attribute this to psychological rather than biological factors; they hypothesize that the mothers who pursued IVF were motivated to have children and dedicated to parenting. As a result, they may have stimulated their children more intellectually than the mothers in the control group.

Cancer

Any drug should be used cautiously, and fertility drugs are no exception. Because ART usually requires large dosages of fertility drugs and other hormones, there has been some concern that women who undergo ART are at increased risk of developing cancer later on in life. The overwhelming majority of studies, however, have found no connection between fertility drugs and cancer. On the other hand, some studies have shown a slight but not necessarily statistically significant increase in ovarian, uterine, and breast cancers. It's possible that those few infertile women who took fertility drugs and subsequently developed cancer might have developed cancer in any case—that whatever caused their infertility in the first place may have put them at risk for cancer.

However, even a slight possibility of a causal link to cancer must be considered when deciding whether or not to pursue ART; and if you do, how many cycles you should be willing to undergo. The possible link underscores the need for judicious use of fertility drugs. You should not take any fertility drugs for more than several months at a time and certainly not for more than a total of six months to a year without careful consideration and discussion with your doctor.

Other considerations

Besides the previous considerations, you and your partner must be comfortable with the medical, financial, philosophical, and ethical issues that are bound to come up during these treatments. You may have faced some of these already during diagnosis, but if you're going ahead with the decision to try the ARTs, they become far less theoretical.

Here are some questions you and your partner should consider before looking into a specific ART program:

- Have we exhausted the traditional less-invasive and less-expensive options?

- What are our chances of pregnancy with these traditional therapies?

- Do we have time to wait for these other treatments to work?

- Can we afford to take the necessary time off from work to undergo ART?

- Are we comfortable with the idea of conception outside the woman's body?

- How many embryos should we transfer?

- What should we do with extra embryos?

- What do we do if I become pregnant with triplets or quadruplets?

- How many ART cycles are we willing to go through?

You may not be able to answer or agree on all of these questions now. Researching these issues and discussing them with your partner can better prepare you for ART.

Choosing an ART program

Once you've talked about the "big issues" surrounding the ARTs, the next step is to find a program that's right for you. Much of the advice in Chapter 5 about finding the right doctor also applies to finding the right ART program. Keep in mind many of the same key elements we discussed in that chapter are critical—especially competency, compatibility, convenience, and last but not least—cost.

Competency is key

When evaluating whether a program's right for you, there are several critical sources of information you should be sure to contact. Both the American Society for Reproductive Medicine (ASRM) and its subdivision, the Society for Assisted Reproductive Technology (SART), issue guidelines for and/or collect information about specific ART programs. You should make sure that the program and its key medical staff are members of these organizations and report their success rates to SART. RESOLVE or another support organization may also be able to provide you with information about specific programs.

Also, check out the programs on the Internet and get their patient information packets sent to you. Be sure to read and evaluate the information carefully. Remember, just because a program has a glitzy promotional brochure doesn't mean it's a good program.

Armed with these patient information packets and the information you obtained on the Internet, you can begin seeking answers to key questions about individual programs. Some of these include:

- Are the doctors board-certified reproductive endocrinologists? (See Chapter 5.)

- What procedures do they do? (IVF? GIFT? ZIFT? Sperm/egg micromanipulation? Donor sperm/egg? Cryopreservation?)

- What is their age limit?

- What is their success rate? (See the discussion about interpreting success rate statistics later in this chapter.)

- What is their multiple pregnancy rate?

- Do they report to SART? (This is also discussed later in the chapter.)

Bright Idea

Check out SART's website at http://sart.org/home.html. Type in your ZIP code and SART will provide you with a list of SART member programs in your area.

Check that the program has on-site labs and monitoring equipment and that they are well staffed. The purpose of the fertility drugs used in ART treatments is to get you ovulating and to increase the number of eggs available for retrieval. Monitoring equipment must be on site not only to look for the right time to get those eggs, but to be certain that you don't develop ovarian hyperstimulation syndrome.

Compatibility concerns

You'll be spending a lot of time—and money—with these programs, to say nothing of the emotional energy you'll be expending. So it's important that you make certain that the program has a good support team of doctors, nurses, social workers, counselors, other patients, and even financial advisors who can help you every step of the way, cycle through cycle of therapy. Again, here are a few basic questions to ask when evaluating an ART program:

- Do I have a choice of doctors?
- How experienced are the doctors? The embryologist?
- Will I be assigned to one or more doctors? Nurses? A team?
- What counseling services are available?

Convenience counts

ARTs require a great deal of time. If you've gone through ovulation induction, you may already have a good idea of what's involved. Ask, "How much time is involved in ART cycles?" "How much work will I miss?" If you must travel a distance to a program, ask, "What accommodations are nearby?" "Does the program help arrange lodging?"

Check out the availability of staff and technicians. Your doctor, embryologists, and clinic *should* have weekend and holiday hours. If you are ready to have your eggs collected near the weekend the program must be ready to retrieve your eggs. Keep in mind, however, that most ART programs have to occasionally close to clean labs, as well as for the staffs' well-earned vacations. You can find out ahead of time when they are closed and plan your own vacation to coincide. But make certain that there will be staff available on call.

Cost considerations

ARTs, as we've said, are very expensive. The cost of just one IVF cycle, complete with ovulation induction, can range from about $12,000 to $18,000. And if you go for more than one attempt, the costs can become prohibitive. Not only do some cycles fail to produce a pregnancy, some cycles are cancelled before they get to the transfer of embryo stage.

Here are some cost-related questions to ask:

- How much does an initial consultation cost? What about pre-cycle screening?

- What does each drug and procedure (retrievals, inseminations, cryopreservation, transfer) cost?

- Do I have to pay in advance? If so, how much?

- What payment methods do you accept?

- Do I pay less if my cycle has to be cancelled before egg retrieval or embryo transfer?

- Is there a shared-risk policy or "money back guarantee"? (This is discussed in Chapter 17.)

- Is a financial office/manager available to help submit insurance bills?

This last point is very important—insurance coverage of ARTs is still a difficult issue, and good financial advice on how to fund your treatments will be extremely important. Chapter 17 further explores financial issues. Also ask how much time you need to devote to a cycle and how much time you and your partner will need to take off from work.

Compassion comforts

Having a caring, compassionate staff can be important when dealing with the difficult emotional, physical, and financial aspects of ART. Although this may be hard to determine ahead of time, you may be able to get a sense of this by speaking to other patients or calling a support group in your area. Get to know the people who are treating you. Key in on one or two. It'll help to hear test results, whether good or bad, from a familiar voice. And try to have someone with you when you call for test results. It might make hearing disappointing news a little easier, and make sharing good news even more joyous!

Making sense of ART success

When gathering information about a program's success, you'll need to understand what the numbers they tell you actually mean. Ask each program to explain how they calculate their success rates and to define the terms they use. If you don't understand, ask again—and again, if necessary—until you do.

Remember, ART is a multi-step process. Success rates are reported based on individual steps: ovulation induction, retrieval, fertilization, embryo transfer, and implantation. But not everyone goes through all the steps. For example, just because you start a treatment cycle doesn't mean that you'll ovulate, or that eggs will be retrieved or fertilized, or that embryos will form, survive, and be transferred, let alone implant and produce a live birth.

When questioning the program, try to get a sense of their philosophy about procedures. For example, do they transfer

Moneysaver

If you go to an out-of-town program, ask them if they have discounts at local hotels or guest houses.

Watch Out!

Many good programs have long waiting lists, but it's not a guarantee of a program's competency. You should still check out the program. If you're still interested, put your name on the waiting lists of several programs with similar success rates and go to the first one that becomes available.

only the very best quality embryos or do they transfer borderline ones? The answer may give you insight into whether the program is more concerned with doing the procedures than the outcome.

Also, when comparing one program's successes with that of another, make certain you're comparing apples with apples. For example, if you're looking at two programs' reported success rates for embryo transfer, make sure both programs were transferring approximately the same number of embryos.

Interpreting success rates

Here are definitions of the terms used most often to calculate or define ART success rates. Become familiar with them so that you can understand the claims each program makes for itself.

- **Chemical (or biochemical) pregnancy.** In essence, this is an early positive pregnancy blood test result that is relatively common after any type of IVF procedure, as it would be in an unassisted conception. Unfortunately, as also occurs in unassisted conception, many of these biochemical pregnancies don't go on to produce a baby. Don't be fooled by a high biochemical pregnancy rate. It's really not telling you much about how good the program is.

- **Gestational sac pregnancy.** Some programs use ultrasound examination to look for a gestational sac, the fluid-filled structure surrounding an embryo in the uterine cavity early in a pregnancy, and call that a pregnancy. Unfortunately, not all of these pregnancies will go on to produce a baby.

- **Clinical pregnancy.** A clinical pregnancy is one in which the pregnancy hormone hCG level has continued to rise and a gestational sac, a fetal "pole," and a fetal heartbeat are detected during ultrasound examination. This usually occurs during week five or six. Most programs define success in terms of clinical pregnancy per treatment cycle. This figure would include everyone who begins taking fertility drugs whether or not eggs have been retrieved, fertilized, or embryos transferred. Other programs calculate success in other terms—they give the clinical pregnancy rate based on embryos actually transferred.

It's very important for you to get an idea of how many women begin treatment and then go on to retrievals. It'll be an indication of how good a program's ovulation induction protocols are. But remember, clinical pregnancies are still *early* pregnancies, and miscarriages and ectopic pregnancies do occur. Another factor to consider is cryopreservation. A single ovulation cycle might actually be responsible for a pregnancy realized after the second or third attempt at embryo transfer. This means that pregnancies from a single ovulation-induction cycle are increasing.

- **Pregnancy rate per cycle (or per transfer).** These are measures of the number of ART cycles started (or number of embryo transfers) that produce a pregnancy. However, those pregnancies may not result in the birth of a baby because they end in a miscarriage, abortion, or stillbirth. Therefore, "pregnancy rate" is not as accurate a measure of success as "live-birth rate."

- **Live-birth rate.** The single most important figure to look at is the live-birth rate, sometimes called the take-home baby rate. After all, the ultimate goal of any infertility treatment is the birth of a live baby. This is the only true indication of a program's success. This rate should reflect the number of *women* who take babies home, not the number of *babies* brought home. If one woman walks out of the program with three babies, it's still only one success story—not three. In other words, the delivery of two or more babies from the same mother should be counted as one pregnancy and even more importantly, one live birth.

There are, in fact, three ways to use live-birth rate as a measure of success: live-birth rate per cycle, per retrieval, or per transfer. This should be kept in mind when comparing programs. Also remember that the success rates per cycle will be lower than the success rates per embryo transfer, as we explain in a moment.

Live-birth rate per cycle is the percentage of cycles started that result in the live birth of one or more babies. (A cycle starts when a woman begins taking the fertility drugs needed for ART or starts having her ovaries monitored.) This is the most important success rate to know because it tells you the chance the average infertile woman has of having a baby at a particular ART program.

Live-birth rate per retrieval is the percentage of cycles in which eggs were retrieved that result in a live birth. This rate doesn't take into account cycles that were started but then cancelled, so this rate will tend to be higher than the live-birth rate per cycle.

Live-birth rate per transfer is the percentage of embryo transfers that result in a pregnancy. Because this rate doesn't take into account cycles that are cancelled or eggs that fail to fertilize, this rate will tend to be higher than either of the other two rates.

▪ **Cancellation rates.** These may reflect a general lack of success with ovulation induction or the fact that a program accepts more difficult patients who have higher cancellation—and therefore lower success—rates.

Current ART success rates

Under a federal law passed in 1992, the centers offering ARTs are required to report their results to the Society for Assisted

Reproductive Technology (SART). The Centers for Disease Control (CDC) then issues a report of the findings based on collated results from the individual clinics.

The most recent report, the 2002 Assisted Reproductive Technology (ART) Report, was released in 2004 (two years are needed to evaluate the outcome of the cycles). According to this report, there were 428 ART clinics in 2002, and 391 of those programs submitted their results. Those that fail to report their findings are listed by state in the appendix of the report. Their success rates may be low and they don't want to publish them, or they may do too few procedures to collect any meaningful data. In any case, these programs may not be your best bet, and you should be wary about participating in them. In 2002, although 42 percent of transfers resulted in a pregnancy, 34 percent resulted in a live birth. It is the 34 percent birth rate per transfer that is the most meaningful statistic to keep in mind. This means that the average woman who undergoes IVF has greater than a one-in-three chance of having a baby. This is extremely good news, since a fertile couple has only about a 20 percent chance of conceiving each month!

In general, success rates are improving; between 2001 and 2002, the live-birth rate for couples using their own freshly fertilized eggs was about 35 percent, an increase of 4 percent. The increases were even greater (6 percent) for frozen non-donor cycles; and for fresh donor cycles.

The following table shows the 2002 success rates for ART. As you can see, the greatest success, fully 50 percent, is with embryos from donor eggs.

 Bright Idea

You can download the full 2002 Assisted Reproductive Technology Report at www.cdc.gov/reproductivehealth/ART02/index.htm.

Table 10.1: 2002 ART Procedure Average Live-Birth Rates per Transfer	
Overall success rate	34 percent
With fresh nondonor embryo	35 percent
With frozen nondonor embryo	25 percent
With fresh donor embryo	50 percent
With frozen donor embryo	29 percent

Source: Centers for Disease Control, 2004. Assisted Reproductive Technology Surveillance United States, 2002.

In 2002, more than 7,500 transfers involved embryos that had been frozen by a couple in a previous cycle. When fresh nondonor embryos were transferred, the live-birth rate per transfer was 35 percent. When the couple's own previously frozen embryos were used, the live-birth rate was 25 percent. Although frozen embryos don't do quite as well as fresh ones, attempts at frozen embryo transfer have the advantage of reducing the number of ovulation induction cycles you need to undergo. Embryos from donated eggs have an even greater success rate. Fully half (50 percent) of the cycles involving fresh embryos formed from donor eggs resulted in a live birth. The results were lower with frozen embryos from donor eggs (29 percent). (The use of donor eggs is discussed in the next two chapters on third-party reproduction.) The lowest success rate was from frozen embryos from the patients' own eggs (25 percent).

In 2002, 115,392 ART treatment cycles were performed, resulting in 33,141 live-birth deliveries, which produced 45,751 babies. Looking at the percentages, fully 83 percent of the pregnancies resulted in a live birth, and 12 percent ended in a miscarriage.

While the clinical pregnancy rate for fresh nondonor cycles was 34 percent, the live-birth rate per cycle was 29 percent. Most cycles (99 percent) were IVF, and 74 percent of the cycles were carried out with fresh nondonor egg-embryos. Frozen nondonor egg-embryos were used in 14 percent of the cycles, and donor egg-embryos were used in 11 percent of the cycles.

Watch Out!

Be cautious about going to a program that does fewer than 100 cycles each year. The doctors or embryologists may not be as experienced as those in higher-volume programs. On the other hand, programs that see hundreds of patients may not be able to provide you with enough personal attention. Weigh the considerations carefully.

Although IVF continues to be the most commonly performed ART procedure, gamete intrafallopian transfer (GIFT) and zygote intrafallopian transfer (ZIFT)—which are not appropriate for many women—have shown slightly higher live-birth rates per retrieval than IVF. As we mentioned earlier, one explanation may be that women undergoing GIFT and ZIFT have healthier reproductive systems to start with. (See the following table.)

ICSI (see Chapter 9)—which has mainly been used as a treatment for male-factor infertility since the early 1990s—was performed in 53 percent of all IVF cycles initiated in 2002. IVF without ICSI is primarily used to treat female-factor infertility. Although male-factor infertility is notoriously difficult to treat, the 2002 data is very encouraging; it shows that for couples using their own fresh eggs, IVF with ICSI had virtually the same live-birth rate per retrieval (32 percent) as IVF without ICSI (34 percent).

Table 10.2: 2002 ART Success Rates for Couples Using Their Own Fresh Eggs

Procedure	Live Births Per Retrieval	How Often Used
IVF without ICSI	34 percent	46 percent
IVF with ICSI	32 percent	53 percent
GIFT	25 percent	0.2 percent
ZIFT	26 percent	0.5 percent

Source: Centers for Disease Control, 2004.

Factors influencing success

There are several factors that can contribute to the success—or failure—of an ART cycle. Some of the most important ones are:

■ Egg quality

■ Sperm quality

■ The woman's health status

■ Genetic factors

■ The skill of the doctor, the embryologist, and other team members

Some other key issues are the number of cycles one undergoes and the number of embryos transferred. These vary depending on several factors, which are discussed in the following sections. Factors such as age and race cannot be changed. However, the age of the egg can be altered by using a donor egg (see Chapters 11 and 12).

Age matters

Once again, it's worth repeating: The chance of conception and ongoing pregnancy decreases as a woman gets older, whether or not she has a fertility problem. Keep in mind it's chronological age that counts, not how young a woman looks or feels.

There are many reasons why older age adversely affects a woman's fertility. Besides medical conditions that can worsen with time, older ovaries become resistant to natural and drug-induced hormonal stimulation. Fewer and fewer follicles are produced, and FSH levels rise. Estrogen and progesterone levels decline, causing menstrual irregularities and making the uterus less receptive to pregnancy. Finally, older fertilized eggs are less likely than younger eggs to develop normally.

Today, more and more older women are undergoing ART procedures. And ARTs are being tried early in the course of their treatment. According to the CDC, the likelihood of live birth resulting from an ART cycle ranged from 11 to 37 percent, depending on the woman's age and the technique employed.

When the female partner's own fresh eggs were used, the live-birth rate per cycle was 37 percent for women under 35, and 11 percent for women 41 to 42.

Not surprisingly, women under 35 years old using their own eggs had the best success rate—37 percent live-birth rate per cycle. This figure dropped to 31 percent for women 35 to 37, 21 percent for women 38 to 40, 11 percent for women 41 to 42, and 4 percent for women over 42.

The good news is that if eggs from a young, fertile donor are used, your age doesn't have much influence on the outcome; women in older age groups have a significantly better chance of having a baby if they use donor eggs than if they use their own. Indeed, regardless of their age, women who use fresh donor eggs have an astounding 50 percent success rate! If they use frozen donor egg-embryos, the success rate drops to 29 percent.

Racial disparities

A recent study of 75,000 ART patients found that the live-birth rate per cycle using fresh eggs (but not frozen embryos) was lower for African American and Asian women than for Caucasian and Hispanic women. Interestingly, Asian women tended to be significantly older than the other women, but even when compared to women of the same age, Asian women had 11 percent lower success rates than Caucasian and Hispanic women. African American women not only had 21 percent lower success rates than Caucasians and Hispanics, but those who did become pregnant after an ART cycle had higher rates of miscarriage than the other women.

 Bright Idea

When comparing one program's success rate with another's, keep in mind that some programs accept older women or other difficult cases. As a result, their success rates might be misleadingly lower than those of other programs.

The reasons for these disparities are unclear and don't appear to be related to socioeconomic factors. There is evidence that African American women have more uterine fibroids and tubal-factor infertility, but even when considering these factors, African American women, unfortunately, have lower success rates. Asian women have higher rates of endometriosis than other women, which could be a factor in their lower success rates. They also consume large quantities of fresh fish, which may be a factor because of high levels of mercury found in some fish. It's important that African American and Asian women take these factors into account and discuss them with their doctors when considering ART.

Number of embryos transferred

Once you choose a program, there are other important decisions to make, especially how many embryos to transfer. While you may think this is the doctor's decision, that's not entirely true. You should have some input into the decision with a clear understanding of the risks and benefits of having more than a few embryos transplanted.

Most ART procedures rely on fertility drugs, and statistics show that the likelihood of success increases if more than one embryo is transferred per treatment cycle. More specifically, when one fresh embryo was transferred, the live-birth rate was 13 percent. That figure jumped to almost 40 percent when two embryos were transferred, and 38 percent with three embryos. The success rates continue to slowly decline to 29 percent when five or more embryos are transferred. It is frequently the case that when embryo quality declines, IVF programs try to compensate by transferring more embryos. This may explain the decline in success rates with an increase in the number of embryos transferred.

But there's more at stake here than success. As we mentioned earlier, multiple pregnancies are a serious concern when more than one embryo is transferred. In 2002, more than 35 percent of the deliveries from ART procedures in which women used their own fresh eggs were multiple births (32 percent twins and 4 percent triplets or more). This compares with a multiple birth rate of only 3 percent in the general population.

Since 1997, the average number of embryos transferred has declined. As a result, the rate of pregnancies with three or more babies has also declined since then, but the rate of twin pregnancies has remained consistent.

Deciding on the number of embryos to transfer depends on several factors, including the woman's age, the embryo quality, and the availability of frozen embryos. Because the greater number of embryos transferred, the greater the risk of multiple pregnancies, the ASRM issues general guidelines on how many embryos should be transferred in an ART cycle. They do, however, emphasize that each individual program should have its own guidelines based on its patient population and individual patient characteristics. The patients' desires and concerns also should be taken into consideration.

The ASRM issued the following guidelines in 2004 for women undergoing IVF:

■ Women under 35 should have no more than two embryos transferred unless there is some extenuating medical circumstance.

■ Those women under 35 with the most favorable prognoses should consider transferring only one embryo. This includes women undergoing their first cycle who have good-quality embryos and women who have previously been successful with IVF.

■ Women between 35 and 37 with favorable prognoses should have no more than two embryos transferred, and others in this age group no more than three.

■ Women between 38 and 40 with good prognoses should have no more than three embryos transferred, and others in this age group no more than four.

■ Women over 40 should have no more than five embryos transferred.

- When donor eggs are used, the donor's age should determine the number of embryos to transfer, not the age of the recipient.

- Those women who have had two or more failed IVF cycles and those with a less favorable prognosis may have additional embryos transferred.

- Because GIFT involves transferring eggs, not embryos, and not all eggs fertilize, for each of the above categories, one more egg than embryo may be transferred.

Interestingly, Sweden recently passed a national law that mandates that only one embryo can be transferred except when the risk of a multiple pregnancy is very low. Not only did the number of multiple births fall from 23 percent to 9 percent, the pregnancy rate remained about the same.

In the United States, the number of embryos to be transferred is a decision you, your partner, and your doctor need to make together while taking the ASRM guidelines into account. Considering the real possibility of multiple births, you should ask yourselves: "How do we feel about conceiving twins? Triplets? Four or more?" And be sure to also ask yourselves this extremely difficult, emotionally charged question: "What would we do if we're faced with the possibility of fetal reduction?"

Other important decisions to make

The decision of how many embryos to transfer has implications beyond the risk of a multiple pregnancy. One such decision is what to do with any extra embryos that are produced that are not going to be transferred. This may seem like an easy decision, but there are several key factors to consider.

Extra embryos

Extra embryos can be frozen and used again, thus saving you considerable time, expense, and the inconvenience of going through a complete ART cycle. If it turns out your embryos repeatedly fail to implant in your uterus, or you cannot carry a pregnancy to term, you can have your extra embryos implanted in a gestational carrier. (This and other third-party reproductive techniques are discussed in the next two chapters.) Another option many couples choose is to donate the extra embryos to another infertile couple. Yet another option is one of the most controversial ones we discussed in the previous chapter—you can donate your embryos to be used for stem cell research. Many couples who have completed their families choose to discard their extra embryos rather than choose any of these options. As we've mentioned, it's ultimately up to each couple to decide for themselves what to do with extra embryos.

Number of cycles

Another decision you may need to make that might affect your chances of success is how many ART cycles you are willing to try. Just as the chance of conceiving from unprotected sexual intercourse does not increase with each month that a couple attempts to get pregnant, the probability doesn't increase with ART either.

In one study, SART looked at the IVF success rates of 54 fertility treatment programs and found no significant decrease in the success rates for the second and third attempts. In their review of more than 4,000 cycles of egg retrieval, they found that success rates remained almost equal for the first two treatment cycles, and then declined only modestly in the third. It wasn't until the fourth attempt that both pregnancy and delivery rates began to decline significantly. It seems probable that IVF simply wasn't going to work for some of these couples, no matter how many times they tried. So if IVF is likely to be successful, you should know within two or three tries.

 Moneysaver

Be sure to ask the cost of freezing, storing, and thawing embryos. It's important to be aware of the fact that about one in three frozen embryos do not survive thawing.

IVF may not be successful for a variety of reasons, and failure of the embryo to implant is one of the major causes. Ongoing research is constantly refining the ARTs and discovering ways to enhance success rates, some of which were discussed in the previous chapter. In the meantime, for some couples, the chances of success may be considerably improved through third-party reproduction. The next two chapters look into these solutions to infertility.

> **"** Infertility treatments can be very seductive. There's always the promise that this month is different, this is the right month: the timing is better, the sonograms look better, you're feeling better this month than the last. You can lose your perspective very easily. **"**
>
> —Millie, 32

Just the facts

- The ARTs have proven safe for mothers who are properly monitored in both the short-term and long-term.

- Children conceived through the ARTs may have slightly lower birth weights than non-ART children, but are basically very healthy.

- When choosing an ART program, consider competency, compatibility, convenience, and cost.

- There are many different definitions of pregnancy used in reporting success rates, but the most important ones are the live-birth rate per cycle and per retrieval.

- African American and Asian women have lower success rates with the ARTs than Caucasian and Hispanic women.

- Multiple pregnancies can be problematic to the mother and offspring and should be avoided, if possible.

Alternative Solutions

GET THE SCOOP ON...
Evaluating third-party reproduction options ▪
Choosing between pregnancy and parenthood,
and other important considerations ▪ Telling the
child and others ▪ The adoption option

PART VI

Is Third-Party Reproduction Right for You?

Chapter 11

As you well know by now, nothing about having a baby is simple for infertile couples. You may be at the point where you've exhausted many of the conventional options—such as drug therapy and surgery—as well as assisted reproductive technologies (ARTs), and be considering other options. The good news is that reproductive medicine is continually expanding your options to have a child. In many instances, these options may help you have a baby who will be completely genetically related to both you and your partner. However, in a growing number of cases, there are options you can choose that will result in the birth of a baby who is partially genetically related to you or your partner, or—in some cases—to neither one of you.

Tens of thousands of couples—both straight and gay—are turning to third-party reproduction—the use of eggs, sperm, embryos, or a uterus that are donated by someone (the donor) so that you and your partner (the recipients) can become parents. For them, it takes at least three to make a baby. And, as you'll see, depending on what factors are causing your infertility, it could take even four or five different "parents."

Third-party reproduction options

The following are the various third-party reproduction options currently available that involve the ARTs or other fertility treatments. (Although it doesn't involve fertility treatment, adoption is also considered third-party reproduction, and will be discussed later in this chapter.)

- **Sperm donation:** A fertile man donates his sperm to an infertile couple to be used to fertilize the female partner's egg.

- **Egg donation:** A fertile woman donates her eggs to an infertile couple to be fertilized by the male partner's sperm. The female partner carries the resulting embryo.

- **Embryo donation:** An infertile couple donates extra embryos produced through an in-vitro fertilization (IVF) procedure to a second infertile couple; the embryos are carried by that second infertile couple's female partner.

- **Traditional surrogacy (surrogate mother):** A woman agrees to be inseminated with the sperm from the male partner of an infertile couple and to carry the fetus to term for that couple.

- **Gestational carrier (donor uterus or gestational surrogacy):** A woman agrees to carry to term an embryo produced through an IVF procedure using an infertile couple's eggs and sperm. The resulting baby is the biological child of the infertile couple.

- **Egg donation/gestational carrier:** A woman agrees to carry to term for an infertile couple an embryo produced through an IVF procedure using some other woman's donated eggs and the male partner's sperm.

Moneysaver

When contemplating traditional surrogacy or using a gestational carrier, factor in the potential hidden costs: pregnancy and delivery complications, such as a C-section or miscarriage and after care; selective reduction for multiple fetuses; and amniocentesis.

- **Egg donation/sperm donation:** The female partner carries to term an embryo produced through an IVF procedure using donated sperm and donated eggs. (Similar to embryo donation, but the infertile couple does not use extra, unneeded embryos from another infertile couple.)

- **Egg donation/sperm donation/gestational carrier:** A woman agrees to carry to term for an infertile couple an embryo produced through an IVF procedure using some other woman's donated eggs and another man's donated sperm. (Similar to above, but the female partner does not carry the pregnancy.)

The following table graphically shows what's required for third-party reproduction compared with normal reproduction, as well as the number of people involved (including the infertile couple). The range is from three people for such techniques as donor egg and sperm to five people in the case of donor egg, donor sperm, and gestational carrier.

Considering third-party reproduction

As you see, the third-party reproduction options available to you are considerable—indeed, mind-boggling. In general, when considering third-party reproduction, you'll need to confront several important issues, both immediate and long-term. These issues become more complicated as the options themselves become more complex. They include, but are not limited to:

- Personal concerns
- Partner's reactions

Table 11.1: How Many People Help to Make Your Baby?

How Many?	The Couple			Donor Involvement				
	Male Partner's Role	Female Partner's Role					Carrier	
	Sperm	Eggs	Uterus	Sperm	Eggs	Embryo	Eggs	Uterus
Normal conception — 2	X	X	X					
Donor sperm — 3		X	X	X				
Donor eggs — 3	X		X		X			
Traditional surrogacy — 3	X						X	X
Gestational carrier (donor uterus) — 3	X	X						X
Donor egg/gestational carrier — 4	X				X			X
Donor embryo — 4*			X			X		
Donor egg/donor sperm — 4*			X	X	X			
Donor sperm/donor egg/gestational carrier — 5**				X	X			X

* Genetically, the same as adoption, except the female partner carries and delivers the baby

** Genetically and biologically, the same as adoption

- Effects on participants' relationship
- Family and friends' reactions
- Confidentiality issues
- Religious prohibitions
- Legal issues
- Ethical considerations
- Financial costs

Before pursuing any of these options, it's a good idea to discuss it not only with your doctor, but also a counselor, a lawyer, and possibly a religious counselor. They can help you better understand the medical, emotional, social, and legal ramifications of these options *before* you commit to them. Virtually all good donor programs—whether totally private or connected with a fertility treatment center—will offer counseling services. In fact, most programs using third-party reproduction, particularly those involving eggs and embryos, require you, your partner, and the donor to undergo psychological evaluation. If needed, it's worthwhile to go outside the program for additional guidance, as well. You'll probably get a more impartial perspective. Think of it as getting a second opinion, something you're probably comfortable with after having gone through infertility testing and treatment.

We'll explore some of the major issues surrounding third-party reproduction. But these are, by far, not the only considerations you and your partner need to discuss. Joining a support group, such as RESOLVE, is a very helpful way to learn more about how these options might affect you, your partner, and your future child. You may have thought about some of these issues before, and may even have formed some strong opinions. But after actually having experienced infertility—and dealing with the emotional, physical, and financial pains and problems—your views may have radically changed, or still may do so.

Motherhood, fatherhood, and parenthood

Whether we recognize it initially or not, at the heart of the matter of third-party reproduction are the questions: What is motherhood? What is fatherhood? What does it mean to become parents? These are important questions to ask yourself as well as discuss with your partner. The answers will help you separate the social roles of motherhood, fatherhood, and parenthood from the biological and genetic roles of impregnation, pregnancy, and childbirth.

You and your partner should also ask yourselves: Do we want to become pregnant, or become parents? Are we enamored with the idea of pregnancy and the attention it may bring, or do we primarily want to build our family? To help you answer these questions, remember: While pregnancy lasts a mere nine months, parenthood lasts a lifetime.

If you decide not to pursue third-party reproduction—or it's been unsuccessful—you may be faced with another question: When do we stop trying to get pregnant and start trying to become parents? Answering these questions may help you to think about another alternative solution that we discuss later in this chapter—adoption.

Passing on genes

The issue of motherhood and fatherhood revolves around—but is separate from—the issue of genetic and biologic connections. To better understand this, it may help to understand the meaning of the terms *biologic* and *genetic*. These terms are confusing and many people use them interchangeably. But they are not precisely the same thing.

As we mentioned earlier, depending on the third-party reproduction method, your child can be completely, partially, or not at all related genetically to you. Although not linked genetically to you, your child may be linked biologically to you. The same holds true for the donor. For example, in the case of donor eggs or embryos, a child is not genetically linked to you, but is biologically connected through gestation and childbirth.

As we explained in Chapter 4, the term *genetic* refers to genes from the sperm and eggs that are passed on to (inherited by) the child. The term *biological* refers to physiologic functions, as when the female partner—or a donor—carries and delivers the child. So, if you contract with a woman to carry an embryo from an IVF procedure using your sperm and eggs, you're genetically but not biologically related to the child. If you carry an embryo donated by another infertile couple, you're not genetically related to the child, but you are biologically linked or related. However, if the donor is a blood relative, you also have a genetic link to that child, and how strong the link is depends on how close you are, genetically speaking, to the donor. For example, the male partner's genetic link to the child is stronger if his brother is the sperm donor rather than his cousin.

> ❝When I ask myself if I could love a child not genetically related to me, I think about my dog. I love that dog and would do anything for her, and would be devastated if anything ever happened to her. And she's certainly not biologically related to me.❞
>
> —Chloe, 37

Likewise, the female partner's genetic link is stronger if her sister rather than her cousin is the egg donor.

However, in most instances of sperm or egg donation, the donor has no genetic ties to the infertile couple. As a result, third-party reproduction introduces another set of genes into your family gene pool. You should, therefore, examine how you feel about having a child who is not genetically related to you. Ask yourself that all-important question, "How important is a genetic connection with my child?"

Coming to terms

The ability to impregnate their partners and pass on their genes is a very important physical and emotional role for men. This may be because the process of impregnating a woman is the only biologic, not to mention genetic, role they actually have in

pregnancy and childbirth. They may, therefore, equate impregnation and genetic contribution as the only thing that makes
them a father. If they can't "father" a child, they may feel that they
have no other major contribution to make and fear that they
will have no interest in or ability to bond with the child.

Women seem to have an easier time than men looking
beyond the genetic and biologic connection, as well as seeking
parenthood rather than pregnancy as their primary goal. In
fact, the term "to mother a child" refers to the *social*, not *biological*, connection. "To mother" means to care for, nurture, and
raise a child, and has nothing to do with being pregnant, giving
birth, or any other biological function, including breastfeeding.
On the other hand, the term "to father a child" means to get a
woman pregnant and, therefore, refers only to the biologic and
genetic, not social, connection.

It's important to remember that being a parent is more than
just contributing your genetic material. It involves getting up in
the middle of the night for diaper changes, feedings, and fevers.
It means being there for the long haul—long after the moment
of conception has passed.

Another issue to be dealt with is what to call those who donate
their eggs, sperm, or bodies. For eggs and sperm, it's fairly
simple—they're called *donors*. However, it can become a problem
for both the recipients and the offspring when these donors are
referred to as the *biologic* or *real* mothers and fathers. The term
birth mother, or worse still, *real mother*, is especially confusing. As we
mentioned, to mother means to care for a child; in most families,
the woman is the primary person to fulfill that role.

To tell a child who is the result of third-party reproduction or
adoption that some other woman is his or her "real" or biologic
mother, one whom the child has not met, is confusing at best,
and possibly detrimental. In the view of many psychologists, a
child's real mother and real father are those people who mother
and father—that is, parent—that child. To imply they're not the
child's real mother or father is not only untrue, it's an insult.

Bright Idea

We need a less emotionally charged term than *birth mother*. Just like the person who donates an egg or sperm is called a donor, the person who is pregnant with the child and gives birth could be called a *bearer, birther, birth person,* or some other term.

Unfortunately, these terms and labels can lead to or reinforce the rejection many of these children may feel and face. These children must sometimes deal with the fact that outsiders consider the people whom they're closest to, the people who raised them, not their real parents.

Donor or interloper?

Some couples fear that a donor will be an intrusion—emotionally, psychologically, or even legally—on themselves and their relationships. A big barrier to using sperm donors, for example, is the impact on both the male and female partners' self image and self-esteem, as well as their relationship. As we've mentioned before, men tend to equate fertility with virility. It's easy to understand, then, why some infertile men feel that resorting to a donor is unmanly. It poses a threat to some and can have a devastating effect on their egos. To some, the thought of another man's sperm getting their wives pregnant is totally unacceptable. They may feel that their partners are being unfaithful. Others feel their wives have been raped or assaulted.

A woman might also have difficulty accepting the idea of donor sperm. Some may feel that using donor sperm conveys unintentionally to their partners that they don't love them. They might see it as betraying their partners, or even as a form of adultery. After the experience, some women have also described feeling as though they were violated, or raped.

Using donor eggs can produce similar reactions in both partners. Men, too, might unconsciously feel betrayed by their wives. On the other hand, a man who encourages his partner to use donor eggs might give off the message that he doesn't really care about her as a person, but only as a mechanism to produce a baby. A woman may feel she's a failure if she doesn't have eggs. And, because largely older women are using donor eggs, some women may feel they're getting "old and decrepit."

Using a surrogate or gestational carrier can confound these feelings. Seeing another woman clearly pregnant from her partner's sperm can devastate an infertile woman's self-image. She may see herself as less feminine and less desirable. She may even see the surrogate as a threat to her relationship with her partner. Certainly, many couples—whether fertile or infertile—often fantasize about what it would be like when the woman is pregnant. A surrogate or gestational carrier can indeed be a big intrusion on that private dream.

Some doctors mix the donor's sperm with the male partner's on the off chance that the child will be genetically his. Some consider this practice psychologically questionable. It might indicate that the couple—or at least the male partner—doesn't fully accept sperm donation. On the other hand, others feel that it's just a little wishful thinking, so what's the harm. Again, this is a decision that should be made by the couple with the help of a qualified infertility counselor.

In her book *In Pursuit of Pregnancy* (see Appendix B), co-author Joan Liebmann-Smith, Ph.D., describes the experiences of a couple, Eric and Lisa, who decided to use donor sperm. Says Eric about what happened when he was with Lisa while she was being inseminated with donor sperm: "I started to cry. I had a very difficult time with the thought of somebody going into my wife's body who wasn't me. That was my macho part again—I wasn't able to make Lisa pregnant, so I felt like a failure. But I was also crying about all that energy that went into this—a year and a half's worth...and here I was in the room holding my wife, and she was trying to get pregnant and it wasn't by me! I really felt the loss right there."

Lisa also had trouble with the concept of accepting sperm from a man other than her husband: "A few days before the insemination, I absolutely freaked. The idea of foreign sperm was so disgusting. I screamed at Eric, 'How could you want me to do this?' Then I found out when I went to our support group that this feeling passes. I began to think of the donor sperm as medicine, and it clicked. I said, 'OK. If it's medicine, it's all right.'"

Lisa became pregnant after her first attempt with donor sperm. Both she and Eric were ecstatic. Said Eric about their experiences with infertility and donor insemination, "When someone pulled the cord on me and put up a roadblock and said, 'Stop! You can't do that!' we found alternatives. Taking those choices along the road and getting to where we are now has made me feel this amazing closeness to Lisa. This child who isn't even born yet has brought us a whole lot closer than we ever were. It's really a commitment to a relationship. It's really a commitment to life."

Family matters

Some couples find resistance when they discuss third-party reproduction options with relatives. The potential grandparents may feel they'll be cheated out of a "real" grandchild—one genetically linked to them. They may wonder about the future grandchild's genetic well-being. Fearing family objections, many couples don't discuss their decisions with family, at least at first.

Keep in mind that a genetic connection can be a mixed blessing. You have to accept the good with the bad. Many people are under the false assumption that they will only pass on their good genes, and never consider that their offspring may look and act more like their weird Uncle Harry than their beloved Grandpa Fred. Most families are plagued by some genetic conditions that may rarely be discussed—or even thought about—when pursing

 Watch Out!

Some religions do not allow the use of donated sperm. If you think your religion forbids or frowns upon a particular aspect of third-party reproduction, talk to your religious leader and your doctor. There are often ways to adhere to your religious principles and still use these methods.

pregnancy. These can range from such genetically linked disorders as heart disease and various cancers to manic depression and schizophrenia.

For some couples and their families, passing along genes also means passing along the family religion. Some religions, such as Judaism, hold that the child's religion is passed to them from their genetic mother.

Legal considerations

The legal concerns surrounding third-party reproduction are considerable—well beyond the scope of this *Unofficial Guide*. It's best to consult legal counsel to learn the laws governing various types of donor use. (See Appendix C for resources for obtaining information on the legal issues related to third-party reproduction.)

Even with artificial insemination with donor sperm (known as DI or TDI)—the oldest and most widely used form of third-party reproduction—both you and your partner must sign a consent form before the procedure is performed. This consent usually waives your rights to learn the donor's identity. It states your responsibility to care for and support a child who may result from the procedure. In other types of third-party reproduction, it gets even more complicated and confusing. For example, some states forbid paying for eggs or embryos.

You'll need legal counseling to enter into traditional surrogacy, gestational carrier, and egg donation contracts, as well as finalizing parental rights. Indeed, in some types of third-party reproduction you must actually adopt the child. Laws are being written on these matters almost daily, so you must check.

You'll also need to look into what identifying and medical information is available to you, your child, and the donor(s), as well as when and how that information might be accessed. All these matters become even more critical if you know the donor. The bottom line is that even if you think you know the laws in your state, always check with a lawyer familiar with these ever-evolving issues. It's essential that the lawyer be knowledgeable and experienced in this highly complex area of family law and

Moneysaver

Choosing a relative as a donor can save you considerable money as well as provide you with some genetic connection to the child. However, be aware that if you choose a brother or sister as a donor, you may have to deal with sibling rivalry and other unresolved family issues.

reproductive medicine *in your state*. For example, some states accept some types of surrogacy, others don't. In fact, the practice is criminal in some states. Some states don't have any specific laws regarding surrogacy, which leaves you open to all sorts of difficulties down the road. Some states don't enforce laws they already have, which can also be a problem.

When contemplating third-party reproduction, not only do you need to seek legal counseling, but psychological counseling as well by a well-trained professional who, ideally, specializes in these issues. (Chapter 16 has advice on finding mental health professionals.) A lawyer will help you navigate the complex legal systems, while a mental health professional will help you deal with the inevitable psychological and interpersonal issues associated with third-party reproduction.

To know or not to know

One of the most important considerations in deciding to use a donor is whether you want to know the donor and whether you want the donor to know you. Like everything in third-party reproduction, the options are many. Here are just a few:

- **Anonymous donation** (also referred to as *total anonymity* or *closed donation*): You don't know the donor; the donor doesn't know you. For decades, this is the way it's been in the majority of donor sperm uses. You get a profile of the donor, maybe a photograph, but little more.

- **Partial anonymity:** You don't know who the donor is; the donor doesn't know you. But you have limited contact, like speaking on the telephone or by e-mail. This is an option sometimes used when choosing an egg donor to help you feel more comfortable in your choice because you have some (albeit limited) knowledge of the donor.

▪ **Limited anonymity:** In some cases, limited information about the donor is provided, and you both might meet each other. However, no identifying information is exchanged.

▪ **Open:** You both meet and know about each other. This is the situation when arranging traditional surrogacy or for a gestational carrier. It's sometimes the arrangement that happens with egg donation.

▪ **Known:** This is the situation when the donor is someone you already know, such as a family member or friend.

Each option has its pros and cons. In any type of third-party reproduction, you'll get—at the very minimum—a profile of the donor. It will describe the donor's medical history, as well as physical and intellectual characteristics. If you get to talk to or meet the donor you can assess these attributes and qualifications yourself. Of course, no matter whether the donor is well known to you or anonymous, he or she can have financial rather than altruistic motives.

When you know the donor

Dealing with a known donor can be complex. The more difficult aspects—emotional, as well as legal—of third-party reproduction come into play when the party doing the donating is contributing more than impersonal sperm and eggs. The issues may become a little more complicated when an infertile couple who has undergone IVF offers one of their extra frozen embryos to another infertile couple. Moreover, when a woman offers her uterus to carry a child intended for you, the decision, the process, and its ramifications become highly complicated.

While knowing or choosing a friend or relative to be a donor may bring the parties involved closer, it can also cause problems. There can be disputes over childrearing, contact with the child, and even custody. If the donor remains totally anonymous,

Bright Idea

Some donor programs require donors to be married or in stable relationships. If your donor is in an ongoing personal relationship, it's important to know how his or her partner feels about the process to avoid conflict. It's important that the donor's partner—as well as the donor—be psychologically evaluated and counseled.

there's little fear of donor interference in your and your child's lives. After all, you may choose third-party reproduction, but you probably don't want third-party parenting.

There's growing concern over how donors will react after their donation. In the decades since donor sperm has been in use, little attention has been given to the long-term effect of sperm donation on the donor. However, today the increasing use of donor eggs is bringing attention to the social and psychological effects of donation on the donor. Some women who at first felt altruistic about their egg donations have later expressed regret. They feel that they've somehow abandoned their child, or potential child. Because many egg donors have had other children, they sometimes express sorrow at having given up a sibling of their other children.

If you're thinking about using donor sperm or eggs, this is something you and your partner should talk about as well. After all, your child may indeed have half-brothers and half-sisters who he or she might later want to know. This need to know might be fueled if a medical situation arises in which a matched organ donor is needed. Then, of course, there is also the issue of a donor's "children" inadvertently meeting, marrying, and mating one day.

A recent survey of about a dozen women who served as surrogates found they had no regrets about their decisions a decade or more later. But many were disappointed that they weren't able to maintain contact with the infertile couple and child—although they had agreed not to. Some felt betrayed that contact had been abruptly severed either right after the births

Watch Out!

You and your surrogate may disagree on key issues. Be certain to discuss with a prospective surrogate ahead of time your views on amniocentesis and how you feel about pregnancy termination or fetal reduction.

or later. Some women in the survey did, however, maintain consistent or occasional contact with the families.

If a known donor is used, all parties must agree going into the process what their future relationships with the child will be. But even if all agree initially, keeping the circumstances surrounding the conception secret depends on the donor's discretion. Certainly, the donor's psychological, social, and even fertility status might change and affect a previously agreed-upon plan. (It's best to have all agreements in writing and drawn up by a lawyer.)

To tell or not to tell

Ultimately, all couples choosing a third-party reproduction method face two important decisions: what to tell their family and friends, and what to tell their child. With the emergence of the use of donor embryos, in which neither partner is genetically related to the child, these decisions become more complicated.

Many couples conceive babies through donors without anyone except their doctors knowing it. They decide that more harm than good can come from telling family or friends. And it really is nobody's business except the child's.

For many couples whose children were conceived through third-party reproduction, being faced with the inevitable question "Where did I come from?" takes on an entirely new dimension. As society becomes more conscious of family history, these questions also take on expanded meaning. There is considerable evidence that it's best to tell children of donors about their genetic fathers and mothers when they're old enough to understand. Most therapists who specialize in infertility believe that family secrets are always bad and can backfire. Secrecy, many psychologists believe, can only lead to shame.

When a child is born from a donated embryo or through the use of a surrogate or gestational carrier, the issues can become more complicated—and more difficult to explain to a child—as more people are involved in making a baby and more closely involved with an actual child.

Deciding who, what, and when to tell must be left ultimately to the couple. Joining a support group and/or seeking counseling from someone who specializes in the unique social and psychological issues surrounding third-party reproduction is imperative. After grappling with these issues most couples do come to a satisfactory decision.

The adoption option

If you decide not to use a donor or surrogate—or you have used a third-party solution unsuccessfully—you may want to consider another form of third-party reproduction: adoption. It's usually not something you even want to think about initially, but after months or years of not conceiving, adoption usually becomes a real alternative to consider. Often, one partner comes to this conclusion before the other, and more often than not, it's the female partner. This is bound to cause considerable conflict in the marriage, as we discuss in Chapter 14. Indeed, adoption is perhaps the most emotionally charged issue infertile couples face.

Losing the chance to have a genetic connection to a child is very difficult for most couples to accept. Most look forward to having children that resemble themselves and their families. Many unrealistically think of children as a way of passing on positive family traits, as well as the family name. What they tend to forget about are all those skeletons in the family closet.

 Bright Idea

If you're thinking of private adoption, send a letter or e-mail about your quest for a baby to everyone in your address book, and ask them to forward it on to all their acquaintances. If you can, include a loving photo of you and your partner. Be sure to include all doctors and lawyers you know; they often have the inside line to potential babies up for adoption.

When considering adoption, it's a good idea to discuss with your partner how each of you feels about having—or not having—a genetic connection to a child. Reread the section earlier in this chapter about passing on genes. You should ask yourselves, "Could we love a child not related to us?" If the answer is "Yes!" or "Maybe," it may be time to start looking more seriously at the adoption option. If the answer is "No," adoption is not right for you—at least, not at this point.

As we mentioned, women are usually more open to adoption—as well as the other third-party solutions—than men are. Indeed, they often contemplate the possibility of adoption well before their partners even consider it a viable option. One reason: Because women undergoing infertility treatment usually go through more both physically and emotionally than men, it might be somewhat easier for them to give up the idea of having a biological child.

Opposition to adoption

The decision to adopt is a very personal one, and it's not for everybody. If you or your partner feel strongly that adoption is not for you, it's better to realize it sooner rather than later. Some men—and women—are adamantly opposed to adoption from the get-go, and refuse to even discuss the issue. Some people are opposed to adoption because they can't be guaranteed a "normal," healthy child.

> **❝** After about six months [of fertility treatment], adoption shifted to something one could possibly do while still trying to get pregnant. Then, when I decided it wasn't worth trying to conceive any more, adoption became the *only* option. **❞**
>
> —Carol, 31

Most of us assume that we'll produce healthy, beautiful, intelligent children. But keep in mind, none of us can be assured any of those traits—much less a "perfect" child—even if we undergo preconception genetic testing and amniocentesis. Not every genetic, medical, or physical defect—not to mention psychological problems—can be screened for prenatally. And, there is absolutely no guarantee that your or your partner's best family traits will be passed on to your offspring, and that the worst ones won't be.

But it's not just concern about adopted children that prevents some from wanting to adopt. For those men who see infertility as a reflection on their masculinity, adoption is extremely stigmatizing—perhaps even more so than the use of donor sperm, which is typically and easily kept secret. On the other hand, for some men, adoption is proof positive to the outside world that they could not get their wives pregnant. Once they adopt, they can no longer pretend that they are childless by choice.

Adoption also represents giving up to some couples. But remember, adoption is really just an alternative way of building a family. And if you do decide to start pursuing adoption, remember that this decision is not written in stone—at least, not yet. Unlike pregnancy, you always have the option of changing your mind until you actually have a baby in your arms and all the legal papers are signed. Of course, until the papers are signed the pregnant woman can also change her mind. But most of the time things work out, and most couples who do adopt are thrilled with their decision; after all, they get to become parents of a longed-for child.

Misconceptions about adoption

If you're still undecided about adoption, you and your partner might try writing down what each of you sees as the pros and cons of adoption. Then compare notes. It may also help to look at two of the common myths about adoption:

- **As soon as I adopt, I'll get pregnant.** This is one of the most persistent—and annoying—myths about adoption. Adoption guarantees you a baby, not a pregnancy. Studies, in fact, have shown that the number of infertile women who conceive after adoption is the same as the number who pursue other options. One reason the myth persists is that you're unlikely to hear anecdotes about someone's friend who adopts and doesn't get pregnant—it doesn't make very interesting cocktail party conversation. So if you're considering adopting because you think it may lead to a pregnancy, you're probably adopting for the wrong reasons *and* setting yourself up for disappointment.

▪ **There are no healthy newborns of my own race available for adoption.** This is also untrue. There are many healthy newborns of all races available through agencies, private adoption, and foreign adoption. You'll find more information about these sources of adoption in Appendix C.

Further considerations

Deciding to adopt is just the beginning of the decision-making process. Here are some other adoption-related issues you may confront:

▪ Should you adopt through an agency or pursue private adoption?

▪ Should you look into foreign adoption? If so, which countries?

▪ Should you adopt a child of another race?

▪ Should you adopt an infant or an older child?

▪ Should you adopt a handicapped child?

▪ Should you have a closed adoption or an open one in which you meet the woman who gives birth to your child?

 Bright Idea

If you're considering adoption, work with a lawyer who specializes in adoption. Adoption lawyers are not only the most qualified to help you with adoption, but also because they're on the front lines, they often hear about pregnant women who need to put their babies up for adoption.

- If you do have an open adoption, should you have an ongoing relationship with the woman who gives birth? Should you allow your child to have an ongoing relationship with her?

Like infertility treatment, you need to take control of the situation and learn all you can about your various options. It will take time, effort, and a lot of research. But the payoff is finally having your longed-for child. In fact, most couples can find the type of child they want to adopt within a few years, at most.

While adoption isn't a cure for infertility, it's certainly a cure for childlessness and the pain it causes. Adoption helps you put infertility behind you while opening up a whole new world of parenthood, as this woman happily discovered:

"I really feel better at this point having stopped (infertility treatments), because we really feel we've done all we could do. Just this last week I began to have hope for the future. I'm forgetting the names of the fertility drugs. I don't know—or care—what day of the month it is. I used to

> **❝**I walk around feeling blessed. I have a feeling that if there is a God, He said, 'Make these people infertile, because they deserve a special child and I have a special kid in reserve for them.' And that special kid is our daughter, Lili.**❞**
>
> —Roy, adoptive father

know everything so well. I'm sure that's because we're so close to adoption—it's like something else to put our minds to.

I feel like I'm playing house, but I'm thrilled. I've been collecting cradles and rockers and little baths and I've been knitting little baby things. And I don't even know when the baby is going to arrive. It could be next month. It could be the summer. It could be the fall. But now I feel it's legitimate and reasonable to make plans, because we're going to have a baby!"

Just the facts

- Third-party reproduction options include donor sperm, eggs, embryos, and uteri, as well as surrogacy and adoption.

- You can build a family by having a child who is only partially—or even not at all—genetically related to you or your partner.

- The laws regarding third-party reproduction vary tremendously from state to state; be sure to work with a lawyer who is well versed in this area.

- Most experts agree that children of third-party reproduction should be told the truth about their origins, but the decision to tell others is strictly up to you and your partner.

- Women usually consider adoption before men do.

GET THE SCOOP ON...
Sperm, egg, and embryo donation ▪ Surrogates
and gestational carriers ▪ Choosing a program ▪
Screening donors and surrogates ▪ Some
important questions to ask

Pursuing Third-Party Reproduction

Chapter 12

In the previous chapter, we looked at the various third-party reproduction options available and how up to five people can be involved in "making a baby." What these various options entail can be confusing, to say the least. In this chapter, we'll clarify what specifically is involved in the various third-party reproduction options, as well as how to go about pursing them.

In the following scenarios we will illustrate how each of these third-party reproductive technologies may help you, and discuss some of the problems that might arise.

Sperm donation

Sperm donation was the first and still is the most commonly used third-party reproduction method. It's been an option for thousands of couples over the last six decades. Couples choose sperm donation in a variety of circumstances, but in every case, the problem is that the male partner can't contribute useable sperm. The following are the major indications for using donor sperm. The male partner has:

- No sperm, a low sperm count, or poor-quality sperm
- A nonreversible vasectomy
- A serious genetic disorder or is a carrier of one
- Undergone unsuccessful sperm aspiration
- Undergone unsuccessful intracytoplasmic sperm injection (ICSI)
- Long-standing unexplained infertility

Sperm donation typically involves three participants: the sperm donor and the infertile couple. Single straight and gay women—as well as lesbian couples—are increasingly using donor sperm to achieve a pregnancy.

Scenario #1: John and Mary have been trying to conceive for three years. But John has severe male-factor infertility due to an ejaculatory duct obstruction from a past infection. He has undergone surgery and sperm aspiration, and Mary has undergone artificial insemination with John's sperm, as well as in-vitro fertilization (IVF) with ICSI—all to no avail. John and Mary opt to use John's brother, Don, as a sperm donor.

Scenario #2: Henry and Sally want children, but both Henry's aunt and brother died in their 40s from Huntington's disease, a rare, hereditary, degenerative disease that the couple didn't want to risk passing along to their child. Because Henry has a 50 percent chance of passing the gene for Huntington's disease on to his offspring, he and Sally decide to use anonymous donor sperm.

What to Expect: Donor sperm insemination is very similar to artificial insemination with a husband's sperm, with a few exceptions. The donor's sperm must be collected and frozen for at least six months to allow the donor to be retested for communicable and deadly diseases. Donor inseminations are typically performed via *intrauterine insemination (IUI)*, which increases the chance of success. They can also be used as part of an ART procedure.

The Pros:

- You pass along the female partner's genetic makeup to your child.

- The female partner has the chance to experience pregnancy and childbirth and the male partner has the opportunity to share in it.

- Even if you use an anonymous donor, you can usually pick some characteristics, like hair or eye color, with the hope that the child will look more like the both of you.

- It's one of the least invasive and safest solutions to male-factor infertility.

- It's not very expensive unless done as part of an ART procedure.

- Unless you tell, no one will know you've taken this route to conception.

The Cons:

- Your child gets half of his or her genes from someone other than the male partner.

- If you don't know the donor, you don't really know their complete medical and family histories.

- There's always a remote risk of infection, even if the donor and his sperm are carefully screened.

- As we mentioned in the previous chapter, using donor sperm can create conflicts in your relationship with your partner.

- If a known sperm donor is used, there's a risk that the donor will be overly involved with the pregnancy and the child.

Egg donation

As with sperm donation, the reasons for a couple to use an egg donor can vary, but they all share a fundamental cause: The female partner can't contribute eggs. Some of the reasons are that she:

- Has no ovaries or eggs
- Doesn't ovulate
- Is too old to have any healthy, fertilizable eggs
- Has or carries a serious genetic disease she doesn't want to pass on to her offspring
- Has had unsuccessful ART treatments
- Has long-standing unexplained infertility

Using donor eggs is another example in which three people are involved in "making a baby": the woman who donates the eggs and the infertile couple who receives them. For many couples, donor eggs have replaced the use of surrogate mothers.

Scenario #1: Although Sophia is only 31, she suffers from premature ovarian failure and no longer produces eggs. She is otherwise healthy and wants to experience pregnancy and childbirth, so she and her husband, Anthony, decide to ask her sister, Donna, to be an egg donor. Donna—who has three children of her own—readily agrees.

Scenario #2: Ellen married Steve when she was in her early 40s. Although Steve has children from a previous marriage, they would like to have children together. Ellen, who still gets her period, had tried several fertility drugs to no avail. Because her eggs are apparently no longer fertilizable, they decide to undergo IVF using eggs donated anonymously.

What to Expect: Eggs, which have been donated either anonymously or by a known donor, are fertilized through ART. The donor usually receives fertility drugs to increase the number of eggs she produces and the recipient usually receives hormones to prime her uterus for embryo implantation. The use of fertility drugs is also important to coordinate timing of the two procedures. Any extra embryos produced may be frozen for future transfer attempts or possible donation to other infertile couples.

Donor eggs are quite successful because they usually come from healthy young women who are likely to have healthy young eggs. In fact, donor egg success rates are about the same or better for older women as ART is for younger women.

The Pros:

- Your child is genetically related to the male partner.

- The female partner experiences pregnancy and childbirth.

- It allows older and even postmenopausal women to have children.

- Extra embryos may be frozen for future transfer attempts.

- If both the fresh and the frozen embryo transfers are successful, the children will be siblings genetically.

- No one needs to know you used an egg donor unless you tell them.

The Cons:

- Both the egg donor and recipient must take hormones to synchronize the egg donor's ovulation with the recipient's ability to implant an embryo. (Of course, if frozen embryos are used, timing needn't coincide.)

- This is a costly option. If an anonymous donor is used, there are the costs of screening and matching the donor with you. Then there's compensation to the donor for her time and inconvenience. (Human eggs can't be sold in this country, but women do receive money for participation in the program and to pay for their expenses.)

- Because egg donation involves ART procedures, there are those expenses—and risks—as well.

- There are legal fees and issues.

- If a known donor is used, there's a risk that the donor will be overly involved with the pregnancy and the child.

Moneysaver

Consider freezing any good quality embryos produced from donated eggs—or your own. This will reduce the cost of another round of fertility drugs and egg retrieval costs.

Embryo donation (and sperm/egg donation)

Embryo donation is another fairly recent development that has only been possible since the availability of IVF programs and cryopreservation. It's one of the few options available for those couples who cannot use their own sperm or eggs—because of severe male- or female-factor infertility or genetic reasons—but still want to experience a pregnancy. It's also an option for couples who may have good quality sperm and fertilizable eggs, but still cannot produce a viable embryo.

Embryo donation involves four people: the three who are biologically involved—the sperm donor, the egg donor, and the female partner who carries the baby—and the male partner, who will be socially, emotionally, and financially involved as the future father. Others use embryos donated by other infertile couples. These are usually couples who have undergone ART, frozen their excess embryos, had a successful pregnancy, and decided to donate the frozen embryos to another couple. Sometimes couples find their own egg and sperm donors who don't know each other. This is often referred to as sperm/egg donation.

Scenario #1: Both Debbie and Ben have fertility problems. She is 42 and has an elevated FSH, which indicates a diminished capacity to produce eggs. He has severe male-factor infertility. They do, however, want to experience pregnancy and childbirth, so they opt to use donated embryos.

Scenario #2: Joshua and Hannah are both 28 and have no apparent fertility problem. However, they both are carriers of the Tay-Sachs gene, and there is a high probability that their biological child would inherit the deadly disease. Because abortion is out of the question for religious reasons, they decide not to risk having their own child. Their ART program has a frozen embryo available from an infertile Jewish couple who are not Tay-Sachs carriers.

Scenario #3: Karen and John are both 40. John underwent treatment for testicular cancer when he was 30, didn't bank any sperm before therapy, and is now sterile. Karen no longer ovulates. They want to experience pregnancy and childbirth, but decide against using a donor embryo. They reason: "We don't want our child to have half-brothers or half-sisters he or she doesn't know. And, besides, it's risky. What if the half-siblings want our child to know them and track us down? And, if something happens to our child, would they try to gain custody of him or her?" Although what they feared rarely happens with donor embryos, Karen and John chose an anonymous sperm donor and an anonymous egg donor.

> 66 The thing that is really important is to raise a child. It isn't the most important thing that the child be physiologically mine. In fact, I've been thinking of some of the advantages for it not to be mine—I wouldn't be responsible for its defects. 99
>
> —James, 29

What to Expect: The recipient will be the only one to undergo a medical procedure. The egg donor will go through an IVF cycle. She must take hormones in advance to prepare her uterus for embryo transfer.

The Pros of Embryo Donation:

- The female partner experiences pregnancy and childbirth.
- Donation costs may not be very high because you won't have to pay the medical and other expenses of finding a sperm and egg donor.
- The program will have extensive medical data on the couple who donated the embryo.

The Pros of Egg/Sperm Donation:

- The female partner experiences pregnancy and childbirth.

- You eliminate the possibility that an infertile couple who no longer has a need for their embryos has second thoughts.

- Any extra embryos produced can be frozen for your use in future transfer attempts.

- If you do have a baby from donor eggs and sperm, and become pregnant with the leftover frozen embryos, the siblings will genetically be full brothers or sisters.

The Cons of Both:

- You and your partner are not genetically related to the child (unless one of the donors is a relative).

- You'll have to take strong hormones to help prepare your uterus for embryo implantation, an ART procedure.

- It can be costly because of the hormones and egg retrieval.

- You'll need legal counseling because laws governing embryo donation—and sperm and egg donation—differ from state to state and you must have explicit prior approval from the donors to use the embryos.

Traditional surrogacy

The third-party options just discussed allow the infertile woman to become pregnant and give birth to the child, whether or not the child is genetically related to her. However, many infertile women either cannot become pregnant even with donor eggs or embryos or cannot hold a pregnancy long enough to carry it to term. One of the first and still most controversial third-party solutions for these women is traditional surrogacy. This option involves three people: the infertile couple and the woman who carries the fetus. The male partner is the biological father, and the surrogate—who carries the baby to term—is the biological mother. The female partner, who has no genetic connection to the child, becomes the legal mother.

Watch Out!

Make sure your surrogate signs an agreement not to have sex during the cycle you want her to conceive with your partner's or chosen donor's sperm. There is always the risk that a surrogate might have sexual intercourse and become pregnant by someone else.

This option is appropriate for women who do not have functioning ovaries or viable eggs, *and* who have uterine or other problems that prevent them from carrying a pregnancy to term.

Scenario #1: Desiree had premature ovarian failure when she was 28, which means she doesn't produce eggs. Her husband Antoine, 30, really wants a child who is genetically related to at least one of them. Since his sperm are fine, the doctor recommends surrogacy, which is legal in their state. Through an agency recommended by their doctor, they find a woman they both like who agrees to be a surrogate.

Scenario #2: George and Sally married in their mid-40s. Since Sally wasn't ovulating, they tried egg donation, but each embryo transfer ended in a miscarriage. When their physician suggests traditional surrogacy, they reject the idea of using a stranger, fearing getting embroiled in a custody battle. Instead, they ask Martha's younger sister, who already has three children, to be the surrogate, and she agrees.

What to Expect: The woman who agrees to be your surrogate will be inseminated with your partner's sperm, usually by intrauterine insemination (IUI). She may or may not be given fertility drugs. She will carry the baby to term and turn it over to you after childbirth.

The Pros:

- The child is genetically related to the male partner.
- If the surrogate is a blood relative of the female partner, the child is genetically related to her as well.

- This does not involve any particularly invasive or expensive medical procedures unless the surrogate needs to take fertility drugs.

- You can follow the surrogate's progress throughout the pregnancy.

The Cons:

- The female partner is not genetically or biologically related to the child unless the surrogate is related to her.

- It can be quite expensive because it involves locating a suitable surrogate and paying her legal fees and medical care.

- There is the possibility that the surrogate will bond with the child during pregnancy or childbirth and wish to keep him or her. A custody battle might ensue.

- Other complicated psychological and legal issues can be involved.

Gestational carriers

There are cases in which the male partner's sperm are healthy and the female partner can produce perfectly viable eggs but she cannot carry a pregnancy to term. In this situation, one option is to turn to a gestational carrier, which some prefer to call a donor or host uterus. This option is also sometimes used for unexplained infertility after failed attempts with conventional treatments and ART. There are three people involved in this option: the infertile couple and the woman who carries and delivers the child.

Scenario #1: When Jose, 25, asked Maria, 22, to marry him, she told him she could never have children because—even though she has ovaries—she was born without a uterus. Jose said he didn't care; they could always adopt. Around the time they were ready to have children, Maria saw a TV special about gestational carriers called "A Womb for Rent." She and Jose decide that this would be a great solution for them since by using her own eggs and Jose's sperm the child would be genetically theirs. Their doctor refers them to an agency that handles gestational carriers.

Scenario #2: When Lisa was 34, she became pregnant with her child, Christie. However, Lisa almost died because she developed a severe form of high blood pressure called *preclampsia,* suffered an uncontrollable hemorrhage, and had to have a hysterectomy. She and her husband, David, want Christie to have a brother or sister. They ask Lisa's favorite cousin, Laura, if she'd carry a baby for them. She says yes.

What to Expect: The female partner takes fertility drugs to produce multiple eggs, and then undergoes IVF to produce embryos. If there are any, extra embryos can be frozen for future attempts. The gestational carrier takes hormones to prepare her uterus for embryo implantation, and the embryos are then transferred to her uterus by IVF.

The Pros:

- The child has both the male and female partners' genetic makeup.

- You can follow the gestational carrier's progress throughout the pregnancy.

- You can freeze extra embryos that aren't transferred during IVF.

The Cons:

- There may be extensive and expensive legal counsel to handle the complicated issues involved.

- This is very expensive because both women take fertility drugs or hormones, and both undergo IVF.

- The IVF procedure and embryo transfer must be carefully synchronized. Both the female partner and the gestational carrier must be available in the same place at the same time.

 Bright Idea

If another woman has carried and delivered your child, you still may be able to breastfeed. La Leche League can help you learn how to produce at least some milk through manual stimulation of your breasts (see Appendix C).

Gestational carrier with sperm donation

This is similar to gestational carrier situations just discussed, except that in this case, because of severe male-factor infertility, a sperm donor is needed to create the embryo that is implanted in the gestational carrier's uterus.

Gestational carrier with egg donation

When the female partner cannot contribute eggs or use of her uterus, but her partner has good quality sperm, the couple can use a gestational carrier who becomes pregnant with a donor egg. This is an offshoot of traditional surrogacy and a pairing of two third-party reproduction methods.

Scenario #1: John and Mary are anxious to start a family, especially since Mary has just successfully been treated for uterine cancer. Unfortunately, the treatment involved removing ovaries along with her uterus. Mary's best friend, Gerry, offers to carry the child for them as a gestational carrier. But because Gerry is 42, everyone agrees it would be too risky to use her eggs. They decide to use an anonymous egg donor, since they all feel that would be less complicated than involving another friend.

Scenario #2: Paul and Karen are in their mid-30s and have been trying to have a baby for 5 years. Karen's had three miscarriages, all occurring during her second trimester. They don't want to risk another miscarriage and aren't sure if there's a genetic component to her miscarriage. Her doctor suggests using a gestational carrier. They'd like their child to be as closely related to them as possible, so they decide to use eggs donated by her sister, Ellen. Because Ellen doesn't wish to go

 Moneysaver

When you're figuring out the costs of third-party reproduction, don't forget to factor in any travel costs for the donor, surrogate, or gestational carrier.

through a pregnancy and childbirth—she has twin toddlers of her own—they go to a surrogacy center and find a gestational carrier.

In the first scenario, instead of Gerry being inseminated with John's sperm and carrying the fetus to term, eggs from an anonymous donor, Ann, are used. In Paul and Karen's case, they chose a family member as the donor, but still turn to an agency for their gestational carrier. In either case, this option involves four people: the infertile couple, the woman who donates the eggs, and the woman who carries the fetus.

What to Expect: This is similar to a gestational carrier, except an egg donor rather than the female partner takes the fertility drugs and undergoes IVF. As in the previous options, the gestational carrier must take hormones to prepare her uterus to accept an embryo transfer. The egg donor goes through a full IVF cycle.

The Pros:

▪ The child is genetically related to the male partner.

▪ If the donor is a blood relative of the female partner, the child will be genetically related to her as well.

▪ You can follow the gestational carrier's progress throughout the pregnancy.

The Cons:

▪ This is very expensive not only because both women need fertility drugs or hormones and both must undergo part of an IVF cycle, but also because you must find and pay for the egg donor (if anonymous), as well as for the gestational carrier's medical and legal expenses.

▪ Because so many people are involved, the chances of medical, legal, and psychological complications are considerably increased.

Gestational carrier with sperm and egg donation

When an infertile couple cannot produce either viable eggs or sperm, or they have a genetic disorder they don't want to pass on to their offspring, they can opt for embryo donation. However, in some of these cases, the female partner doesn't have a functioning uterus, and cannot—or should not for medical reasons—carry a pregnancy to term. The solution that most couples would choose under these circumstances is the same one that's been used for centuries: adoption. However, some couples are not willing to go the adoption route and want to somehow be involved in a pregnancy. In those cases, they can use donated sperm to fertilize donated eggs via IVF, and then transfer the embryos to a gestational carrier.

Scenario #1: Bill and Jean are in their early 30s. Bill is a paraplegic and Jean had a total hysterectomy several years ago. They don't want to adopt because they want to have some input on the creation of their child. Neither electroejaculation stimulation nor sperm retrieval have yielded viable sperm. They carefully choose an anonymous sperm donor. Jean's sister is willing to be the gestational carrier, but she experiences infertility problems that are overcome using donor eggs. They find an anonymous egg donor.

Scenario #2: Andrew and Sandy have been trying to conceive for 10 years. They've exhausted all their options—including IVF, GIFT, ISCI, and even acupuncture and herbal medicine. Andrew's last sperm count indicated he was virtually sterile, and Sandy, who's in her late 40s and has diabetes, was told by her doctor that it would be too risky for her to become pregnant. They don't want to adopt because they are determined to have a genetic connection to their child. Andrew's brother offers to donate his sperm and Sandy's cousin says she will donate her eggs, but she doesn't want to go through a pregnancy. A local agency finds a gestational carrier for them.

Watch Out!

Regardless of your age, if you use an egg donor who is over 34 and you become pregnant, you should plan to have amniocentesis and/or other prenatal tests. Donors who are 35 and older are at increased risk of passing on a serious genetic disorder.

What to Expect: Virtually the same medical processes are involved as in the gestational carrier with egg and sperm options. The only difference is the egg and sperm come from donors rather than the infertile couple.

The Pros:

- You can pick each donor involved, including the sperm and egg donors and the gestational carrier.

- Having one or more of the donors related to you provides a genetic connection.

- Having one or more of the donors known to you provides an added bond to the experience.

The Cons:

- Unless a donor is related to you or your partner, the child will not have any genetic link to either of you.

- It's expensive because of all the medications for the egg donor and carrier, and the IVF procedures for both.

- It's also expensive because you must arrange for three types of donation—sperm, egg, and uterus—as well as for the services and care of the egg donor and gestational carrier.

- Because of the many people involved, coordination of the medical procedures may be very difficult.

- Because three donors are involved, the risk of legal complications is high.

- Because three donors are involved, psychological complications may be multiplied.

A summary of the options

If you're confused, it may help to review the third-party reproduction options currently available. The following table summarizes the various options and what needs to be contributed by the donor and/or the infertile couple.

Third-Party Option	What's Needed
Sperm donation	Donor's sperm, partner's egg, partner's uterus
Egg donation	Partner's sperm, donor's egg, partner's uterus
Embryo donation	Donor's sperm, donor's egg, partner's uterus
Traditional surrogacy	Partner's sperm, surrogate's egg, surrogate's uterus
Gestational carrier	Partner's sperm, partner's egg, surrogate's uterus
with sperm donation	Donor's sperm, partner's egg, surrogate uterus
with egg donation	Partner's sperm, donor's egg, surrogate's uterus
with egg and sperm donors	Donor's sperm, donor's egg, surrogate's uterus

Finding a program or agency

By now, you may have decided one of these options seems right for you. If so, the next step is to find the appropriate doctor and program to help you through the many medical, psychological, and legal steps involved in making the final decision and plans to use these approaches.

Many of the same principles we mentioned in Chapter 5 on finding a fertility specialist and in Chapter 10 on finding an ART program apply when looking into a third-party reproduction program. Your or your partner's fertility specialist is a good place to start. You can also contact the American Society for Reproductive Medicine (ASRM) and RESOLVE, the national organization for infertile couples. (See Appendix C for contact

Moneysaver

When choosing a donor or surrogacy program, check out various programs around the country on the Internet and request information packets from them. Then compare the prices and the services they offer.

information on these and other recourses for information about third-party reproduction.)

Ultimately, the program you choose depends on what your medical needs are, as well as what you're ready emotionally to pursue and what you can afford financially.

Third-party reproduction programs

For convenience, it helps to look at the third-party reproduction options as two broad categories: *donor gametes,* which are sperm, eggs, and embryos; and *surrogacy,* which includes traditional surrogacy (surrogate mothers) and gestational carriers. How much involvement you'll need from your fertility specialist, ART program, and/or donor or surrogacy agency depends on the third-party reproduction method you choose. Here's a brief rundown of the options:

- Sperm donations are used widely and can be handled routinely through many infertility specialists and centers. They might have their own sperm banks or have working relationships with one or more sperm banks. However, as we mentioned in the previous chapter, some couples prefer to use a relative or friend as a donor.

- Egg donations are handled medically through ART centers, which may or may not have a program in place to find a suitable donor for you. If they don't, finding an egg donor can be arranged through private agencies (see the following section). As with sperm donation, you may prefer to use a relative or friend who has agreed to donate her eggs.

- Embryo donations are only handled through ART programs. They have the frozen embryos on hand and they do the transfers. They should assist you and the donor in all the necessary medical and legal paperwork.

- Surrogacy—which can be more complicated because it may involve a combination of sperm, egg, or embryo donation—is typically handled by both ART and surrogacy programs. Some agencies are specially set up to match a surrogate or gestational carrier with an infertile couple. Some of these programs also provide services to find donor eggs. Even if you have a prospective surrogate in mind, these agencies can help with the legal paperwork.

Private agencies

There are private agencies working independently from ART programs that will assist infertile couples in many of the steps surrounding third-party reproduction—in particular, egg donation and surrogacy arrangements. While their services vary, they often can:

- Maintain donor lists
- Screen donors
- Act as intermediary between the donor and recipient
- Work with medical centers chosen by the donor or recipient
- Coordinate legal services for both the donor and recipient
- Arrange legal and medical appointments, travel arrangements, and disbursement of fees

The agency should be set up to help coordinate the medical aspects of the donation (psychological testing; screening; and arrangements for ovulation induction, egg retrieval, IVF, and embryo transfer), as well as draw up the legal contracts between you and the donor.

If you find a donor or surrogate on your own, you'll have to coordinate all medical and legal aspects involved. In addition, if you choose your own donor, you'll be having contact with him or her. Working through a private agency—though more expensive—covers many of these issues and allows the option of some anonymity—at least in the case of sperm and egg donations.

Screening and other guidelines

The ASRM has guidelines for gamete donation, including sperm, egg, and embryo. Be certain the donor sperm and egg clinic—whether physician based, hospital based, or commercial—is following ASRM guidelines for monitoring and testing donors. The American Association of Tissue Banks (AATB) has established standards for tissue banking, including tissues used in reproductive medicine. They inspect and accredit member tissue banks, similar to what's done for blood banks or clinical laboratories. Check that the tissue bank you or your program uses is accredited by the AATB.

> ❝We talked about having a child first by adoption or donor sperm and then worrying about whether I could father my own child at some future time.❞
> —Nick, 32

In accordance with federal and state regulations, all sperm and egg donors must be screened for genetic diseases, hepatitis B and C, sexually transmitted diseases (STDs), and HIV. (You can get a list of these tests from the ASRM or AATB.) Many banks also run other blood chemistry tests and tests for other genetic and infectious diseases. Many of these tests are based on an evaluation made by a clinical geneticist of a potential donor's risk of carrying medical and hereditary diseases. You probably want to make sure that all sperm donors are screened, for example, for cystic fibrosis carrier status. Other potential donors are screened, based on their genetic background, for breast and ovarian cancer (BRCA-1) gene mutations, Tay-Sachs disease, sickle cell anemia, and thalassemia. Depending on the test and the program, tests are done initially and then tests for infectious diseases are repeated every six months. Some programs retest more frequently.

Watch Out!

All third-party reproduction options involve important and potentially explosive pyschological and legal issues. They all require careful psychological and medical screening, as well as psychological and legal counseling.

HIV

Only frozen sperm that has been quarantined for at least six months can be donated through an anonymous program in this country. This allows donors to be retested for antibodies to HIV, the virus that causes AIDS, which may not develop or be detected for several months after a person's exposed to the virus.

In addition, some programs will perform more sophisticated HIV testing using *polymerase chain reaction (PCR)*. PCR can actually test for the virus inside cells months before HIV antibodies are seen in blood or semen. Testing potential donors with this method can eliminate donors before specimens are procured.

Because freezing eggs is ostensibly experimental, screening egg donors for HIV is a problem. While the risk of HIV transmission is low, it nonetheless exists. The program should be screening potential donors for disease before they are accepted. Once accepted and chosen to be a donor, they should be retested. But, as we mentioned before, it can take six months before HIV antibodies are detectable. There's no way to guarantee that the eggs retrieved today are from a donor who wasn't exposed to HIV last week.

In unusual cases, recipient couples decide to have the donor eggs retrieved, fertilized in an IVF procedure, and any embryos frozen. The donor can be retested six months later, and, if given a clean bill of health, the embryos are transferred. Remember, however, that frozen embryo transfers are not as successful as fresh ones.

Infectious diseases

ASRM guidelines require that donor embryos be quarantined for at least six months so that the potential donors can be tested for infectious diseases before the embryos are transferred to the recipients. However, in some situations donor testing may not be possible; for example, in a postmortem donation. (An infertile couple may have specified their willingness to have extra frozen embryos donated upon the death of either or both of them.)

Physical characteristics

Most of these programs will provide you with patient profiles that allow you to closely match the donor's physical characteristics (such as eye color, and hair color and texture), ethnic and racial background, and even occupation, special interests, and skills, with that of the male or female partner. To help you pick a sperm donor offering the best chance to have a child that resembles your family, some sperm banks allow you to submit your picture. The staff will rank the resemblance of the donor's with your photo and the characteristics you've outlined.

Important questions to ask

The decision to go with a gamete donor—or surrogate—should not be taken lightly. In addition to the previous considerations, you'll of course want to know what the donor program's success rate is and what the costs—and hidden costs—might be. (See Chapter 10 for more on interpreting success rates.) There are

---

 Bright Idea

A donor—even if he or she is a family member—should be retested for communicable diseases after six months. Such diseases as STDs, AIDS, and hepatitis may not be detectable in blood tests when first exposed. Don't assume because the donor is a relative you know his or her sexual history.

Watch Out!

It's not only the donor or surrogate who should be tested for HIV and other infectious diseases. The donor's or surrogate's partner as well as the recipient and his or her partner should also be tested.

also some other important questions you should ask a sperm or egg donor program:

- Do your donors have children themselves?
- Do you limit how many times a donor's sperm or eggs will be used? If so, how many?
- Are these limits confined to specific geographic areas or do they apply nationally?
- Do you limit how many stimulation cycles a donor undergoes? If so, how many?
- If a successful pregnancy ensues, can we use sperm or eggs from the same donor for another pregnancy?

The following are questions you should ask of programs or agencies that provide the services of surrogates or gestational carriers:

- How much experience does your center have working with surrogates and gestational carriers?
- Do you have specially trained counselors to work with the surrogates and/or carriers?
- Do you have a legal staff with contract experience?

If you're going to be using donated embryos, you should ask:

- What is your success rate using frozen embryos?
- Are the embryos you use the product of an infertile couple's eggs and sperm, or were the eggs and/or sperm donated by paid donors?
- What are the charges for embryo thawing, transfer, cycle coordination and documentation, and infectious disease screening of both recipients and donors?

As you unfortunately know by now, no infertility treatment is guaranteed to get you pregnant, no matter what its reputation among patients and doctors. So, it's important to know how a program handles things when events don't go as planned. You should ask:

- What are my costs and liabilities if no eggs are retrieved from the prospective donor?
- If eggs are retrieved, but we do not get pregnant, can we change donors?
- If so, how much will it cost?

If you use a surrogate or gestational carrier you'll have another series of questions, including:

- If the gestational carrier fails to get pregnant, what are our options?
- What are our financial and legal responsibilities?
- What happens if an amniocentesis test result comes out abnormal?
- Will the carrier have an abortion and, if so, who pays for it?
- Who is responsible if the child is born abnormal?
- Who will raise and care for the child?

If none of these third-reproduction options appeal to you, it may be time to reconsider adoption or even consider the possibility of choosing childfree living. Rereading the sections in the previous chapter on pregnancy and parenthood, and adoption may be helpful. Childfree living is discussed in Chapter 16.

 Moneysaver

Besides medical treatment, your partner and your donor and/or surrogate will need to undergo some psychological counseling, and you'll need help with legal documents. Going to a program that provides all these services can save you both time and money.

Whether or not you choose to turn to third-party reproductive options, you may be considering or curious about some of the alternative solutions, such as acupuncture and herbal remedies. In the following chapter, we look at some of these alternatives that seem promising, and some that don't.

Just the facts

- Although each has its pros and cons, sperm, egg, and embryo donations may be successful options for many infertile couples.

- Using surrogates and gestational carriers are options for women who cannot physically carry a pregnancy to term.

- Programs and agencies should provide psychological and legal counseling as well as their donor or surrogate services.

- Donors, surrogates, and gestational carriers must be periodically screened for HIV and other infectious diseases.

- Before pursuing third-party reproduction, there are many important questions you need to ask both the program and the donor or surrogate.

GET THE SCOOP ON...
Non-traditional vs. traditional treatments ▪
Vitamin therapy, herbal remedies, and other
natural treatments ▪ Considerations when
choosing a CAM provider

Complementary and Alternative Solutions

Chapter 13

Some of the newest approaches to infertility treatments have their roots in some of the oldest forms of medicine—ancient Eastern cultures dating back thousands of years. These nonconventional medical treatments are commonly referred to as *alternative medicine*. Alternative medicine usually refers to treatments used *in place of* conventional medicine. *Complementary medicine* and *integrative medicine* are the terms used by medical professionals to describe alternative treatments used *in conjunction with* conventional medicine. To simplify the issue, the term CAM (*complementary and alternative medicine*) is now being used by most health care practitioners and researchers.

Complementary and alternative medicine (CAM)

Whatever it's called, CAM is becoming recognized as a legitimate component in the management of many conditions, including infertility. Increasingly, researchers and doctors are realizing that alternative medicine is more than just aphrodisiacs and fertility statues. They are catching up with consumers in their acknowledgment of the potential benefits of CAM for many conditions. In very recent years, several medical publications, including the prestigious *Journal of the American Medical Association* (JAMA), have called for manuscripts on CAM, and in the late 1990s JAMA's editorial advisory board selected alternative medicine as one of the top three subjects for future journal issues.

A staggering number of Americans, an estimated 74 million people or 36 percent of adults in this country, are current users of CAM for various conditions. These figures don't include an additional 26 percent who use prayer for medical reasons, which is now considered a CAM. One in three people in the United States use CAM on a regular basis. In fact, more visits are made to CAM providers than primary care physicians! On the other hand, most CAM users do so in conjunction with conventional medical treatments. CAM users are spending an estimated $36 to $47 million a year on such treatments as acupuncture, chiropractics, homeopathy, herbs, or other therapies that fall under the CAM umbrella. Studies show those who are most likely to use CAM are women, people with higher education, those who have been hospitalized in the past year, and former smokers.

> 66 Infertility patients are a vulnerable group that often seek a non-medical solution for their failure to conceive.... CAM may be addressing a need that is not fully met by traditional medical practices. 99
>
> —Catherine Coulson and Julian Jenkins, *Journal of Experimental & Clinical Assisted Reproduction* (2005)

Spawned by thousands of anecdotal reports and a growing body of legitimate study results—and a Congressional mandate—the National Institutes of Health (NIH) established the U.S. Office of Alternative Medicine in 1992 to help formalize research on the use, safety, and effectiveness of a broad range of nonconventional therapies. Now called the *National Center for Complementary and Alternative Medicine (NCCAM)*, it has an annual budget of more than $40 million. NCCAM currently funds CAM research at 10 research centers across the country. More than 300 complementary and alternative medicine therapies have been documented in the United States, which NCCAM groups under these four domains:

- **Biologically based practices.** These involve the use of various substances found in nature. Included are the use of herbs, special diets, homeopathy, and mega vitamins.

- **Energy medicine.** This is the use of energy fields. This category includes acupuncture, light therapy, magnetic fields and biofields, electrostimulation, and electroacupuncture.

- **Manipulative and body-based practices.** These involve the movement or manipulation of various parts of the body. This category includes acupressure, chiropractics, osteopathy, massage therapy, Alexander technique, reflexology, and therapeutic touch.

- **Mind-body medicine.** This domain involves various techniques that attempt to enhance the mind's ability to affect bodily functions and relieve symptoms. These include stress management, hypnosis, imagery, tai chi, qi dong, yoga, and prayer for health reasons.

The most commonly used alternative medical treatments in this country (not counting prayer) are deep breathing, meditation, chiropractics, yoga, massage, special diets, and the use of natural products.

 Bright Idea

The Internet is an easily accessible, quick source of information about CAM. You might want to start with NIH's NCCAM website at http://altmed.od. nih.gov. They also have links to many other legitimate CAM Internet sites.

CAM and infertility

While there are no national statistics on how many infertility patients seek CAM treatments in the United States, if the national average holds true, at least one in three do. Surveys of infertile men and women in other countries also confirm that many use CAM as an adjunct to conventional infertility treatment. A survey in England published in 2005 found that almost 32 percent of infertile women used CAM. Most of the women used reflexology, acupuncture, or sought nutritional advice. Of those women who used CAM, 13 percent said it helped them psychologically and 33 percent said it helped them to relax, but only 10 percent thought it had been helpful for their infertility problems.

The survey also found that only about 13 percent of men used CAM, and most of those who did used herbs or sought nutritional advice or spiritual healing. However, a recent survey of infertile men in Canada found a higher CAM usage (31 percent). The majority of the men were taking antioxidant vitamins or minerals such as zinc, selenium, and vitamins C and E.

The American Society for Reproductive Medicine (ASRM) has published articles in their journal, *Fertility and Sterility*, on CAM practices such as acupuncture, yoga, and stress reduction; and RESOLVE offers fact sheets and other information on stress reduction, naturopathic medicine, and acupuncture. Other CAM practices that are popular among people with fertility problems are relaxation techniques, yoga, support groups, herbal medicine, and homeopathy. It's been estimated that there are over 100 different CAM treatments for infertility and miscarriages.

 Moneysaver

Check ahead of time to see if your insurance policy covers CAM visits. Increasing numbers of insurance companies are now paying for visits to CAM practitioners such as acupuncturists, homeopaths, naturopaths, and chiropractors.

Unfortunately, most of these treatments have not been adequately studied or evaluated.

In the following sections, we will briefly describe some of those CAM treatments used to treat infertility that have—at least to some extent—been evaluated or reported on in medical journals with regard to the treatment of infertility problems. We want to stress that the following is for informational purposes only, and we are not recommending any of these methods. While some practices—such as acupuncture—have proven safe for most people when properly done by trained professionals, others may not be, or may be counterindicated in your particular case. So if you are considering trying CAM, be sure to discuss it with your physician first. Be aware, however, that not all doctors are knowledgeable about or open to CAM. If this is the case with your doctor or he or she is opposed to CAM, you may want to consider having your CAM provider talk to your doctor. Or bring some literature on the CAM you're planning to use with you to your next appointment.

Acupuncture

Acupuncture is an ancient Chinese medical system that has been practiced for over 3,000 years in the East. Practitioners of Chinese medicine believe that disease disrupts the flow of healthy energy, called *qi* and pronounced "chee." Acupuncture is used to correct the imbalance of energy flow by stimulating acupuncture points on the body with very thin needles, heat (moxibustion), massage, electrical stimulation, and occasionally herbs.

Acupuncture became popular in the United States in the early 1970s among both consumers and physicians. According to the FDA, approximately one million Americans spent approximately $500 million on acupuncture each year. There are approximately 15,000 practicing acupuncturists in this country alone, and over 4,000 of them are physicians.

While acupuncture is most often thought of as a method of pain relief, it has many other applications, including the treatment of infertility. According to Chinese medicine, infertility

Watch Out!

Acupuncture needles can spread dangerous infections, including the HIV virus. Make sure your acupuncturist uses single-use disposable needles from sealed packages. This will reduce the risk of infection.

can be caused by such conditions as "deficient blood," "cold womb," and "weak kidney energy," and practitioners of Chinese medicine believe that acupuncture and herbs can successfully treat these conditions. A 1997 review article of CAM therapies published in *Obstetrical and Gynecological Survey* reported one study in which infertile women who had undergone acupuncture were found to be more likely to become pregnant and have fewer miscarriages than a control group. In another study, conducted in Israel and published the same year in the *Archives of Andrology*, acupuncture was found to improve sperm motility in subfertile men.

To find a physician trained in acupuncture, as well as more information on the subject, check out the website of the American Academy of Medical Acupuncture at www.medical acupuncture.org.

Vitamin and nutritional therapy

We all know vitamins and minerals are essential to maintaining good health. Research is increasingly being conducted on the preventive and curative effects of certain vitamins and minerals. For example, a study on sperm motility and vitamins in infertile men was conducted in Scotland. The results, which were published in the *British Journal of Urology* in 1998, found that supplements of selenium improved sperm motility in some subfertile men, and as a result, increased the chances of successful pregnancy in their partners. Selenium is found primarily in whole grains and eggs, and is also available as a supplement. Be careful: Doses greater than 200 mcg can be toxic.

Vitamins and minerals such as vitamin E, vitamin C, vitamin B_6, vitamin B_{12}, and zinc are purported to enhance fertility in both men and women. Zinc and vitamin B_6 have been reported to be especially useful for male infertility and impotence. Antioxidants in general are believed to protect sperm from toxic damage.

Some encouraging new research in Italy has found evidence that *carnitine*—an amino acid (the basic building block of protein)—may improve sperm maturation, motility, and count. Concentrated forms of carnitine are found in both the epididymis and sperm. The food sources of carnitine are primarily meats, especially mutton and lamb.

Certain foods such as soy products, flaxseeds, and yams contain natural estrogens. They have been used to treat menopause and may also prove to be a useful adjunct to the treatment of infertility.

The results of studies on many other vitamins, minerals, and other nutrients are just starting to come in, and not all have been tested. So claims of effectiveness should be taken with a grain of salt. And remember, just because something is "natural" doesn't mean that it's safe. Some natural products are extremely toxic in high—or even low—dosages.

Be sure to check with your fertility specialist before taking vitamins or minerals because they can interfere with other medications you're taking. It's a good idea to discuss the dosage as well.

Herbal medicine

Herbs and plant derivatives have been the basis for medical treatments for thousands of years. According to the Bible, Rachael, who poignantly lamented, "Give me children or else I die!" finally conceived after eating mandrakes, a root that is shaped like a man. (Mandrake roots are a member of the nightshade family and can be poisonous, so don't try this at home!)

About half the medications used in Western medicine are plant based. These include many of our most accepted, effective, and popular drugs such as aspirins, digitalis, cascara, and the taxanes, a group of anticancer drugs. These drugs are tried and true and have been through rigorous testing in animals and humans.

Many herbs have been purported to be beneficial for infertility and other conditions, but most have not yet gone through the necessary research trials to prove them safe and effective. But this is rapidly changing, with government funds being poured into evaluating the safety and effectiveness of these herbal remedies. Time—and testing—will tell. In the meantime, since definitive proof is still lacking for most, they should be used with caution. Because of potential adverse reactions, and because some herbs can interfere with other medications you might be taking, it's important to discuss any herbs you are planning to use with your doctor or fertility specialist first. The following are a sampling of herbs for infertility that have been tested to some extent and are purported to be helpful.

- **Ho shou wu,** a Chinese herb that is used to treat female infertility, has been demonstrated to be effective in animal studies.

- **Chasteberry or chaste tree** (*Vitex agnus catus*) has been shown to affect the secretion of progesterone and estrogen production and may help in correcting hormonal imbalances.

- **Dong quai** (*Angelica sinensis* or *Chinese Angelica*), another Chinese herb, is also known as the "queen of female herbs" and "female ginseng." Often used with other herbs, dong quai is said to balance and nourish the female reproductive system.

 Watch Out!

Some popular herbs can damage your reproductive cells or cause other adverse reactions. California researchers found that high doses of echinacea, ginkgo, and St. John's Wort had adverse effects on eggs, and St. John's Wort caused mutations in sperm cells.

Moneysaver

To avoid wasting your money on herbs and vitamins that may not work—or may even be counterproductive—check out the Mayo Clinic's website for information: www.mayoclinic.com/findinformation/druginformation/index.cfm.

- **False unicorn root** (*Chamaelirium luteum*) has one of the best reputations among herbalists for enhancing fertility, and is often used to treat ovarian dysfunction and prevent miscarriages. It has also been used to treat impotence.

- **True unicorn root** (*Alertris farinosa*) is another herb that has been said to help prevent miscarriages and impotence.

Homeopathy

Homeopathy was developed 200 years ago by Samuel Hahneman, a German physician and chemist. Homeopathy is a form of medicine that uses highly diluted doses of medicine usually derived from herbs, plants, and minerals to stimulate the body's own defense mechanisms to cure various disorders.

Most homeopaths in the United States are medical doctors who attend four years of regular medical school and then specialize in homeopathic medicine. Homeopathy is also popular with other licensed medical professionals, especially naturopaths, acupuncturists, chiropractors, physicians, nurses, dentists, and veterinarians. There are three recognized accredited schools of homeopathy that can train these health professionals in three- or four-year programs. However, not all homeopathic training programs require that the student have prior medical training. Several professional organizations certify or license homeopaths, who are referred to as Doctors of Homeopathy (D.O.H.).

Homeopathy claims to be useful in the treatment of endometriosis, and in helping to shrink both cysts and fibroids, although fibroids are said to take longer to treat. A recent pilot study in Germany found evidence that homeopathy might help

Bright Idea

For more information on the training and licensing of alternative medical professionals, check out the American Medical Student Association website at www.amsa.org/humed/camresources/alt.cfm.

improve sperm counts in infertile men. Homeopathic treatment for these conditions should be done through an M.D. or Doctor of Osteopathy (D.O.). The only professionals licensed to practice homeopathy in all 50 states are M.D.s and D.O.s. And self-treatment should be avoided.

Naturopathic medicine

If you're interested in pursing a CAM treatment for infertility but are not certain which one would be best, consider seeing a naturopathic doctor (N.D.). Naturopathic medicine, while having its roots in ancient medicine, was developed in the United States about 100 years ago by Benjamin Lust, a German physician immigrant. Naturopathic medicine focuses on prevention and treating the whole person through the healing power of nature. N.D.s use a wide variety of natural treatments including homeopathy, nutritional and vitamin therapy, acupuncture, ayurvedic (Indian) medicine, Native American medicine, herbal medicine, and stress management.

There are more than 1,000 licensed naturopathic physicians in this country. Only two schools in this country, however, are presently accredited: Bastyr University of Natural Health Sciences in Seattle, Washington; and National College of Naturopathic Medicine in Portland, Oregon. Bastyr is one of the research sites funded by NIH's Office of Alternative Medicine. N.D.s from accredited schools undergo four years of medical studies similar to what standard medical schools require.

About 70 insurance companies in the United States cover treatment by licensed naturopaths. At present, coverage for naturopathic medicine is mandatory in two states: Washington and Connecticut. (See Chapter 17 and Appendix E for more information on insurance coverage for infertility treatment.)

Licensing and certification

If possible, always consult a practitioner who is licensed, or at least certified. All 50 U.S. states license chiropractors; 35 states license massage therapists; 41 states license acupuncturists (acupuncturists who are medical doctors are automatically licensed); and 10 states license naturopathic practitioners. Ayurvedic medical practitioners in India have training requirements similar to those of an M.D. in the United States; however, there is no formal licensing or certification for ayurvedic medicine in this country.

Stress reduction

Since the 1960s when Harvard researchers found that relaxation techniques could lower blood pressure, the mind-body connection has been looked into with growing acceptance.

A 1998 study, for example, found that group therapy seemed to help improve the chance of pregnancy among a group of infertile women. Group therapy and support groups provide invaluable information, motivate members to make positive decisions about their treatment, and steer members toward the best doctors and most effective treatments. All of these factors, rather than the therapy per se, are likely to result in higher pregnancy rates.

As we have pointed out many times in this book, stress is often the result of infertility, but there is very little evidence that it is a significant causal factor in infertility. You can't just "relax and get pregnant," but relaxing certainly doesn't hurt—on the

 Watch Out!

Some people put N.D. after their names after completing a mail-order course in naturopathic medicine, but lack the necessary training to effectively and safely treat many conditions. Make sure you check out an N.D.'s credentials just as you would the credentials of any medical practitioner.

Alternative Medicine Acronyms
(for Licensed and Certified Professionals)

A.P.—Acupuncture Physician

B.A.M.S.—Bachelor of Ayurvedic Medicine and
        Surgery

C.A. (C.Ac.)—Certified Acupuncturist

C.A.M.T.—Certified Acupressure Massage Therapist

C.C.H.—Certified in Classical Homeopathy

C.H.—Certified Herbalist

C.Hom.—Certified in Homeopathy

C.M.T.—Certified Massage Therapist

C.P.H.T.—Certified Practitioner of Homeopathic
        Therapeutics

D.Ac.—Doctor of Acupuncture

D.C.—Doctor of Chiropractic

D.H.M.—Doctor of Homeopathic Medicine

D.O.—Doctor of Osteopathy

D.O.H.—Doctor of Homeopathy

D.O.M.—Doctor of Oriental Medicine

H.M.D.—Homeopathic Medical Doctor

L.Ac.—Licensed Acupuncturist

L.M.P.—Licensed Massage Practitioner

L.M.T.—Licensed Massage Therapist

L.N.—Licensed Nutritionist

L.N.C.—Licensed Nutritionist Counselor

M.Ac.—Masters of Acupuncture

M.H.—Master Herbalist

M.O.M.—Masters of Acupuncture and Oriental
        Medicine

N.D. (N.M.D.)—Naturopathic Doctor

O.M.D.—Oriental Medicine Doctor

R.Ac.—Registered Acupuncturist

R.Y.T.—Registered Yoga Teacher

contrary, it can help keep you fit to meet the physical and emotional challenges of infertility diagnosis and treatment. And relaxing may just help you do the things necessary to increase your chances of conceiving. Relieving stress can increase your desire to have and/or ability to have intercourse. It can also make it easier for you to undergo unpleasant and invasive tests and treatments such as hysterosalpingograms, laparoscopies, and IVF. When people are under less stress, they are more likely to remember to take their medication at the right time, and to have sex at the right time.

Stress reduction and relaxation techniques can also help you in your everyday life, going through a pregnancy or adoption, and dealing with a newborn, and later, toddler and teenager. And there certainly are no contraindications for or negative side effects from stress reduction. It can be used as an adjunct to any medical treatment, no matter what your diagnosis is.

> ❝Yoga and meditation can help women experiencing the challenges of infertility...meditation and relaxation can help increase the clarity of the mind, maintain healthy body chemistry, and give patients the patience to undergo the rigors of infertility treatments. ❞
>
> —H. K. Khalsa, *Fertility and Sterility* (2003)

Should you go the alternative route?

If you're considering trying one of the previous or some other CAM therapies, here are some things to keep in mind:

- Before starting CAM therapy, be sure to tell your doctor to ensure that it won't interfere with other nutritional supplements or medicines your doctor has prescribed.

- Find a CAM provider the same way you would any other medical provider—by taking the time to check out all your options and caregivers. Start by reviewing Chapter 5 on finding the right doctor.

■ Many people without specialized training and credentials claim to be experts in alternative medicine. Make certain you carefully check the credentials of any CAM practitioner you go to (see the Alternative and Complementary Medicine Resources in Appendix C).

■ As mentioned earlier, try to choose a licensed or certified CAM provider. Many practitioners of nonconventional medicine must be licensed and belong to professional organizations that set practice standards.

■ Find out where the practitioner trained and whether he or she completed the training program. Also find out what, if any, professional organizations she or he belongs to.

■ Try to get information about the training institute or program—such as whether it's accredited—in order to ascertain its legitimacy.

■ Interview the practitioner. Ask: "Do you have a working relationship with conventional doctors in your area?" "Are you affiliated with a hospital?" "What experience do you have in working with infertility patients?"

■ Talk to some of the practitioner's or clinic's patients. While testimonials should be taken with a grain of salt, they do give some indication as to the effectiveness of a practitioner, from at least the patient's perspective.

■ Try only one CAM at a time. More than one approach can be counterproductive.

■ If a technique doesn't work within a few months, don't continue it. Of course, a CAM therapy such as yoga, which helps you in general, doesn't need to be abandoned. Regardless of its direct effectiveness in resolving your fertility problems, keeping your mind and body healthy and relaxed is probably the best thing you can do for yourself.

Just the facts

- Complementary and alternative medicine (CAM) is receiving increasing attention and becoming recognized as a legitimate component in the treatment of infertility.

- Some studies of acupuncture have found that it may be helpful for both male and female infertility.

- Recent studies have found that some vitamins and herbs can enhance fertility in men and women.

- Stress reduction can help you cope with the emotional and physical pain of infertility treatment, as well as increase your chances of conception by helping you make the right decisions.

- Legitimate CAM providers should be trained, licensed, or certified just like conventional health-care providers.

The Social, Emotional, and Financial Sides

PART VII

GET THE SCOOP ON...
And the doctor makes three ▪ Scheduling sex ▪
How to avoid and resolve conflicts ▪ Gender
differences in coping ▪ Keeping the lines of
communication open ▪ Making sure your
relationship stays strong

The Infertile Couple

Chapter 14

Infertility is a major life crisis that can wreak havoc on the best of relationships. But it doesn't have to. In this chapter, we'll look at some of the common problems infertile couples face, some solutions to those problems, and some ways to forge a stronger relationship from the adversity that infertility issues often cause.

...And doctor makes three

When you first decided to have children, it may have crossed your mind that a baby—at times—might come between you and your partner, especially in the bedroom. It probably never occurred to you, however, that it would be your *quest* for a baby that would disrupt your sex life. And it also probably never crossed your mind that a doctor would become involved in the most intimate areas of your life, telling you when to have sex, when not to have sex, how often to have sex, and sometimes even *how* to have sex.

When sex—normally a private, personal matter—becomes scheduled, and part of a medical diagnosis and treatment, the results can be disastrous for the couple. Prior to infertility, most infertile couples have normal, happy sex lives. But infertility can put an end to all that, at least temporarily.

The doctor's involvement in an infertile couple's sex life usually starts when the doctor asks the man to produce, by masturbation, a sperm sample for semen analysis. On the surface, this request seems innocuous enough. But many men are embarrassed, annoyed, and even humiliated by this apparently simple but critical request. Their partners, on the other hand, tend not to have much sympathy for their feelings. After all, they themselves have to go through invasive and sometimes painful diagnostic procedures, while all the men have to do is masturbate, something that is actually pleasurable. Said one woman, "What's the big deal, jerking off into a jar? But he resents showing up late to work because of it. He says that it make him feel more tense at work, and that he feels tense enough already."

The reality is that most men do resent being told by their doctors that they have to masturbate. Indeed, this is probably the first time that they've been ordered to do something that many as youngsters had been taught was "wrong." But periodically throughout infertility treatments, doctors will need to ask for sperm samples for re-evaluation. Some men get used to it; others get increasingly bothered by it.

> **❝**I knew things were screwed up in our marriage when my husband was giving me shots and the doctor was giving me sperm!**❞**
>
> —Chloe, 37

Unless a donor is being used, the man also has to produce sperm for medical procedures such as artificial insemination and in-vitro fertilization (IVF). If he refuses to cooperate, he can ruin the couple's chance of a pregnancy for that entire month. And every month counts, especially for older women. It's understandable, then, that women often become furious when their partners balk at producing semen.

Men find it especially humiliating when a female receptionist or nurse requests a sperm sample. Said one man, "When the nurse handed me the jar, everyone in the waiting room knew what I was going in the bathroom to do. I was so embarrassed!" Some men find it very difficult to "perform" and are grateful when the bathrooms are equipped with adult magazines or other incentives.

If your partner gets upset about or refuses to produce a sperm sample, here are some things you can do to ease the situation:

- **Be sympathetic.** Tell him you understand how difficult this is for him, and you appreciate his cooperation—and contribution.

- **Don't pressure.** It will only anger him and make things worse.

- **Provide a "helping hand."** Offer to accompany your partner when he has to produce a sperm sample. He may appreciate the help, and it can be fun for both of you.

- **Lighten up.** Try to see the humor in the situation. Others certainly do. Check out www.fertilityplus.org/faq/humor/ihumor.html, a website that deals with infertility and humor. But keep in mind that your partner may not see any humor in the situation, at least at first.

Sex on schedule

As the infertility work-up and treatment progress, your doctor will very quickly become privy to your love life. As part of your medical history, he or she will need to know how often you have intercourse, when, and what positions you customarily use. If you haven't already done so, the doctor may first ask you to keep a basal body temperature (BBT) chart for three months (see Chapter 3). Your doctor will also want you to mark the days when you and your partner have intercourse. When doctors ask a couple how frequently they have intercourse, many couples are tempted to exaggerate, which can be counterproductive. It's very important for your doctor to have an accurate record of when and how often you have sex; this information can be extremely helpful for diagnostic purposes.

Bright Idea

Medications usually prescribed for erectile dysfunction, such as Viagra or Cialis, often work wonders for performance anxiety. Sometimes just having the medication in the house as a safety net can help.

Your doctor is also likely to tell you to have intercourse on certain predetermined days each month, right around the time of ovulation. So much for spontaneity! For awhile, at least, your sex life will no longer primarily be dictated by love, affection, or sexual desire, but by your doctor, the thermometer, and your ovulation prediction kit. It's no wonder scheduled sex often leads to sexual and other problems in the relationship.

Scheduled sex is also part of the postcoital exam. To do a postcoital exam correctly, your doctor will tell you to have intercourse on certain days around ovulation. As we mentioned in Chapter 6, a postcoital exam requires that the couple have sex the night or morning before the exam.

Because of all this pressure to perform on demand, it's not unusual for men to have bouts of impotency and to begin to have trouble achieving or maintaining an erection. And scheduled sex takes its toll on women as well. Many infertile women find they have difficulty reaching an orgasm, or are totally uninterested in sex for anything except procreation. One woman described her sex life like this: "I think my husband knows that I'm lying there thinking, just deposit the sperm and leave. Which is all I'm interested in. I'm not interested in sex anymore. I'm interested in conception...If I could take a little pill in the morning instead of having sex, I would rather do that—that would be wonderful."

Scheduled abstinence

Just when you've come to terms with scheduled sex, you might find yourself confronted with another problem—scheduled abstinence. There are times throughout a treatment cycle when a doctor might tell you not to have sex at certain times. As we mentioned in Chapter 3, some doctors may feel that abstaining a few days before ovulation can build up your partner's sperm count if it's low. On top of that, if you do conceive, your doctor may tell you to abstain for the first few weeks or even months of the pregnancy because of concerns about possible infection.

Surviving scheduled sex

After going through month after month of infertility, sexual intercourse can start to feel like a futile effort. When conception continually fails to occur, sex is often seen as the culprit, even if the problem is unrelated to intercourse. So sex becomes not only a routine and sometimes difficult chore, but dreaded and unsatisfying, too. As one woman put it, "You're going through the motions of something that time and again has been proven clinically to be unsuccessful. Unless you have absolutely no brains and no sensibilities or sensitivities, you've got to be affected by all that negative reinforcement."

Scheduled sex combined with the mood changes caused by both fertility drugs and continued

> **66** Scheduled sex made us the best of friends and, for a very long time, very lousy sex partners. **99**
>
> —Wendy, 38

failure to conceive can't help but adversely affect a relationship. Sexual intercourse—a once spontaneous act of love and sexual desire—can become a chore, a duty, a medical prescription often devoid of any feelings of sexuality or even affection. Said one frustrated woman, "There was very little making love. It was mostly making babies."

You might be concerned that things will never be the same again sexually. But there are things you can do to try to put the spice back into your sex life. First and foremost, concentrate on making love, not babies. Try to do things a bit differently. Use your imagination, be adventurous, do anything that will help

Bright Idea

If your partner is having sexual problems, you may find it helpful to become more subtle, seductive, and even secretive when you're ovulating. Even if your partner catches on, you have nothing to lose.

you separate sex from conception. Here are some suggestions that seem obvious but are worth mentioning because they might appeal to you both:

- Experiment with different positions.
- Have oral or other nonprocreative sex when you're not ovulating.
- Have sex when you're not ovulating.
- Have sex in places other than the bedroom.
- Wear sexy underwear—both of you!
- Rent X-rated movies.
- Read sexy novels in bed.

Fertility fights: whose fault is it, anyway?

Sex is not the only aspect of the couple's relationship to suffer from infertility. Couples are likely to fight over any number of issues related to infertility—and sometimes over issues that are not so related. One woman described how infertility affected her, her husband, and their marriage:

"My husband started getting depressed about the fact that the news was getting worse and worse. He was also starting to see that my patience and psychic energy to continue was being used up. I was starting to consider all the options—everything from continuing trying to never having children. He was very angry that I was no longer so committed to trying to conceive, that there was the possibility of my quitting. He became very hostile to me and criticized everything that I did. My hair was parted in the wrong place. I served too much soup or too little soup. He was constantly criticizing me. I was really aware that he was really angry at me, but I don't think I was aware, at that point, of how angry I was at him. When we finally sat down and talked about it, all those complaints translated into 'You're not dealing with this the way I would do it.'"

> **❝**You're forced to have sex to try and impregnate your wife...and it becomes a chore—sometimes it's a pleasant chore, sometimes it's not...the recreational aspects become minimal and the procreational aspects become huge.**❞**
>
> —Gordon, 30

To help avoid conflict and fights with your partner, it's important to respect each other's differing reactions, actions, and emotions. Here are some hints for maintaining a peaceful relationship during this stressful time:

- Don't blame each other...or yourself.
- Don't hurt each other's feelings.
- Talk it over. Be open with each other about your feelings, concerns, and limits.
- Empathize with each other.
- Be a united team. Keep in mind that the two of you are striving for the same goal: a family.

When couples fight, they commonly blame, insult, and accuse each other of all kinds of things. At some point, you may find yourself blaming your partner for the way he or she deals with infertility—or for being infertile in the first place. This might be especially tempting if your partner has the primary fertility problem, such as blocked tubes or a low sperm count. But even if you are the one with the primary problem, you may still

Watch Out!

Sometimes sexual problems can rapidly escalate, jeopardizing a couple's relationship. If you're having serious sexual problems, consult a sex or family therapist as soon as possible.

find reasons to blame your partner, perhaps for waiting too long to try to conceive, or waiting too long to call an infertility specialist. Some people become so convinced their partners are to blame they start fantasizing that if they had been with someone else, they'd have many children by now. Others even fantasize about having an affair with someone more fertile. Fortunately, most people don't act upon these fantasies. The reality is that you may not be any more likely to conceive with another partner than the one you're with now. One woman described her temptations this way: "I have thought in my really dark moments that maybe it's just my chemistry with my husband that's not working out. Maybe I should contact an old boyfriend or something. Not for an affair, not for kicks. But just for the right sperm, in my search for this master sperm that can find its way to this very obviously elusive egg."

Blaming your partner will not get you any closer to a pregnancy, and can only hurt your relationship. Your partner probably feels guilty enough as it is, and doesn't need to be reminded of his or her contribution to your fertility problem.

Both partners, in fact, are likely to have some feelings of guilt and self-blame about their fertility difficulties, regardless of who has the primary medical problem. They may blame themselves for something they did in the past—such as having had an abortion, an affair, or numerous sex partners—and feel that infertility is their punishment for their past "crime." They may even offer their partners a divorce out of guilt over not being able to please them by giving them the one thing they want: a baby.

Blame, whether it's directed toward oneself or one's partner, is counterproductive. It doesn't bring you closer to achieving a pregnancy, and it certainly doesn't help the relationship. Guilt and blame can only lead to depression, anger, and tension, when what is really needed is unified action.

How men and women cope with infertility

Most of the relationship problems infertile couples have are the result of the differences in the way infertility affects each partner. Each is likely to have different emotional reactions and coping styles. For example, one may become despondent, pessimistic, and passive while the other may be more optimistic, see infertility as a challenge, and take charge of the situation. Or one may wish to talk about it endlessly and join a support group while the other prefers to remain silent on the subject and shuns all association with other infertile couples.

There is no right or wrong reaction to infertility, as long as your reaction doesn't hurt either of you or your chances to conceive. Each person has a right to deal with infertility in a way that helps him or her cope. Each one also has to respect and understand the other's emotional reaction and coping methods to avoid conflicts and arguments. But this is easier said than done. Each partner's differing reactions to infertility can't help but cause some friction and fights. Being aware of potential problem areas can help you avoid them, or at least lessen their impact.

While we prefer to avoid sexual stereotyping, many reactions to infertility are, in fact, gender related. For example, most women believe that infertility is both emotionally and physically harder on them than on the man, and most men agree. The reality is

> ❝It made us both angry that Mary wasn't getting pregnant. She was hurt, worried, and depressed. I was just plain angry...I was angry at myself or Mary or the doctor or whatever, and it spilled over into everything.❞
>
> —William, 28

that men can better distance themselves—both emotionally and physically—from the infertility than women can. Said one woman about her husband's response to infertility, "He's like the stereotype of a man who is able to suppress it all, and goes to work...it just doesn't have the same meaning and terror for him."

Not only does infertility tend to have a greater personal and biological impact on women than on men, but women also have a more difficult time putting infertility out of their minds. This may be because women are ultimately the ones who will or will not become pregnant and give birth. Because of the emotional and physical involvement in their infertility treatment, women tend to think about it, talk about it, and obsess about it more than men do. Most men only think about it when they have to, such as in the doctor's office or when they're actively involved in a diagnostic or treatment procedure. A common result is that men become angry with their partners for making infertility a focal point of their lives, and women get angry with their partners for being or seeming to be uninvolved, unsympathetic, and uncaring.

Obsession

If a man feels overwhelmed by his partner's preoccupation with infertility, he may become angry, withdraw, or even belittle her for what he sees as a useless obsession. This has the potential to explode into huge arguments. To avoid these arguments, it's important to understand why infertility is likely to become a major preoccupation, if not an obsession, for most women, but not for men.

Women tend to obsess about infertility because its diagnosis and treatment quickly become an integral part of their everyday

---

 Bright Idea

If you find you're fighting a lot or can't resolve the problems in your relationship, consider joining a couple's support group. Or if you prefer, see a family therapist who has some expertise in treating infertile couples.

lives. As we have seen in previous chapters, infertility treatment for women requires frequent doctor appointments and close monitoring of her menstrual cycle. So even if a woman tries to forget about her infertility, she has constant reminders: Every morning the first thing she might do is put a thermometer in her mouth. Every time she goes to the bathroom, she may look for menstrual blood or check the quality of her cervical mucus. Every time she and her partner make love, she wonders if it worked this time, or whether they were wasting time and sperm because she was not ovulating. "It's with me every single day. I wake up with it, I go to sleep with it, and I think about it literally 50 times a day. It is always with me. I dream about it. It's night and day, and day and night, seven days a week ever since this began," said one woman. Another woman explained, "For three years it's been a constant, like my heartbeat." On the other hand, men—even those who are diagnosed as having a fertility problem—do not have these constant reminders of their infertility.

Withdrawal symptoms

Because of all the attention women pay to infertility, many men become angry, resentful, and emotionally withdrawn. If the man has the primary fertility problem, he may also feel guilty that he can't impregnate his partner and might become even more emotionally distant or upset.

When a man retreats emotionally, his partner is likely to feel rejected first, then angry. She might lash out and accuse him of not caring about her and their future family. She'll most likely feel that he's uninvolved and unsupportive and she'll long for both a child *and* her partner. As a result, she may become even more preoccupied with infertility and withdraw from her partner, perpetuating a vicious cycle.

Helping him get involved

Many women are upset not only by their partners' apparent lack of interest in infertility, but their lack of involvement in their medical treatment. Said one woman, "I felt he wasn't as

Moneysaver

One way to involve your partner in your treatments *and* save money is to have him give you your hormone shots. And playing doctor can be fun!

concerned about infertility as I was, that I was doing most of the work. I was the one who had to go to the doctor. I was the one who had to get the injections. I was the one who had to make the appointments, and call the doctor, and get follow-up and get the lab tests, and schlep him there. And I was the one who kept bringing it up for discussion, like when should we think about adoption? Or when should I change doctors? Or should I have the laparoscopy?"

One way for a woman to help counter this problem is to find ways to involve her partner more in their infertility treatment. Perhaps the best way to do this is to bring him with you to your fertility specialist whenever possible. Most women, in fact, prefer to have their partners accompany them to the doctor's office; while many men would rather not have their female partners go with them to a urologist.

Although it may not always be necessary for medical reasons, it's reassuring and helpful to have your partner there for emotional support. This is especially true when you have to undergo treatment or tests that are invasive, potentially painful, or anxiety provoking; or when the test or treatment results are critical in determining your chances of conceiving; or when important decisions must be made concerning treatment and other fertility-related matters.

The problem is that many men do not see their ongoing presence at doctor appointments as necessary, much less desirable. While most men are cooperative about going to the doctor when it's absolutely necessary, many resist and then resent it when they believe it's not essential to be there. This, too, can cause tension, as one woman discovered: "Each time I needed him to come to the doctor with me, I'd have to fight for it. I'd say, 'Remember, tomorrow we're going to the doctor.' And he'd say, 'Oh, I forgot. I have a meeting.' And I'd say, 'I'd really like you to come with me.' And he'd say, 'Oh, okay, all right. I'll cancel the meeting'—this whole big martyr shtick."

Talking it over...and over

Throughout this book, we've urged you to think about some of the steps you might be taking on your journey through infertility diagnosis and treatment. We've encouraged you to explore the ramifications of your options and to talk over your views with your partner. We've also pointed out that it's not unusual for your feelings to change as you move through the treatment process. Keeping the lines of communication open, then, is a key to avoiding the myriad problems that infertility can cause. Each partner must try to understand and accept the other's feelings, as well as keep the discussions going. You need to talk about infertility with each other: what it means to each of you, what concerns you have, and what it's doing to your relationship.

When one woman and her husband finally sat down to talk about what they were going through, it was a revelation to her. He told her, "You know, last night when you told me that you'd gotten your period, I felt like you stabbed me. And I realized that even though you accuse me of not being concerned about it, I really am. In fact, I'm so concerned that I can't even deal with it. It's really hard for me." And they both started to cry.

For most women, talking about infertility helps them cope. In general, women are more comfortable talking about feelings and discussing personal issues than men are. Unfortunately, sometimes a woman's need to talk about fertility problems can

 Bright Idea

Ask your partner to watch TV shows or movies with you that deal with infertility or adoption. They can be just the icebreaker you need to get a discussion going on these topics. But don't push it.

alienate her partner. For him, talking about infertility may be an unwelcome and seemingly constant reminder of his failure to get his partner pregnant.

To talk or not to talk?

Men tend to find the topic of infertility quite boring, while many women find it infinitely interesting. This is similar to the different ways men and women discuss pregnancy and child-birth. In fact, infertility can create the same kind of jealousy that a newborn does in many relationships. The man feels excluded and unneeded when his previously attentive partner focuses solely on the baby. During infertility treatment, a man might feel that his partner's yearning and quest for a baby is interfering in their relationship. He may resent the child even before it's conceived.

A woman's need to talk about infertility treatments and options with her partner can cause misunderstandings and conflicts in a relationship. Some men find it particularly upsetting when their partners call them at work. Although infertility is probably the last thing a man wants to discuss at the office, his partner may have to call him to discuss a test result, or to schedule an appointment for an insemination, or for comfort after bad news.

Many women complain that their partners are also reluctant to discuss infertility with friends or relatives, and this often becomes another area of conflict. Some men even forbid their partners to talk about infertility with anyone. Some women cope with infertility by making it the focus of their lives; they don't hesitate to reveal their infertile status to virtually all their acquaintances, and many strangers. Many men, on the other hand, try to ignore or deny their infertility. Said one woman, "My husband found infertility very embarrassing, and I guess he felt emasculated. So he wouldn't talk about it. He would rather have people assume that if we didn't have children, it was because we didn't want children."

Fruitful discussions

Discussing infertility with your partner is not just an idle obsession, it's a necessity. As we have seen in previous chapters, many medical decisions must be made which ideally involve the consent and agreement of both partners. These include everything from which doctor to see, to when to change doctors, to trying IVF, to stopping treatment and pursuing adoption.

Infertility forces couples to confront issues and make decisions they never thought they'd have to make. Discussing these issues together will help you avoid making decisions with which your partner might not agree, such as the importance of family and a biological connection to a child. Depending on how much you agree or disagree with each other, these issues can either help or hinder your pursuit of having a child.

Here are some questions you should ask yourselves and each other:

- What is more important to us, becoming pregnant or becoming parents?
- Are we giving in to pressure from our parents or in-laws to produce grandchildren?
- Are we willing to sacrifice anything—money, even our relationship—to achieve a pregnancy?
- Can we love a child who is not biologically ours?

Infertility requires constant evaluation and reevaluation of the situation to determine how much you can take medically, emotionally, and financially. It's also a good idea to periodically ask each other—and ideally your doctor—the following questions:

- Should we change doctors?
- Should we consider third-party reproduction?
- Can we afford this?
- Should we stop trying?
- Should we consider adoption or child-free living?

Bright Idea

Set aside a specific time each day to discuss fertility issues with your partner. Put a limit on the length of these discussions. Knowing they won't—or can't—go on all night will make them more productive...and less onerous.

While these questions can lead to arguments, they can also lead to a better understanding of your own and your partner's feelings and beliefs about these very important issues. Remember, it's not so much the answers to these questions that are important; over time, you and your partner are likely to change your minds on some of these issues. The main thing is to talk to each other and keep the lines of communication open. We go into more depth about each of these important issues in other chapters.

Fertility rights

We saw what can go wrong in a relationship as a result of fertility problems. Now let's see what can be done to set things right while you're waiting to become parents.

As much as you long to have children, now's a good time to take advantage of your freedom. You and your partner can do things together you probably won't be able to do very often once you do have children. Doing special things together can also help keep your relationship happy, exciting, and alive. And you won't have to worry about child care or paying a babysitter. Here are some things you might be interested in doing now:

- Take a break from infertility treatment and scheduled sex.

- Take a vacation: Go somewhere that doesn't allow children, such as a honeymoon-type resort or health spa. This will help you realize there is more to life than children.

- Spend a weekend away at a charming bed and breakfast or fancy hotel.

- Go to a romantic city, such as Paris, Venice, or the place you went to on your honeymoon or first date.

- Go on an adventure vacation where children are unlikely to be, such as a hiking, biking, or rafting trip.

- Go to the movies. Not those cutesy G or PG movies, but romantic, sexy, R-, or even X-rated movies. Not only will you be less likely to see children, but the movies will most likely be about adult topics.

- Have an adults-only dinner party at your home. Choose the couples carefully so discussions won't revolve around children or infertility. Consider having a gourmet potluck or wine-tasting dinner party.

- Eat out in romantic, child-unfriendly restaurants.

- After a romantic dinner, watch a romantic or X-rated video.

Long-term effects

Infertility is likely to have some lasting effects on your relationship, both good and bad. Unfortunately, some couples do split up as a result of infertility. Said one woman whose marriage was breaking up, "After five and a half years of temperature charts and trying and anticipation, infertility really caused stress in the marriage and we're breaking up. Not just because of infertility, but it definitely contributed."

How you resolve your fertility problem—the options you ultimately choose or don't choose—will certainly have an impact on your relationship. The good news is that infertility can bring you closer together rather than pull you apart, especially if you follow the advice in this chapter and seek help when you need it. Infertility can help couples gain a deeper understanding of—and new respect for—their partners. Said one woman, "I think our relationship is stronger, our mutual respect for one another is greater, our love is certainly deeper, and it's a whole different relationship than when we started. And probably a much better one. Going through this process put a real strain on the marriage. But I can't imagine another thing happening in our marriage that we wouldn't be able to deal with, having survived and experienced this together."

Many couples find that by confronting their fertility problems together and finding mutually satisfying solutions, their relationships are, indeed, strengthened. And the positive effects can last for years. Ten years after her infertility experiences, one woman, who had adopted two children, said: "We feel like we came through a storm and we're closer for it. We've gone through things that other couples never have and survived. That brought us closer together. We no longer take anything for granted with ourselves or our kids."

Just the facts

- At times, your doctor may tell you when to have sex—and when not to.

- Scheduled sex can wreck havoc with a couple's sex life and relationship.

- Women often cope with infertility by talking and obsessing about it while men tend to avoid the topic.

- You can avoid and resolve conflicts if each of you openly discusses your feelings about infertility and respects each others' opinions.

- Going to the doctor together and making joint decisions about your treatment can not only help strengthen your relationship, but can bring you closer together.

GET THE SCOOP ON...
Revealing your infertility to others ▪ Dealing
with other women's pregnancies ▪ Managing your
career and infertility ▪ How infertility can
positively affect your career

Living and Working in the Fertile World

Chapter 15

A s we saw in the previous chapter, infertility can wreak havoc on a couple's relationship. But it can also have unexpected effects on your relationships with friends, relatives, and co-workers. For example, you may feel differently about—or even resent—your friends who are pregnant or have children, and they may treat you differently as well. You may find some friends and relatives very comforting to be around, and others very annoying.

Coming out

Infertile couples not only have many medical decisions to make, but social ones as well. Perhaps the most challenging one is deciding who to tell, who not to tell, and how much to disclose about your infertility. While some people are very open about their fertility problems, others are extremely cautious about telling their friends, relatives, or co-workers. Many people feel infertility is stigmatizing, embarrassing, and too personal to discuss with others. Others may want to talk to their friends and family about it, but their partners object. Most often, it's the male partner who feels uncomfortable when a couple's infertility is made public—many men feel threatened by infertility because they associate it with impotency. For them, talking to others about infertility is tantamount to admitting to sexual problems, even if this is not the case. Disclosing your infertility, therefore, must be a very carefully thought-out decision that each of you has to make both as an individual and as a couple.

Asking yourself—and your partner—the following questions can help:

- What can be gained by telling that person?

- What are some of the possible negative ramifications of telling—or not telling—that person?

- Is that person likely to hear about our problem from someone else?

- Can we trust that person to keep our fertility problem confidential?

- Is that person sensitive and not likely to make upsetting remarks?

Once you decide who to tell, you still have to decide how much to disclose, and when to do it. Some people, for example, only reveal that they have a fertility problem when they undergo a surgical procedure or have a miscarriage. Again, there's no hard and fast rule. You have to do what's best for you and your partner.

When you do tell people about your infertility, it's hard to anticipate their reactions. Everyone has his or her own personal baggage about reproductive issues. Some will respond with sympathy, some with indifference, and some with embarrassment. Said one woman who was a psychiatric social worker, "I went slowly telling people. I did total 'psychosocials' on everyone before I told them, and I only told people who I knew would give a very supportive response. But it didn't always happen." Some are pleasantly surprised by how supportive their friends

Watch Out!

If you let others know about your infertility, you open yourself up to unsolicited advice, unwanted pity, or even insulting remarks. On the other hand, if you don't tell someone, you open yourself up to being questioned over and over about when you're going to have children.

and relatives are when they mention their fertility problems. "I had been afraid to tell [my family] partly because they have never been supportive of anything that I have ever done in the past," explained one man. "I was afraid they'd blame me for it, that I would be seen as defective." It turns out that his mother had assumed they didn't want children. So when he told her they were having fertility problems, it was a big relief, and she turned out to be very supportive.

Strained relations

While many infertile couples find their friends and relatives very sympathetic and supportive, others complain about insensitive and unsupportive responses. One man describes what happened when he told an old friend: "I told him we were having fertility problems and he said that when he wanted to get his wife pregnant, he'd knock her up right away! I was really pissed off. When they did finally try, he turned out to have a major fertility problem. What poetic justice!"

Even comments that may be well intended can hurt. In fact, you may find there is very little anyone can say that you would find comforting. If the listener is too sympathetic, you may feel patronized. If, on the other hand, the listener makes light of your problem, and says, "You'll see, it'll all work out," you may see that person as unsupportive and insensitive.

Unsolicited advice

You may find it irritating to receive unsolicited advice from friends and relatives, or even strangers. They might give you advice on everything from what doctor to see, to what fertility drug to take, to what sexual position is best. How do you handle this? It's probably best to thank them for their interest and say that you've already researched the subject and have carefully chosen a doctor whom you trust, and that you're taking your doctor's advice on the subject.

Insensitive comments

You might find it even more annoying when the advice and remarks imply that the infertility is somehow your fault. People are quick to blame women, especially, for causing fertility problems. They might tell a woman it's her fault for waiting too long, without knowing or understanding the reasons why she delayed childbearing. Other insensitive comments you might hear are: "Just relax and you'll get pregnant," "Take a vacation and you'll get pregnant," or "Adopt and you'll get pregnant." As we mentioned in previous chapters, there is no scientific evidence supporting the notion that stress causes infertility—and that relaxing, taking a vacation, or adopting a child will cure it. But these are perhaps the most persistent and annoying myths about infertility.

Another thing that might drive you up a wall is when people make negative comments about having children, such as, "You're crazy to want kids; kids are a pain in the butt." Remember that your friends and relatives mean no harm by these comments. Although remarks such as these are usually intended to comfort you, they unfortunately can really hurt.

Family gatherings can present a real challenge. There are always nosy relatives asking you questions. But insensitive questions and comments are not limited to relatives. As we have seen, friends, even if they mean well, can be incredibly insensitive and annoying as well.

Some people feel it's best to ignore these comments. Others find that the best way to handle these comments is by anticipating them and preparing responses ahead of time. You can pretty much anticipate that your prying Aunt Sadie will say something

Bright Idea

Try role-playing with your partner and take turns being the one who makes the insensitive or obnoxious remark. The other has to come up with a good retort. This can be an extremely useful, not to mention an enjoyable, exercise.

like, "When are you going to stop being selfish and make your mother a grandmother?" or your Cousin Charlie will say something obnoxious such as, "Obviously, you guys don't know how to do it right. Want me to give you a lesson?" You might, for example, say to Aunt Sadie: "We very much want a family but we're having fertility problems, and it pains me to talk about it." As for Cousin Charlie, you can laugh it off, walk away, or you may be tempted to joke, "From what I hear, you wouldn't know where to begin." But be careful not to get into a one-upmanship contest; it may escalate into an argument.

Depending on how you feel about such people, and your future relationship with them, your response can be polite, humorous, sarcastic, or blunt. Many people prefer the blunt approach because it acts almost like shock therapy, and tends to stun and silence the person. One woman tried several approaches until she found one that worked for her: "At first when people asked me if I was going to have children, I used to say, 'We're trying.' Later I just said, 'We're infertile.' And then I got to the point where I would say, 'I'm barren.' I did it on purpose because when you say that you're trying, they ask you four thousand questions, but when you come out and say, 'I'm sterile' or 'I'm barren,' they just shut up!"

What if someone asks you about having children and you don't wish to disclose your infertility? Perhaps the person asks, "So, when are you having kids?" Two possible responses that don't give any details but are still polite are "Why do you ask?" and "We'll let you know when it happens."

The fertile earth

Most women with fertility problems are hypersensitive when it comes to anything to do with pregnancy, especially the pregnancies of others. Finding out about a friend's or a relative's pregnancy can be especially disturbing. How the news is conveyed can make a difference. The following woman described what happened when she was awakened at night by a phone call from an older cousin who already had two children: "My cousin said, 'I just wanted to let you know before you heard from your mom, I'm pregnant.' And I said, 'Oh, congratulations. You must be really excited.' I was totally appropriate, but it was really hard for me. When I got off the phone there was sweat dripping down my arms. Later I realized how angry I was at her. She didn't have to phone me up at night. She could have written me a letter three days before she told the family...it would have been much better for me to read it so I didn't have to react. Because what am I going to say to her? 'You bitch! Don't you have enough already?'"

While the pregnancy of a friend or relative may be the last straw, not being told about a friend's or a relative's pregnancy can also be devastating. It may make you feel patronized and even more inadequate and vulnerable than you already feel. The thought that your friends find it necessary to shield you from the truth implies you're incapable of handling it, and that can make you understandably furious. As one woman explained, "There were people in the family who became pregnant and I wouldn't be told about it, and that really started driving me crazy. I felt that people shouldn't make the decision for me."

Seeing mothers with their small children—whether you know them or not—can be an upsetting experience for infertile women, especially women who have had miscarriages. You may, therefore, want to avoid gatherings and places where pregnant women, babies, and toddlers may be present. It's not just that their presence can cause problems; these mothers and about-to-be mothers may not understand your lack of enthusiasm about their condition or children. While being around babies and small children is hard for many, you will probably find that the hardest situation to bear is being around pregnant women. Infertile women seem to have, as one woman put it, tunnel vision for pregnant women. Because of this, they tend to feel that the whole world's pregnant but them. Being among pregnant women often makes infertile women feel like failures. You may ask yourself why you can't succeed at something these other women seem to do with ease.

Someone else's pregnancy can cause feelings of jealousy, rage, inadequacy, guilt, and even hatred in infertile women and some men. Seeing a friend's pregnant partner can make an infertile man feel inadequate and pose a challenge to his masculinity. And many infertile women have violent fantasies toward pregnant women. According to one woman, "A pregnancy was devastating to me—it destroyed me. I didn't want anything to do with pregnant women. I had fantasies of them having miscarriages, or still-born or deformed babies. I wanted their pregnancies to fail so that they would be failures like I was." After a while, her husband also started having the same feelings, with some exceptions: "I wanted to punch pregnant women right in their big fat bellies. But I also felt happy when someone who had really struggled with infertility became pregnant. They were more deserving."

> 66 Infertile women should avoid events that they can foresee are tailor-made to devastate them. 99
>
> —Barbara Eck Menning, founder of RESOLVE

Some women are confused or embarrassed by these feelings. As one woman put it, "I feel that I have a personality flaw, that my misfortune shouldn't color the way I relate to other people. But it does. I can't stand being near pregnant women. It does me in."

If you have these negative feelings and violent fantasies about pregnant women, remember that you're not alone. And fantasies can't cause harm. However, if you do feel tempted to act out these feelings, consider seeing a therapist, ideally one who specializes in working with infertile couples (see Chapter 16).

To go or not to go

One sure-fire way to avoid these negative, hostile feelings is to avoid being around pregnant women if at all possible. If this sounds anti-social or weird to you, ask yourself, "Why should I put myself in a painful situation in which I have nothing to gain?" Protecting yourself from pain is not selfish, it's sensible.

Holidays such as Christmas, Hanukkah, Thanksgiving, Easter, and Passover—not to mention Mother's Day and Father's Day—can be especially painful times for infertile couples. These are holidays that families celebrate together and are often child centered. It's virtually impossible to avoid the topic of having children at such occasions. They're also difficult to avoid, unless you have a really good excuse. So if a holiday or other occasion is coming up that you'd love to avoid, plan to take a vacation at that time. Being away is one excuse most people understand.

Probably the worst social situations for most women with fertility problems are baby showers, christenings, and other celebrations that definitely revolve around babies. Having to observe, and, even worse, participate in, the celebration of a pregnancy or new baby can be traumatic. When you get an invitation to such an event, it may seem like a no-win situation—if you don't go, you may feel guilty. If you do go, you'll probably regret it because of the emotional pain it causes you.

 Moneysaver

If you are invited to a baby shower, get a few friends to chip in to buy the gift. Not only can you save money, but by pooling your money, you can get a nicer gift. As a bonus, you might be able to get someone else to do the shopping for you and to present the gift at the shower.

Bright Idea

Because of strained relationships with the fertile world, you may find it easier to pursue friendships with other infertile couples. If you don't know other couples in your situation, you'll meet them by joining infertility support groups.

Realistically, if you don't go to your friend's shower, it won't be the end of the world. After all, the party is about her and her baby, not you. She'll be so distracted by the party, the gifts, and everybody else, she may not even notice your absence. If it's a "true" friend with whom you have shared your infertility problem, she should understand.

If you're still having trouble deciding whether or not to go to a baby shower, child's birthday party, or other potentially painful event, ask yourself these questions:

- Is my presence essential?
- Will my absence really make a difference and ruin the event?
- Will the guest of honor suffer more by my absence than I will by my presence?
- Is it worth several hours of emotional pain just to spare a friend a brief moment of disappointment?

If you decide not to go, don't feel guilty about it. Going through infertility, perhaps more than most other conditions, requires that you protect yourself emotionally. The following woman described what happened when she went to her niece's first birthday party right after her second miscarriage: "I felt like, well, it's my sister. But when I stepped in the house I knew I had made the wrong decision. I was crying inside and just holding myself together. That's all I could do. It was dumb of my sister not to think it through; I think I would have. She had lots of mothers there with their babies. I decided I would never go through that again. It's my life, and it's too painful. I feel right now that I come first. I will not subject myself to people who are pregnant or have small children. If they don't understand, it's their problem, because I don't care right now. But that will pass. And if those friendships don't last, I don't care."

If possible, you should take care not to hurt the other person's feelings. Be honest with your friend. Simply explain that you're in the midst of infertility treatment, and that while you're thrilled for her, you're unhappy with your situation, that being at a baby shower with a lot of people would make you extremely uncomfortable, and that you're sure she'll understand. If she doesn't understand, she's not a good friend.

There will be times during infertility treatment when you need to put yourself first. Give yourself permission to do that without feeling guilty about it. It's not selfish, it's a matter of survival—of getting through the process intact. The good news is that you won't feel this way forever. Once you resolve your infertility—through a pregnancy, adoption, or decision to remain child-free—you most likely won't continue to be plagued by these hostile feelings toward pregnant women. Said one woman who adopted a baby, "Adoption brought an immediate and instantaneous relief to all these feelings of wanting to kill, take out a knife and stab every pregnant woman." And another woman described how she and her husband were flying home with their newly adopted baby, when a pregnant woman got on the plane: "I turned to my husband and said, 'She's pregnant and we've got ours!' It was really a nice feeling."

Also, if you do choose to continue your quest for a child—through a pregnancy or adoption—you and your long-awaited child will likely be the guest of honor at at least one of these celebrations. And if an infertile friend doesn't want to go, you'll know just how she feels and let her off the hook.

Pregnant co-workers

Being around pregnant friends, relatives, and even strangers are situations you can potentially avoid. The problem becomes more complicated when you have no choice, such as at work, and the pregnant woman is your co-worker, or worse still, your boss. You have to act professionally regardless of whatever feelings you may have of jealousy or hostility. And you certainly cannot avoid going to work. Having to work with pregnant women can put a tremendous strain on your relationships with them—relationships that normally require objective professionalism.

At work—as in social situations—some people think it is best not to tell infertile women about co-workers who are pregnant. But this usually backfires since a pregnancy cannot be hidden for long. One woman, an assistant manager of a boutique, was extremely upset because her boss did not tell her that she was pregnant. What made it worse for her was that all the other employees were told, even the part-time ones. "I was the last person at work she told, so I was very angry with her. I said, 'I really think you should have told me—even if knowing would upset me—if for no other reason than because I am your assistant manager.'"

Job interference

Women undergoing infertility treatment have many other work-related issues to deal with besides pregnant co-workers. Infertility can mentally and physically interfere with your work. There are times, for example, when you'll have to call the doctor from your job for test results or for specific instructions about medications. It may be difficult to find a private phone so that you won't be overheard.

It's especially difficult to concentrate on your work and carry on as usual when you get distressing news. Hiding your reactions and emotions is also not easy, as this graduate student discovered: "My doctor said to call him for the results of my second pregnancy test at three o'clock. I was in the middle of interviewing a woman for a research paper and couldn't find a private phone, so I used one in the room. The nurse told me my hormone levels weren't rising as they should be, indicating a possible miscarriage. I started to shake and cry. I was really embarrassed and couldn't complete the interview."

Watch Out!

Make certain that if you get insurance coverage for your infertility treatment through your company insurance, they won't disclose your condition to your employers. Unfortunately, if your employer finds out you're trying to get pregnant, it may negatively affect your career.

Regardless of whether or not you have a private office, there may be occasions when you may not be able to hide your emotions or your fertility problem. The following teacher wound up having to tell her co-workers about her infertility: "There are times when I'm in my office and I'm crying or I have my head down and I'm hysterical. One time, however, I fell apart during a meeting and began to cry, so I had to tell them why."

If you feel that the emotional aspects of infertility are interfering with your work—or any aspects of your life—it's best to consult a therapist. Chapter 16 tells you how to find therapists who are experienced in working with infertile couples.

Telling women you trust at work about your fertility problem can be helpful for some, but it's not always an option. Many women feel strongly about keeping their infertility a secret on the job.

Risky business

Many career-minded people find that infertility has a dampening effect on their enthusiasm for their jobs. Job performance can be adversely affected and careers put on hold, making career advancement—and satisfaction—extremely difficult. Said one woman, an editor: "I've done very bad work in the last six months. I've barely been functioning. I'm no longer committed to my job. My work has gotten sloppy. The kind of work I do is creative, but when I'm depressed nothing is generated."

Diagnosis and treatment often require that a woman take time off from work for doctor appointments. Many women complain that juggling work schedules and doctor appointments is disruptive and stressful, as this urban planner discovered: "I haven't been able to work full time ever since the beginning of this. How can you, when you're taking off for this and that and the other thing, and going three times a month for artificial inseminations, and then this time for blood tests and that time for postcoital tests? I don't know how anyone can work full time and actually do all these tests, and then take off for a laparoscopy here and surgery there."

Because most people do not want employers and co-workers to know about their fertility problems, getting away from work—especially when it involves leaving early or missing important meetings—can be very difficult. "I had to lie all the time," said an executive. "It was tremendous pressure...and I always felt guilty about it."

Taking a lot of time off for doctor appointments doesn't usually sit well with bosses, and raises the issue of whether or not you should tell them about your fertility problem. Admitting to being infertile is also an admission of planning a pregnancy. You may be legitimately concerned that the knowledge of your planned pregnancy could jeopardize your job. Many employers are upset when employees become pregnant because pregnancies cost companies time lost to maternity leave and money spent on insurance benefits. As a result, it can cost you your job. Although this constitutes discrimination and is illegal, unfortunately it does happen.

However, if you don't tell your boss or supervisor, he or she may wonder why you're leaving work and going to the doctor so often, possibly even worrying that you have a life-threatening

 Watch Out!

Even though part-time jobs make it easier to fit in doctor appointments, they may not be great for your career. Not only do they pay less, they tend to be less secure, less prestigious, and less likely to carry medical insurance than full-time jobs.

disease that you are trying to conceal. You have to weigh all the pros and cons very carefully about disclosing your infertility status at work.

If your job involves travel, you have the added difficulty of not only fitting in doctor appointments, but scheduled sex as well. One woman, a publisher, turned down one job in favor of a less desirable one because the first job would have required travel during ovulation. But another woman, a public relations executive, was lucky enough to work for a company that would fly spouses in for "conjugal relations," which she carefully planned to coincide with her ovulation.

You can work it out

Every job situation is different, as is every boss. When making work- and career-related decisions, you have to weigh many factors and decide what's realistic, appropriate, feasible, and ultimately best for you and your career. Here are a few ideas that may work for you:

- Ask for a flexible work schedule that would allow you to periodically come in early and work late, or vice versa.

- Ask if you can work part time for a limited period of time.

- Ask about working at home. With home computers and the Internet, more and more people are able to telecommute successfully.

- Try to schedule your appointments during your lunch hour or on weekends whenever possible.

The waiting game

Infertility involves a lot of waiting...waiting for doctor appointments, test results, ovulation, an open slot at an IVF program, an adoption to come through, and on and on. As a result of all this waiting, many people have to, or at least believe they have to, put their lives on hold.

For many women, it's very often their careers that they put on hold while they wait for a pregnancy or baby that may or may

Moneysaver

When changing jobs, try to choose a job with a medical plan that covers infertility treatments.

not appear. They may not look for new opportunities or new jobs because any month now they may conceive. They may postpone major career moves or turn down great jobs just to stay in a job they hate but find convenient, as did the following woman, a lawyer: "I kept expecting to get pregnant, and that's why I've kept this job. I don't like what I do, and I need to go job hunting and get a new job. On the other hand, if I get pregnant, I'm in a wonderful position because I can take time off. I can walk to work and would be four blocks away from my baby. If I'm going to have children, I'm working at the perfect place. So I keep delaying doing anything about it."

By postponing positive career moves, you can wind up without either the job or the child of your dreams. The following physician took a nonprestigious job at a city hospital because, as she explained, "I thought that if I had a child it would be a really good job for me, but the job sucks, and I don't have a family. So now I'm angry at myself because I never should have made a decision based on something I had no control over."

Working through your problems

While infertility often has a negative effect on work and careers, many women find their jobs and careers help them deal with their infertility. They find that their work helps keep them sane while going through the process of infertility treatment—that being able to throw themselves into their work and careers helps them forget about infertility, at least during working hours. Said one woman, a teacher: "One of the things that really surprised me when going through infertility treatment was how much my work meant—how much a support and a lifeline it became."

Work is also a place where your worth is determined by hard work and achievement, not by whether or not you pass a pregnancy test. For some, work also helps to compensate for not having a baby, as this woman, a fundraiser, discovered: "The result of all my frustration and disappointment was that I got more involved in my job. It was a way to try to forget. I worked longer hours. I wanted to be productive. I wanted to produce a baby but I couldn't so I decided to produce a body of work. I just worked harder and harder, and was very successful. So it was nice. It paid off."

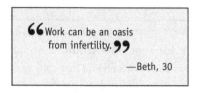

❝Work can be an oasis from infertility. **❞**

—Beth, 30

The type of work you do may also have some impact on both the way you cope with infertility and the way you cope with your job. While some people with fertility problems may find working with small children difficult, most seem to derive pleasure from it. As one woman who worked with young children explained, "I think I have an advantage working with children—it does take a certain amount of maternal feelings, even though it's on a professional level. It's enjoyable and I'm in an enviable position. I think it's more enjoyable for me than it would be to be an aunt or visit a friend's child. When I have these kids, they are my kids."

Keep in mind that you have a lot to gain by getting involved in your job. It can be a positive distraction, give you a sense of accomplishment, and help you feel more in control over your life. Make the most of it and it will probably pay off professionally and financially.

Infertility can also have a positive effect on your career in unexpected ways. For example, some people—especially those in the helping professions who come in contact with people with fertility problems—find that their experiences with infertility help them deal more empathetically and effectively with their clients. "I've been able to help a lot of people pursue adoption or pursue infertility treatment," said an internist who ultimately adopted two children. "Not that I would wish an illness upon a doctor or other medical professional, but I think illnesses or physical problems help people be better doctors, nurses, or whatever."

Infertility can also affect someone's career choice. Some put so much time and energy into infertility that they decide to make a career out of it. For example, one woman, a career counselor who adopted a child, started a successful side business in counseling women on adoption. Another woman, a social worker who was president of a local affiliate of RESOLVE, broadened her practice to include infertility and adoption counseling after she adopted a child. And many of the books about infertility and adoption, including this book, are written by people who have experienced infertility firsthand.

Just the facts

- Not everyone needs to be told that you have a fertility problem; tell only those who need to know and who you think will be supportive.

- If other women's pregnancies are causing you emotional pain, avoid gatherings and places where pregnant women, babies, and toddlers may be present.

- Although it can difficult to concentrate on your work and carry on as usual, there are ways you can avoid having infertility issues interfere with your job.

- Many women find their jobs and careers help them deal with their infertility in unexpected positive ways.

GET THE SCOOP ON...
Common emotional reactions to infertility ■
Regaining a sense of control ■ Taking time to
mourn ■ Joining self-help organizations and other
coping strategies ■ Infertility counselors vs. traditional therapists ■ Choosing to be child-free

Surviving and Resolving Infertility

Infertility is considered a major life crisis, and for good reason. As we have seen in the past two chapters, infertility can have an adverse effect on an individual's self-image, sex life, relationships, and career. And, like all major life crises, infertility has serious emotional consequences for the individuals involved. Most couples feel they're on an emotional roller coaster, with ups and downs that seem to follow those of their temperature charts. If you ask couples with fertility problems what the worst part of their ordeal is, most will say without hesitation it's the emotional toll it takes on their lives.

A multitude of losses

Barbara Eck Menning—founder of RESOLVE, the national organization for people with fertility problems—described the predictable emotional responses most people have to infertility: surprise, denial, isolation, anger, guilt, a sense of unworthiness, depression, and grief. These feelings are

Chapter 16

mainly due to the myriad losses a person with fertility problems suffers—the loss of control over one's life, the loss of a normal sexual relationship with one's partner, and perhaps most important, the loss of the dream of having a child of one's own.

Loss of control

Loss of control is especially hard to accept for those who are used to being in control over their lives. Many talk about how, until they experienced infertility, they always felt in control. As a result, they're not used to failure, as the following woman explained: "I always accomplished what I wanted. I wanted my own apartment, I had it. I wanted my own life, I got it. I wanted to support myself in a style to which I had become accustomed, I did. I wanted boyfriends, I had them. I wanted to get married, I got married. All of a sudden, a major thing, and I'm not getting it. I cannot believe it. It never occurred to me that I wouldn't get what I wanted."

Infertile men and, probably more so, women, also tend to experience a loss of control physically as well as emotionally. Their bodies are not doing what they're supposed to be doing. Rather than making love to make a baby, they're having physical procedures done that may be painful, not to mention embarrassing.

The physical loss of control can be especially difficult for women and men who are used to being in control of their bodies. They most likely have spent years controlling their fertility by carefully choosing and using contraception to avoid an unwanted pregnancy. Now they find that their fertility is out of their hands.

Loss of self-esteem

Feeling out of control of your life can profoundly affect your self-esteem. Whether infertility primarily involves failure to impregnate your partner, failure to conceive, or failure to carry a pregnancy to term, infertility ultimately is the failure to become a mother or father, at least biologically. As a result, your self-image and self-esteem may suffer. Indeed, people with fertility problems often use words like inadequate, incomplete, flawed, defective, and damaged goods to describe themselves.

Loss of positive sexual identity

Many men see infertility as a negative reflection on their masculinity. For them, infertility spells impotence. They equate fertility with virility. Women, too, often have a similar reaction and equate fertility with femininity. As one woman explained: "It's a reflection on my womanhood. I don't feel very womanly because my image of being a woman is to be a parent, a mother. I measure myself a lot against other women whom I see with children and with careers, and with family life. And somehow I don't feel I'm as good as they are."

> 66 It's an ego-battering experience. I don't feel as pretty, and I certainly don't feel as fertile or as feminine. 99
>
> —Sarah, 28

While men do not carry any outward signs of their fertility or infertility, women do—the pregnant belly is proof positive of being fertile. And while not being pregnant doesn't convey to the outside world that a woman is infertile, many people do associate pregnancy and biological motherhood with being a complete woman.

Not being able to do what most other women can—become pregnant and give birth—can distort a woman's sexual identity. Said one woman, "Sometimes I feel like I have a caricature of a woman's body. That it's sort of too feminine on the outside and it's no good on the inside."

Regaining control

When people feel that they have lost control of their reproduction, they often try to compensate—or overcompensate—by taking control of their bodies in other ways. They may shift their focus from fertility and try to change their external appearance. For example, men may try to enhance their outward signs of masculinity by taking up sports or bodybuilding.

Attempting to lose weight is another common means of gaining control of one's body. As one woman put it, "I felt very unhealthy; my body wasn't doing what it was supposed to do. So I joined exercise programs and I joined a weight-reducing program. This was all because I wanted to control my body, which was out of control." However, as we mentioned earlier, being excessively thin can itself interfere with conception.

Others change the way they dress to conform to the stereotypical images of masculinity and femininity. Men may grow beards and start wearing work clothes, and women may start wearing frilly, flowery, feminine dresses. "For a long time I really did feel like less of a woman," one woman admitted. "I went through a period of wanting to look very, *very* feminine. I stopped wearing pants. I let my hair grow long." But her behavior didn't last very long. She resolved her feelings of inadequacy and came to the following realization: "Not being able to have a baby doesn't make you any less womanly than having a baby makes you more womanly. What it is to be a woman is really socially, not biologically, defined."

To help you separate fertility from masculinity and femininity, keep in mind that hundreds of thousands of men and women are voluntarily sterile. They choose to have vasectomies and tubal ligations—whether or not they've ever had children. In fact, men who have vasectomies tend to be considered quite "macho." And women who've had their tubes tied are certainly not considered unwomanly. Nonetheless, these men and women are, in fact, totally sterile.

Some people are able to use their experiences with infertility to gain more insight and a deeper understanding of what it really means to be a man or woman, and a mother or father. They realize, like the woman above, that neither the ability to reproduce nor a biological connection to a child is necessary to adequately fulfill those roles. In fact, one woman said she felt that infertility actually made her feel *more* like a woman. "I really have had to come to grips with what it means to be a woman," she explained. She was able to come to the realization that the physical processes of pregnancy and childbirth were not what defined womanhood or motherhood.

Mourning your losses

Resolving the emotional issues surrounding infertility and coming to a realistic understanding of parenthood doesn't come easily. First, you need to accept that you're infertile. That involves going through a period of grieving for the many losses you suffer because of infertility. This doesn't mean that you'll never conceive or that you're at the end of the road and giving up. It just means that you acknowledge your condition.

Grief and mourning—and the tears that often follow—can be cleansing and healing. Grieving can help you come to terms with your infertility. Once you grieve about your losses, you can better make rational decisions not only about what to do next, but how and even whether you're going to continue to try to build a family.

Because of the losses it involves, many experience infertility as a kind of death—the death of the dream of possibly having their own children and the death of children who might never be. The fertile world doesn't always understand this type of death and the need to mourn. As one woman poignantly explained, "It's not as if an actual person has died. So you can't get the kind of support you'd like, as you would if someone died. I don't know how to explain to people that this child in me, who never existed, died."

For those who have had miscarriages, the equation of infertility and death is even more real. But even though miscarriage is actually the death of a fetus, some people, including doctors, don't see it as such. They don't understand the depth of the couple's despair. Couples who have miscarriages are often told that miscarriage is nature's way of getting rid of a mistake, and they could always get pregnant again. Telling a couple who just experienced a miscarriage that the child they conceived was nature's mistake can add insult to injury. To them miscarriage is the actual death of their child, and treating it like a death, not a mistake, helps them cope and carry on. In fact, many couples hold private services to help them mourn their lost child. Some find that burying items such as baby booties or performing other rituals can be especially helpful in recovering emotionally from this trauma.

> 66 The physical pain of surgery is over in a few days, but the emotional pain lingers on and on. 99
>
> —Debbie, 31

Survival strategies

As you can see, people react to infertility in many different ways. There are also many different coping mechanisms available to help people deal with the various emotional crises of infertility. One of the most common coping mechanisms is seeking the support of others.

Many infertile people turn to their partners, friends, and family for support and comfort. It's not unusual for them to reach out to different people at different times, as this woman described: "There were times when my husband was an anchor for me, and at other times my mother has been very good. At other times it's been my nephews; just seeing two normal children playing and having a marvelous time is a reaffirmation of what you want to do when you get discouraged. At other times it's been work—being able to say I have other things that make me important. Other times it's been me. And permeating this whole experience has been a religious orientation."

Spiritual support

Some men and women with fertility problems find religion or other forms of spirituality a major source of support and consolation. They may find the spiritual meaning of religion or the familiar rituals comforting and helpful. While some may turn to organized religion and prefer to worship as part of a group at a church, synagogue, temple, or mosque, others seek solace in a more personal, inward spirituality and prefer to pray alone silently. Some may pray for a pregnancy and child, and some use prayer to help them resolve infertility in other ways, as this woman did: "I felt that I should try to be more religious, more accepting. I pray a little more, a little harder, and more sincerely to try to be more accepting of what will be, just accept what God has destined for me. I've never prayed for a baby. To this day, I've never prayed, or lit a candle, or done a novena for a baby. I have prayed for strength. God knows we need a lot of that going through this process. I've prayed for insight to make good decisions for us."

Turning to religion for support, strength, and guidance may be a new experience for some. They might be quite surprised to find themselves being religious for the first time, as did the following woman, who had always regarded herself as an agnostic and viewed religion as a crutch: "I became more Jewish about this for a while. I thought that would help. I was wearing a *chai* around my neck for a year because that was a symbol for life, and I thought if you wore a *chai* you'd get pregnant. Going to Israel was another part of the Jewish year."

And some may develop a religion of their own design to suit their own spiritual needs. For example, one woman who was born Jewish and then became an atheist said that when things got really bad, she went to a church, lit candles, and spoke to Jesus. "It helped because I just felt like I was trying basically to get a feeling that there was something outside myself helping me to cope with this," she explained.

Self-help organizations and support groups

Virtually everyone with a fertility problem needs others to talk to who can relate to their situation. But it's not always easy to find people who can really understand what you're going through, much less talk about infertility. As we saw in previous

Moneysaver

Joining a self-help organization and/or going to a support group will cost considerably less than seeing a private therapist.

chapters, your partner isn't always available, able, or willing to discuss infertility issues. And, unfortunately, those in the "fertile world" often lack empathy and understanding about the subject. The good news is that there are self-help organizations and support groups available in many communities.

There are several ways you can find support groups; contacting RESOLVE and/or the other consumer organizations listed in Appendix C is a good place to start. Your doctor's office is also likely to have a list of local support groups. The Internet and the Yellow Pages are also good options.

Self-help groups and organizations can be extremely useful for anyone with a fertility problem—whether just beginning the diagnostic and treatment phases, in the midst of treatment, or thinking of stopping and pursuing alternative solutions. Indeed, becoming a member of such organizations and/or joining an infertility support group is probably the single best thing you can do for yourself to help you deal with the social, emotional, and medical issues related to infertility.

People join these self-help organizations and support groups for a variety of reasons. Some want to get information about fertility specialists or specific infertility treatments. But most do so for emotional support. They may not know anyone else with a fertility problem and want to meet people going through the same difficulties. One woman, for example, explained that she joined a support group at the fertility clinic she attended because her husband had forbidden her to discuss their problem with anyone else and she found it intolerable to be so isolated. Some people join because they're curious to see what other infertile couples look and act like; they're usually amazed that everyone looks normal and healthy just like they do.

Overcoming reluctance

Some people are reluctant to join a support group or attend a seminar or meeting about infertility. If this describes you—or your partner—it may help to think about what there is to be afraid of. In Chapter 15, we discussed a similar situation—being hesitant to disclose infertility to friends and relatives for fear of what they might think about you and say to you. But there's one big difference: Everyone in the support group is in the same boat! They, too, suffer emotionally and physically, have been the victims of insensitive remarks, and have had to live in the sometimes cruel fertile world. It's highly unlikely that they'll be judgmental. On the contrary, they can empathize with you. A bonus of being in a support group is that members often share doctors' names, good and bad experiences, and valuable information about treatments and adoption. You can feel free to laugh and cry together. So you have a lot to gain from being with others with similar problems...and nothing to lose.

By now, you may be eager to join a support group but find that your partner isn't. Women in general tend to be more receptive to joining support groups and self-help organizations than men. So many women take the first step and join a group, and sometimes their partners follow. But sometimes they don't. Organizations such as RESOLVE are still primarily run and attended by women, although more and more men attend meetings and support groups each year.

For those who do attend meetings or support groups, most find it comforting, reassuring, educational, or helpful in some way. Even those who are dragged there tend to come around after they get over their initial anger or embarrassment.

 Bright Idea

If you can't get your partner to join you at a meeting, try to get together with some other couples for drinks or dinner beforehand. It might be just the icebreaker you need to get a reluctant person involved.

Support groups fulfill needs that partners, friends, relatives, therapists, and doctors often cannot. Many say that a major benefit of support groups is finding others like themselves. It's not just an issue of "misery loves company." It's finding people who are nonjudgmental and with whom you can share your problems. Said one woman: "I was astonished to find there were a lot of others like me. I had never discussed this with anyone for a lot of reasons. It was all inside me. The only one I spoke with or cried about this with was my husband. I guess it became too overwhelming and I felt we couldn't help each other anymore. So I started going to meetings."

As we said earlier, a major benefit of being in a support group and/or self-help organization is that you become extremely knowledgeable about many of the medical aspects of infertility. You get the chance to listen to—and have your questions answered by—guest speakers who are often top fertility specialists in your area. You can also hear first-person accounts by their fellow patients.

> 66 It was a relief to meet other people and also to find out that my reactions to the whole thing were not as bizarre as I was being told they were by my husband. 99
>
> —Elaine, 30

Support groups are especially helpful when you're considering resolving infertility through third-person reproduction—such as egg or sperm donation, surrogacy, or adoption—or by choosing to be child-free. The struggles, experiences, and insights of others in similar situations can be invaluable.

Seeking professional help

As good as support groups are, they aren't for everybody. Also, there may not be one in your area. So if you feel you can benefit from emotional or psychological help, and support groups are not the answer, you may want to consider seeing a therapist. Seeing

Watch Out!

If you're seeing a therapist who objects to your joining a self-help or support group, find a new therapist. A good therapist is likely to welcome such a positive move.

a therapist does not necessarily mean you need to be in long-term therapy or analysis. Many people are helped by short-term therapy.

Individual psychotherapy or psychological counseling are common ways people get help dealing with short-term crises, as well as long-term problems. You might just need help in getting over the emotional upheaval of infertility and sorting through the pros and cons of the various options available to you. You may also decide that seeing a couple's or family therapist can be helpful in resolving the infertility-related issues—and other pertinent issues—in your relationship.

If you're not sure whether or not you should see someone, the Mental Health Professional Group of the American Society for Reproductive Medicine (ASRM) provides the following list of symptoms or situations that *might* indicate that you should see a therapist:

- Persistent feelings of sadness, guilt, or worthlessness
- Social isolation
- Loss of interest in usual activities and relationships
- Depression
- Agitation and anxiety
- Increased mood swings
- Constant preoccupation with infertility
- Excessive discord in your relationship with your partner or others
- Difficulty concentrating and remembering
- Confusion about treatment options

- Change in appetite, weight, or sleep patterns
- Increased alcohol or drug use
- Thoughts about suicide or death

Keep in mind that you're likely to have experienced many, if not all, of these symptoms at some point in the course of your infertility diagnosis and treatment. But you may need the help of a therapist if these symptoms persist over an extended period or if any of them are extreme or interfere with your life and daily functioning.

Infertility counselors

If you've decided you should seek professional help for infertility, you now have to find the best person for you and your situation in the same way you would go about finding a fertility specialist (see Chapter 5).

There are many different types of mental health professionals who might consider themselves infertility counselors. They can be psychologists, psychiatrists, psychiatric social workers, family therapists, marriage counselors, nurses, and pastoral counselors. The main thing to remember is that they should be professionally trained and have credentials in their field of mental health—and equally, if not more importantly—that they have specialized training and knowledge in the field of infertility. They need to understand the physical as well as emotional aspects of infertility.

Infertility counseling is a relatively new profession, and there is no uniform training. Ideally, an infertility counselor has undergone some training in reproductive medicine by working

---

 Watch Out!

Some therapists claim to be infertility counselors because they see infertility patients as an untapped market of educated and affluent potential clients. As with all health professionals, you should check their credentials *and* their experience.

Moneysaver

Make certain the therapist you're seeing is fully licensed in your state. Your insurance company may not reimburse you for sessions unless he or she is.

closely with fertility specialists, in a fertility clinic, or by attending postgraduate medical as well as psychological courses. Many infertility counselors are mental health professionals who have experienced infertility themselves. Some have training and some don't. It's up to you to find out what training and experience—if any—a therapist has. And it goes without saying that a therapist should be licensed in your state. Your fertility specialist or IVF program may have their own counselors or support groups, which can be very helpful and convenient. But make sure that the therapist is looking after your best interest, not that of her employer or fertility program.

One good way to find an infertility counselor is through your local affiliate of RESOLVE. You can ask your doctor or fertility clinic if they work with an infertility counselor or if they can recommend one in your area. You can also contact the ASRM's Mental Health Professional Group mentioned earlier and ask for their membership list. The membership list will not, however, give you information on a member's qualifications—you'll have to check that out for yourself. But membership in ASRM at least shows a special interest in infertility.

Here are some questions you should ask about the infertility counselors you're considering:

- What degree do they have and where did they get their training in therapy? Your therapist should have a minimum of a Master's degree, usually in psychology, social work, or counseling, from a reputable graduate school.

- Are they licensed to practice therapy? Being licensed as a mental health professional guarantees that a therapist has had postgraduate training.

Bright Idea

If possible, interview a few infertility counselors before settling on one. Choose this person carefully, because he or she can have a profound effect on both your emotional life and the decisions you make about infertility and your pursuit of parenthood.

- What experience in infertility counseling have they had? Have they worked closely with a fertility specialist or in an ART program? If so, for how long? Make sure the therapist has worked with a reputable doctor or program, or has had some training in infertility.

- What percentage of their practice is in infertility? It's probably better to see an infertility counselor who devotes at least half of his or her time to treating people with fertility problems.

- What professional organizations do they belong to? Besides being a member of ASRM's Mental Health Professional Group, the therapist should be a professional member of RESOLVE. Membership in these organizations is an important indication of the therapist's interest and dedication to the field of infertility. Belonging to other mental health organizations is also important.

- Have they personally experienced infertility? This question is tricky. In general, therapists don't divulge information about their personal histories. But many make an exception in the case of infertility counseling. While it's not necessary that a therapist has had a fertility problem to help couples cope with the emotional aspects of infertility, it can be helpful. Adequate training, experience, and sensitivity are probably more important. But *as long as therapists are able to remain objective,* they may be able to draw on their own experiences to help you make decisions about various treatment options, adoption, and even child-free living.

As you can see, it may not be easy to find a therapist who's trained in the physical and emotional aspects of infertility and can truly understand infertility in a nonjudgmental way.

Traditionally trained therapists can be very helpful for many emotional problems, including some of those related to infertility. However, most therapists are not trained to deal with the unique issues infertile individuals or couples face. Therefore, they may not adequately understand the emotional and medical aspects of infertility that people with fertility problems face.

Blaming the victim

One of the most frequent complaints people with fertility problems have about traditional therapists is that they, like many uninformed people in the fertile world, tend to believe that stress, ambivalence, and other psychological factors are major causes of infertility. By emphasizing stress, these therapists are, in effect, blaming the victim. This can be not only painful and counterproductive, but confusing—especially if you're being treated for a specific, diagnosed physical problem.

Being told that you're infertile because of unconscious factors or stress can make you feel guilty and more depressed—not to mention more stressed—than you already are. One therapist told a woman who had a diagnosed ovulatory problem, "Your mind is very powerful. It could be that this is a case in which the harder you try the more difficult conception becomes." Her therapist had, like many who do not understand infertility, jumped to the conclusion that ovulatory problems were the result of psychological problems.

 Watch Out!

Be aware that some therapists or counselors who've had infertility problems themselves might be living out unresolved issues through you and their other patients. Rather than being objective, they may give you advice based on their own bad experiences.

Moneysaver

Massages are one of the best stress busters you can find, but they can be expensive. Rather than pay for one, you and your partner can give each other massages. It's also a nice way to be physically close without the pressure to conceive.

As we've mentioned several times in this book, even if you have unexplained infertility, there is little evidence that stress is a significant cause. There is some evidence that stress can interfere with ovulation in certain cases. But it's virtually impossible to determine if and when ovulatory problems may actually be the result of stress. In addition, the woman in the previous example—like most women being treated for ovulatory problems—was taking fertility drugs. So even if her therapist was correct and stress was a factor, it wouldn't matter since fertility drugs more than compensate for the possibility of an emotionally induced anovulation.

Millions of women living under extreme emotional, physical, or financial stress manage to conceive with ease. In fact, in some of the poorest countries with the worst living conditions, such as India, China, and parts of Africa, overpopulation—not underpopulation—is a major problem.

Rather than being the cause, stress is probably the most common emotional side effect of infertility. Relieving stress in any way possible is a good idea. In fact, although it might seem contradictory to what we said earlier, relieving stress might help you conceive, at least indirectly. The less stressed you are, for example, the more likely you'll want to have sex. Depending on the cause of your fertility problem, the more frequently you have sex, the better your chances to conceive. And the less stressed you are, the more likely you'll be to make positive decisions about your infertility treatment and other options.

Deciding that enough is enough

At some point, the emotional, physical, and financial stresses of infertility may get to be so overwhelming that you say, "Enough is enough!'" Or you may have pursued all the options medically and socially acceptable to you and your partner. If you're at this point, you have three choices:

▪ **Take a break.** You may want to take time off from treatment, and, at least temporarily, get on with your life. Taking time off from treatment gives you time to reflect on your situation and review your options more objectively. It also can be physically helpful, since taking fertility drugs and/or undergoing invasive treatments can take their physical, as well as emotional and financial, toll. Many doctors insist their patients stop taking fertility drugs for several months to give their bodies a chance to get back to normal. In fact, it's not unusual for patients to conceive during a break from fertility drugs. Again, this is not because they're under less psychological stress (although that may be a positive side effect), but because their bodies are under less physiological stress from treatment.

▪ **Revisit your other options.** You may decide to reconsider one of the donor or surrogacy options, or adoption. What seemed out of the question to you or your partner a year or even a few months ago may now not seem like such a bad idea. This is when being in a support group can be extremely helpful. Being able to talk to others who are struggling with these issues, or have done so in the past, can give you invaluable insights as well as information.

Start doing more research on the options that seem most appropriate and appealing. It might help to first reread Chapters 11 and 12 about third-party solutions, including adoption. Then turn to Appendixes B and C to find Internet sites, books, and organizations that can provide you with more information about these options.

▪ **Consider child-free living.** You and your partner may decide that you want to put infertility totally behind you and get on with your life. This, for most couples, means choosing to be child-free, unless, of course, you already have children living with you. In that case, you may choose to accept your family as it is and stop trying to have or adopt another child.

Childless by chance...or choice

Some infertile couples who previously considered themselves involuntarily childless ultimately decide to be child-free. After putting so much time, energy, and money into trying to have a baby, this is a difficult choice for many infertile couples to make. However, choosing to be child-free can be a positive choice for some couples. In fact, that's why we prefer the term *child-free*, an active term with positive connotations, to *childless*, a passive term with negative implications.

> **66** Contraception was our declaration of independence from the cycle of hope and despair and for us the final step in being child-free. **99**
>
> —Jean and Michael Carter, *Sweet Grapes: How to Stop Being Infertile and Start Living Again*

An estimated 14 percent of couples in the United States today are childless, and many of them are childless by choice.

Choosing to be child-free, like choosing to adopt, can be a positive decision that means you are taking control over your life and moving on. While you didn't have control over your previous state of childlessness, you can now take control of the situation.

Choosing to be child-free doesn't mean giving up. After all, living a child-free life is what you've probably been doing for quite a long time. Before this whole infertility mess happened, you and your partner were probably very happy together without children. You can continue to be happy together...just the two of you. Michael Carter, who co-authored *Sweet Grapes: How to Stop Being Infertile and Start Living Again* with his wife, Jean Carter (see Appendix B), wrote the following about their decision to remain child-free:

Childfree means that we have taken the strength we found in our struggle with infertility and turned that strength toward making our lives good again. It means taking advantage of the benefits that can come from not having children....To me...the most important part about the childfree option is that it offers a message of hope to all of us who are infertile: even if you don't end up with a child, you and your spouse still have the potential for a happy, productive life together. It says that two can also be a good size for a family.

—quoted in RESOLVE Fact Sheet,
"Childfree Decision-Making," by Merle Bombardieri

Talking points

Couples want children for many reasons, some reasonable and some not so reasonable. In trying to decide if you should continue to pursue pregnancy, look into adoption, or remain childfree, you might want to go back to the basics and ask yourself why you want to have children. Understanding your motives—both the rational and irrational ones—can help you make the right decision for yourself and your partner. Ask yourself—and your partner—the following questions about your motives regarding both pregnancy and parenthood:

- Are you pursuing this to please your partner? Your parents? Your in-laws? While your partner's wishes are key, the wishes of your parents or in-laws should not influence your decision. If your partner, however, wants children and you don't (or vice versa), that's a serious issue that may be helped by seeing a family therapist or marriage counselor.

- Do you want a child in part because you want to relive your happy childhood? Or conversely, are you trying to rewrite your unhappy childhood and right what your parents did wrong? Whether your childhood was happy or sad, remember, no two children or childhood experiences are ever alike. Your child will be a totally different person and will grow up in a totally different family environment. Probably your parents, like most, decided to raise you differently from the way their parents raised them! And, as much as we'd like to, we can't guarantee our children will have a happy childhood.

■ When you picture your child, do you picture a sleeping infant, cuddly baby, or a chubby-cheeked toddler? If so, remember, the early years go by very quickly and parenthood goes way beyond babyhood. Can you picture yourself parenting a precocious pre-adolescent or a temperamental teenager? Or what about a handicapped child? There is no guarantee that your child will look like one of the babies in television commercials.

■ Are you trying to fill a void? Do you want a child because you're bored with your life or job? Raising a child will certainly keep you busy—it's time-consuming and can be all-engrossing. But, as any parent will tell you, much of parenting is boring and tedious. And there's no paycheck at the end of the week. Remember, while you can quit a job you don't like, you're a parent for life. Also, it's unfair and unrealistic to expect a child to fill a void in your life.

■ Do you want children so you won't be alone when you're old? By now, you should be well aware of the fact that things don't always go as planned. Having children certainly is no guarantee that you will live to a ripe old age. And even if you do, your children may have other plans for where and how they live.

■ Do you want children because all your friends are having them? Or because you think you'll lose all your friends who have children because you won't have anything in common with them?

Bright Idea

Try to spend some afternoons, evenings, or weekends, if possible, alone with friends' or relatives' children of various ages. It will give you a more realistic sense of what it's like to have children.

There are no right answers to these questions. They may all apply to you to some extent. However, if any one of them is your *primary* motive, perhaps it should give you pause.

Ambivalence

It's normal to feel ambivalent about any major decision. In fact, you or your partner may have been ambivalent about having children in the first place. But once you got caught up in pursuing pregnancy, you may have lost sight of that original hesitation, and the reasons for it. If you or your partner were initially undecided, it may help to recall some of the reasons for that. Another thing you can do that you might find very helpful is for each of you to make two lists—one of the pros and cons of having children, and the other of the pros and cons of being child-free. Not only will this exercise provoke a lively discussion with your partner, it can further clarify each of your desires, beliefs, and concerns about having children.

Child-free living is obviously not for everybody. If you're uncertain—and you probably are since you've devoted so much time, energy, and money into trying to have children—you should read as much about the subject as you can. Try to find a support group for child-free couples or couples seriously considering this option. Join chat rooms on the Internet. Try to observe and talk to as many child-free couples as you can. Ask them about the issues that concern you. Said the following woman about the child-free marriage of her recently widowed aunt and uncle: "My aunt and uncle were one of the happiest couples I've ever known. Because an ectopic pregnancy ruined her tubes, my aunt could not have children. However, they loved surrounding themselves with their nieces, nephews, and friends' children. But more than that, they loved being together and were totally devoted to each other. Up until the day my uncle died, at the age of eighty-two, they acted like newlyweds. Does my aunt have any regrets? Only one: that she outlived her beloved husband."

Remember, if you have a child, there's no turning back, but if you do make a decision to remain child-free, it's not written in stone. You can change your mind down the road and look into other options, especially adoption and foster parenthood. Most couples, however, who do make the decision to remain child-free are happy with that decision and stick with it. Indeed, research shows that child-free couples are just as happy as couples who have children. While they may have moments of regret, we all have those moments about every decision we make, including the decision to have children.

The need to nurture

One of the reasons people want to have children is to fulfill their maternal or paternal need to nurture. But couples waiting to conceive or adopt—or even child-free couples—can fulfill their need to have children involved in their current lives, be they nieces and nephews, children of friends, or children in their community. In fact, volunteering to work with children, especially underprivileged children, is a wonderful way to help them and yourself.

You can volunteer to...

- Be a reading or math tutor at your local school.
- Be a Big Brother or Big Sister.
- Be a mentor in an after-school program.
- Be a Scout leader.
- Be a Little League coach.
- Be a Sunday school teacher.
- Work with homeless children.
- Work with children with AIDS.

- Work with handicapped children.
- Be a foster parent.

Another way to fulfill your need for nurturing is by bringing pets into your life. Dogs, cats, and other pets require care, nurturing, and affection—and you get plenty of affection in return. And if you do decide to continue pursuing parenthood, you can have both a child and what every child longs for—a family pet.

Just the facts

- Feeling a loss of control and loss of self-esteem are common reactions to infertility.

- Taking charge of your fertility treatment can help you regain a sense of control.

- Infertility is akin to the death of a dream; allow yourself time to mourn.

- Infertility counselors are specifically trained to deal with the emotional, social, and other consequences of infertility, while most psychotherapists do not have this training.

- Joining a self-help organization or support group is one of the best things you can do to survive and resolve your infertility.

- Child-free living is a reasonable option for many couples.

GET THE SCOOP ON...
Treatment costs ▪ Infertility insurance ▪
Understanding your policy ▪ What's covered and
what's not ▪ Financial strategies ▪ State mandates

Money Matters

A s you have seen in the previous chapters, the diagnosis and treatment of infertility has made major strides over the past 20 years. As a result, the majority of infertile couples today who seek treatment will succeed in having their own children. The bad news is that many couples cannot afford the necessary treatment. According to RESOLVE, out of the 5.4 million infertile couples in the United States, only 2 million are getting treatment, and the high cost of treatment is one of the major reasons why more couples don't seek help. Many of those who do pursue treatment wind up making tremendous financial sacrifices. But for most of those who succeed, the sacrifices were well worth it. Still, there are ways to lessen the financial burden, and this chapter will help you do just that.

The costs of treatment

Like so many aspects of infertility, the costs of treatment—and insurance coverage for those costs—can be highly unpredictable and a bit of a crap shoot. In addition to your diagnosis and treatment options,

Bright Idea

Take all your insurance documentation to your first appointment. If you've got your policy information at your fingertips, the office manager or billing supervisor will be better able to help you work out the best way to approach your insurer for reimbursement.

the costs depend on such factors as the part of the country in which you live, how many competing programs are in your area, the laws in the state in which you live, and which insurance policy you have. And the actual charges for treatment vary from program to program.

While it's impossible to predict what your total costs will be, by breaking down the treatment programs into component parts, it is possible to come up with an estimate of the kind of money you're looking at having to pay. No matter what form of treatment you ultimately decide upon, you will have to undertake an initial consultation. This may cost anywhere from $150 to $400, depending on where you live.

After the initial consultation with the doctor of your choice, you'll have to undergo a basic infertility work-up (see Chapter 6). The work-up itself consists of a variety of tests, from screening for infectious disease to ultrasound and laparoscopy. Each test adds to your overall costs, as the following table shows.

Sometimes additional blood tests may be required—to measure hormone levels during ovulation or during the luteal phase—and these will add from $45 to $100 to your bill, per test. Keep in mind that your particular case may not require every one of the tests included in the basic work-up. It's best to go into the process knowing what the possible costs are, however. The total can range considerably, from about $3,000 to over $10,000, depending on what diagnostic procedures are required, as well as where you have the work-up done.

Table 17.1: Average Costs Associated with the Standard Infertility Work-Up

Test Type	Average Price Range
Blood test	$200-$600
Hormone testing	$180-$1,500
Semen analysis	$150-$300
Ovulation test	$0 if done by basal body temperature charting; $40-$100 if done with an ovulation induction kit
Ultrasound	$125-$200
Ultrasound (pregnancy)	$175-$375
Endometrial biopsy	$75-$375 for the biopsy; $50-$150 for lab analysis
Postcoital test	$300-$400
Hysterosalpingogram	$400-$600
Cannulization of Fallopian tubes	$800-$1,200
Laparoscopy	$600-$1,200 for anesthesia; $1,400-$3,500 for hospital stay; $4,000-$8,000 for surgeon's fees
Hysteroscopy	$1,000-$2,500

If the basic work-up fails to disclose any abnormalities in your reproductive functions or those of your partner, further testing is indicated. These advanced tests can run from $200 to $400 for a hemizona assay or a sperm penetration assay. Some doctors may order antibody testing, which can cost from $75 to $100 per test; and immunological testing, which can cost from

$1,000 to $2,000. Obviously, in both the basic work-up and in the advanced testing phase of your infertility treatment, it may be necessary that some tests be run more than once, further increasing treatment costs.

Fertility drugs

In addition to the cost of the tests themselves, medications may be required. For ovulation induction—the most commonly recommended treatment for infertility—the drug clomiphene citrate (Clomid or Serophene) is prescribed, at an average cost of $20 to $55 per ovulatory cycle. In some cases, clomiphene citrate is replaced by, or prescribed in conjunction with, human menopausal gonadotropin (Humegon or Repronex), or other medications such as Metrodin (an FSH frequently used with clomiphene), which can cost as much as $75 per dose.

Drug prices can also vary tremendously and have a major impact on your total cost of treatment. Since you will need to take anywhere from 15 to 40 doses during a single ovulatory cycle, the monthly cost of the medication can range from $800 to $2,500.

Fertility drugs are available at a discount, especially through online pharmacies. We again caution you to be very careful if you decide to purchase your drugs online; be sure to buy from websites with the Verified Internet Pharmacy Practice Sites (VIPPS) seal of approval, which identifies licensed Internet pharmacies. You can also find out if an online pharmacy is a

---

 Moneysaver

If possible, charge all your drugs and fertility treatments to a credit card that offers frequent flyer miles. You can then spend those hard-earned frequent flyer miles on a well-deserved vacation.

Watch Out!

Some patients sell their extra medication on the Internet. This is both illegal and potentially dangerous for both buyer and seller. Fertility drugs must be properly refrigerated and stored. There is no guarantee that someone's left-over drugs are safe or even the same drug you use.

licensed pharmacy in good standing with the National Association of Boards of Pharmacy at www.nabp.net.

Don't buy drugs from foreign or off-shore suppliers; there is no way of knowing whether or not they are safe and effective. The drug you get may be different from its American counterpart, it may have expired, or it may even have been contaminated. Also, there is no quality control or dosing standard, and no guarantee that it will be shipped properly and safely. And last but not least, it's against the law, and the Food and Drug Administration (FDA) can confiscate your drugs. For more detailed information about buying drugs online, check out the websites for RESOLVE at www.resolve.org and the FDA at www.fda.gov/oc/buyonline.

Monitoring ovulation

As we discussed in Chapter 7, if you take fertility drugs, your physician must monitor you through the ovulatory cycle to avoid hyperstimulation syndrome. The costs of monitoring not only can be quite high, they can be very unpredictable. It depends on which drugs you take and for how long, as well as on how many ultrasound scans (at $75 to $200 per scan) or blood tests (at $45 to $100 per test) you need.

Intrauterine insemination (IUI)

If your doctor recommends that IUI be performed during the ovulation induction cycle, you'll be looking at a further series of charges. These are broken down in the next table.

Table 17.2: IUI Costs per Ovulatory Cycle

Procedure	Purpose	Average Price Range
hCG injection	Triggers ovulation	$20-$40
Laboratory preparation of sperm	Prepares sperm for insemination	$75-$250
IUI procedure	Insemination of sperm into the uterus	$225-$400
Progesterone suppositories or daily progesterone injections	Luteal phase support	$40-$120

Surgical costs

If you and your doctor have decided that you will need surgical intervention, the costs of infertility treatment rise dramatically. Depending on the condition requiring treatment, total fees for surgical intervention can range from about $3,000 to $18,000. The following table gives a breakdown of these costs for common surgical procedures used to correct infertility.

Surgical intervention is obviously more costly than outpatient procedures for a number of reasons. The most significant cost factors are the surgeon's fees and the cost of the hospital stay, and the latter costs can really mount up if any complications extend your stay. Unaccounted for in the cost breakdown is the recovery time at home, which may be as long as six weeks. If your employer will not provide paid sick leave for an extended absence, you must take into account the lost income you will incur as well.

The ARTs

The ARTs are the high-end infertility treatments. They are also, unfortunately, the least likely forms of infertility treatment to be covered by insurers. These technologies, discussed in detail in Chapters 9 and 10, range from in-vitro fertilization (IVF) to

Table 17.3: Typical Costs of Surgical Treatment for Infertility

Type of Surgery	Hospital Fees	Anesthesia	Surgeon's Fees
Hysteroscopy, myomectomy	$1,200-$3,500	$600-$1,200	$4,000-$8,000
Laparoscopy	$1,800-$5,000	$600-$1,200	$3,200-$6,500
Exploratory laparotomy (includes OR and Recovery)	$4,500-$13,000	$800-$1,000	$4,800-$10,000

gamete intrafallopian transfer (GIFT) and zygote intrafallopian transfer (ZIFT). The cost is even higher if your IVF treatment requires an egg donor or surrogate carrier.

GIFTs will cost as much as IVFs, and then some—they have the additional expense of egg recovery to consider as well. The following table provides a breakdown of the costs associated with the ARTs.

Table 17.4: Breakdown of Basic Costs Associated with ARTs, per Cycle

Procedure	Average Cost Range
IVF	$6,500-$6,800
Ovulation stimulating drugs	$2,000-$5,000
Embryo freezing	$100-$500
Embryo storage costs (often not charged for first year)	$10-$50/month
Frozen embryo transfer (with estrogen-progesterone preparation of the uterus)	$600-$2,000
Donor eggs	$14,000-$20,000

Watch Out!

The cost breakdown for the ARTs presupposes a single cycle—a circumstance that rarely applies to real-life treatments for infertility. A couple can typically expect to undergo ART therapy for at least two or three ovulatory cycles.

When you add the costs of involving a third party in your infertility treatment, prices increase dramatically. At this point, legal fees are added to the medical costs, as are fees for medical and psychological screening of the surrogate. Finally, payments to the surrogate—insurance coverage, medical expenses, and delivery of the child—must be accounted for. The use of a surrogate gestational carrier can cost anywhere from $10,000 to more than $55,000. This is in addition to the costs of the IVF itself.

The insurance debate

As you can see, the costs of infertility treatment are both high and highly variable. And in these days of HMOs and coverage limitations, it can be extremely difficult to find ways to get the treatments you need without breaking the family bank. Some insurers refuse to cover any of the costs associated with infertility treatment. Others restrict their coverage to the basic work-up, or cover only some of the available treatments. If your particular condition is not among those for which covered treatments are appropriate, your insurance is not going to be of much help to you.

When you combine the fact that different carriers offer different means of coverage with the difficulty most of us face trying to understand the contract legalese of most insurance policies, trying to figure out what you can count on for help in paying for treatment can be daunting. This is perhaps the major reason why an estimated 60 percent of all infertile couples never even explore treatment options.

Infertility as dysfunction

The single biggest reason for the difficulty in finding appropriate insurance coverage for infertility treatment is that there are no real standards for it in the health insurance industry. There are also no state or federal agency standards for the regulation of coverage. Coverage disparities can be noted among insurers, as well as among states, which is discussed later in this chapter and in Appendix E.

> **❝**I was afraid I'd wind up with an empty pocket-book and an empty cradle.**❞**
>
> —Mary Ann, 35

Part of the problem is that, in the United States, infertility treatment is largely regarded as a non-necessity. The health insurance industry argues that the costs of covering procedures like IVF would price their overall coverage packages beyond the reach of most buyers of insurance—and the buyers are employers, not individual patients. In the insurers' view, infertility is not a disease—it doesn't threaten life or health—but rather a dysfunction. In addition, they tend to define the expensive, high-tech ARTs as "experimental" rather than as accepted medical practice.

Proponents of coverage for infertility treatment, on the other hand, strictly hold to a definition of infertility as an illness. The American Society for Reproductive Medicine (ASRM) takes issue with the definition of ARTs as experimental, citing a high live-birth rate per IVF cycle (35 percent) that is now even higher than the normal conception rate for healthy couples (20 to 25 percent).

Infertility as disability

One route that has been taken to force coverage from employer-provided insurers has been to attempt to change federal legislation defining infertility as a disability. The Americans with Disabilities Act (ADA) of 1990 contains a provision that "requires reasonable modifications of policies and practices that may be discriminatory." This has been interpreted by some to mean that employers may be required to modify the insurance coverage they offer to include infertility treatments.

Watch Out!

Even if your insurance company covers the cost of IVF, they typically pay only 15 to 25 percent of the costs.

Breaking down the language of the ADA provision, the legal argument for coverage starts with the premise that health insurance is a significant "policy and practice" of employment: It is a standard benefit offered to workers, provided on a contractual basis. While there is no federal requirement that employers *offer* insurance to their workers, once insurance is provided, the employer is required to include coverage of disability conditions unless there is good cause for their exclusion. The limitation of coverage must be based on "sound actuarial data or other legitimate business or insurance justification," writes Gwen Thayer Handelman, associate professor of law at Washington and Lee University School of Law. The denial of coverage, then, can be justified by demonstrating that providing it would be too costly for the employer to bear.

This argument has implications for paying for infertility treatment on two counts, both of which lie at the heart of the debate between insurers and proponents of coverage. These are:

■ Is infertility a disability?

■ Is it too costly for employers to offer coverage for infertility treatment?

Both of these issues are currently being addressed in federal courts and remain unresolved as yet.

The fundamental point of disagreement between insurers and proponents of infertility coverage is whether or not reproduction can be defined as a "major life activity." A disability, according to the ADA, must involve an impairment that impacts upon an individual's ability to engage in one or more major life activities. Unfortunately, the ADA never specifically defined what "major life activity" means. Walking, seeing, hearing, and learning are examples of such activities that have been accepted by consensus in the courts, but other activities, such as procreation, are still disputed. One side of the debate argues that major life activities are only those that have a "public, economic, or daily character." The other side argues that reproduction "falls well within the phrase" and is "central to the life process itself." The ultimate determination as to whether reproduction is a major life activity, and therefore whether infertility qualifies as a disability, remains to be made.

Business as usual

Even if the determination is made that infertility is a disability and thus covered under the ADA, it is possible for employers to refuse to provide coverage for certain disabilities if providing it would be too costly. If the cost of providing coverage would constitute an "undue burden" on the employer, the ADA permits that it be excluded from benefits packages.

The insurance industry—and many employers—make the claim that it is indeed the case that infertility coverage would be too expensive. However, in 1993 a team of researchers provided a study for the Massachusetts Commission on Insurance. The researchers found that infertility treatment costs constituted less than one half of 1 percent of the total medical expenses for the period under study. In terms of dollars and cents, this works out to under two dollars per month per insured. In other words, there were no appreciable increased insurance costs to the consumer.

Until these two issues—infertility as disability, and the cost to consumers of providing coverage—are resolved, there is no likelihood of federally mandated coverage for infertility treatment.

 Bright Idea

Talk to the person who handles insurance for your doctor ahead of time. He or she can not only help you with your claims, but also give you an idea of how much your treatment will cost and what, if any, coverage you're entitled to.

Proponents for coverage, most notably RESOLVE and the ASRM, are actively involved in supporting cases that will provoke definitive court rulings supporting the right of individuals to secure infertility coverage.

Insurers and infertility treatment advocates vehemently disagree on the costs to insurers of offering coverage. You'll see studies cited by both sides, each offering a different perspective on the issue. Check the sources of the studies cited to see if they might to be biased by the opinions or objectives of the group that commissioned their research.

What's covered, what's not

In the absence of a coherent set of industry and federal standards requiring coverage for infertility therapy, couples seeking treatment are faced with a patchwork of policies, plans, and state laws.

Some policies cover diagnostic procedures but won't pay for treatment. Some will cover low-tech treatments, and most refuse to cover such high-tech treatments as IVF. And even when treatments are covered, drugs are often excluded.

So what can you do if you're considering infertility treatment but can't handle the out-of-pocket expense? First, explore your insurance options. If your current plan provides little or no coverage, check to see if you can change carriers, and if there is one available to you that covers more of your costs. And by all means, take a long hard look at your treatment options. If you can't get coverage for the whole treatment regimen, break it down and seek coverage for its component parts.

 Watch Out!

Be creative, but be careful. While you and your doctor's office might have some leeway in describing your condition in order to get insurance coverage, be sure not to commit insurance fraud! It's a felony and can land you in jail!

Type of carrier

The amount of coverage available to you for your infertility treatment will depend on the type of insurance plan you carry. There are four general types of insurance plans:

1. **Commercial companies.** Aetna, Prudential: basic medical plan, major medical plan, or combo.

2. **Nonprofits.** BlueCross/BlueShield: basic and major medical combo.

3. **Self-insurers.** Employers that pay benefits directly: basic and major medical combo.

4. **Provider networks (PPOs)/HMOs.** Require primary care provider who'll authorize your use of a specialist. This type of insurer can be one of four types: Staff Type HMO, Group Type HMO, IPA Type HMO, and Network Type HMO.

The first three types of plans generally have either a deductible (averaging about $250 to $500 per year) or a co-payment (percentage of total) that you are liable to pay. The fourth type of plan usually imposes a co-payment obligation on its insured in the form of a specific dollar amount that is payable by the insured at the time a service is performed.

The coverage offered also varies by state, and state laws often impose different requirements on the various types of insurers. Be sure to determine whether or not your state has mandated infertility treatment coverage, the terms of any such mandate, the type of insurer that issued your policy, and the terms of your insurance coverage. (State mandates are discussed later in this chapter.)

Decoding your policy

There has been a trend in recent years away from the legalese that once characterized all insurance policies, but the contracts are still difficult for most of us to understand. A common mistake made by employees is to confuse the "statement

Moneysaver

If you know that you are likely to go through several ART procedures, consider taking out a private health insurance policy. Even though they are far more expensive than group insurance, the greater coverage private insurance offers can easily offset the increase in premiums.

of benefits" they receive upon their initial employment with an actual copy of their policy. The Employee Retirement, Insurance, and Security Act (ERISA) requires your employer to provide you with a true copy on your request, but you'll probably have to go to your human resources department to pick one up.

Once you've secured a copy of your actual insurance contract, one that is dated for the current year and bears all necessary signatures, it's time to sit down and evaluate the language to determine precisely what kind of coverage you're entitled to. Here's a checklist of what to look out for:

- **Inclusions and exclusions.** Be sure to check to see if infertility services in general, or specific treatments like IVF, are specifically included or excluded.

- **Limits of coverage.** See if there are any specified limitations of coverage. Some policies have a total lifetime limit for all medical coverages, some may specifically place a cap on infertility treatments. Ask if there are any annual or lifetime limitations on infertility coverage, or coverage for a specific treatment such as IVF.

- **Diagnosis.** Carefully check the terms of coverage for diagnostic tests and procedures. Even if your coverage excludes infertility treatment but does not specify that diagnosis is excluded, you should be able to file claims for coverage of diagnostic testing and procedures— these can make up one third of your total infertility therapy costs.

- **Prescription drugs.** If your policy specifies that all of your prescriptive drugs are covered, you may be able to get reimbursed even if your policy specifically excludes infertility treatment.

- **Specific treatments.** Check the specific terms of coverage. Some policies will cover "services to restore reproductive abilities" but exclude infertility treatments that seek to use artificial means to achieve pregnancy. This exclusion means that IVF and IUI won't be covered.

Once you've gotten a good sense of just what your insurance excludes, you're in a better position to start calculating how you're going to handle the costs of your infertility treatment. At this point you have to decide just how much, if anything, to tell your employer and your insurance carrier.

Mum's the word

Because the actual owner of the policy that provides your coverage is your employer, you want to be careful about how much you disclose when you begin infertility treatments. This is especially true if your insurer places limits on your infertility coverage. Remember, your employer can generally change the terms of your coverage at any time simply by contacting the insurer and negotiating new terms or exclusions. If your policy currently provides favorable coverage terms for infertility, but your employer (or insurer) chooses not to accept the liability, tipping either one off on your plans to undergo fertility treatment might easily spur a quick change in the coverage offered, and you might find yourself facing medical costs that you had blithely assumed would be covered.

 Watch Out!

Religious groups are exempt from providing policies to their employees that cover treatments that conflict with the beliefs of the group. For many, infertility treatments fall into the "conflict" category.

There *are* benevolent employers that will willingly provide coverage, just as there are insurers that will pay for your infertility treatments, but unless you know for certain that this is true in your case, you need to take care to protect your financial interests. Until the legal climate has changed to more directly favor the patients over the interests of business, it is probably wise to be discreet about your treatment plans. This will require that you work with the financial advisor or office manager at your treatment center or clinic.

> ❝ The word infertility raises a red flag with insurance companies who see dollar signs go up when they hear the word. They fear that your treatment will cost them thousands of dollars in drugs and IVF, which in fact may be the case. But that's their problem, not yours—unless they refuse to pay. ❞
>
> —From *Getting Pregnant When You Thought You Couldn't* by Yakov M. Epstein and Ilelane S. Rosenberg (Warner, 2001)

For example, if your treatment is billed as a single charge for the total services rendered—let's say, for an IVF—your claim for coverage could quite easily be denied. However, claims for fees covering individual elements of the IVF procedure might easily be covered, if they are billed separately. Your clinic's office manager can prepare individual bills for your various blood tests and ultrasound tests, as they were broken out in the beginning of this chapter. Similarly, if your policy excludes IVF but covers treatment for the underlying causes of infertility, payment for much of the diagnostic treatment, and even the fertility drugs, might be offered without a protest.

Cost-cutting strategies

If your current insurance carrier or HMO has very restrictive policies regarding the coverage of infertility treatment, and your employer provides a list of alternative insurance options,

Bright Idea

If you talk to your insurance company and they agree to cover certain procedures, be sure to get it in writing in case there is a disputed claim later on.

explore the terms of the other carriers on this list. It could be
well worth your while to switch plans to one more lenient in its
coverage. This is best done early on—preferably before you
begin any infertility treatment and your employer learns that
you're seeking such treatment. Let's look at several other ways
that may help you cut the costs of treatment.

Pre-paid ovulation induction

Some programs and insurance companies are offering their
patients who do not have other insurance coverage for infertility the option of pre-paying a set price for their ovulation cycles
at a discount. If the cycle involves more drugs and monitoring
than anticipated, the patient does not have to pay the additional
costs, but if the cycle involves fewer than expected, the patient
receives a partial refund.

Money-back guarantees

Money-back guarantees or refund policies are a relatively new
and growing innovation for financing the ARTs. This typically
involves paying a predetermined lump sum that will cover the
costs of three (or sometimes four) ART cycles. Usually the couple also pays a "premium"—an additional amount that is based
on their chances of conceiving in three cycles. If you become
pregnant, even in the first cycle, the full amount is kept by the
program. If, however, you do not succeed in three cycles, you
will get a full or partial refund, depending on the terms of the
policy. If, for example, you paid a premium, the premium will
not be refunded.

In some cases, refund policies make good sense. But you
have to evaluate the policy based on your own chance of success

Bright Idea

If you're considering a money-back guarantee, be sure to find out if it covers you for a pregnancy or live birth. Live-birth coverage is definitely preferable since a pregnancy can end in a miscarriage.

and financial risk involved. If you are in your late 30s or early 40s, you are likely to pay a very high premium because of your lower chance of success. If you do become pregnant, all well and good. They keep the money and you have your baby. However, if you do not become pregnant, your refund will not include that high premium you paid. Whether or not it makes financial sense is up to you.

Refund policies also give the programs an added incentive to succeed in getting you pregnant. However, this can be a double-edged sword. To boost your chance of success, some programs transfer more than two or three embryos. Unfortunately, this will also boost your chance of a multiple pregnancy along with the subsequent risks to you and your babies (see Chapter 10). Some programs don't offer this option to patients with infertility insurance coverage.

Foreign ARTs

We've emphasized many times throughout this book that relaxing and taking a vacation can't get you pregnant. On the other hand, it certainly can't hurt. And in some cases, traveling abroad may actually help you achieve a pregnancy at a significant savings. More and more couples are choosing to travel abroad for their ART treatments. Drug costs, surgical costs, and hospital costs are all considerably cheaper in many other countries.

In the past, couples from the United States have traveled to Great Britain for the ARTs, where success rates were high and costs low. But recently, their costs have risen too high and couples are now traveling to such diversified countries as Italy,

Romania, Germany, South Africa, and Belgium. Some couples seeking egg donors of their own ethnic backgrounds travel to Israel or the Far East for the ARTs. In addition to being cheaper—in some cases couples get two cycles for the price of one in the United States—you get to travel to some interesting countries. And if you've been charging your infertility treatment to a credit card that offers frequent flyer miles, you can use those miles to pay for your airfare.

There are downsides, however. The ARTs in many of these countries are not nearly as advanced as in the United States, so your chances of success may be compromised. Also, medical standards—not to mention sanitary conditions—may not be on par with the programs in the United States.

Moving

Medical care of all types tends to be far more expensive in major urban centers than elsewhere in the country, so where you live makes a real difference in the costs of these procedures. A simple IVF can range from $3,500 to $11,000, and that's before you add in the costs of ovulation-stimulating drugs. Where you live and where you go for treatment not only can have a significant impact on the cost of your care, but on the likelihood of your being reimbursed. If you have enough time to plan well in advance of seeking treatment, and you live in one of the states that provides no mandate for coverage (or fails to enforce mandates that have been passed by the legislature), you might consider relocating. Massachusetts, for example, has the most patient-friendly legislation mandating infertility treatment coverage, while California and Texas are extremely lax in enforcement of their laws. Most states have no protective legislation at all.

 Watch Out!

States that mandate to offer infertility coverage *do not* require employers to pay for the coverage. You may have to pay for the additional coverage yourself.

State mandates

A few states mandate coverage for infertility treatment in one way or another. But "mandated coverage" means different things in different states. So-called soft mandates—the most common type—require only that infertility insurance be available in theory. Insurance companies in those states only have to *offer* coverage, but they are not actually required to provide it to everybody. "Hard" mandates are a much rarer breed—they require that some form of insurance coverage be offered to the insurance consumer (that's you) as opposed to just the insurance buyer (your employer). But even where coverage is "hard" mandated, lack of enforcement has often meant that insurers feel free to delete it or deny payment. Only two states, Massachusetts and Illinois, actually have put some teeth into their legislation.

- **Mandate to offer** coverage means that the state must offer their clients a policy that covers infertility treatment. The cost for that additional coverage would then be paid for by the employer or the patient.

- **Mandate to cover** means that the state requires that all insurance companies provide coverage for infertility treatment in each policy. The cost of the policies include the cost of infertility coverage.

As of Summer 2005, 15 states have passed laws that require insurers *to either cover or offer coverage* for infertility diagnosis and treatment. The 15 states with legislation that addresses the full range of infertility treatments vary widely to the degree in which they mandate coverage and enforce the laws that currently appear on their books.

 Moneysaver

Many states require that you document a longstanding (two- to five-year) condition of unexplained infertility in order to be reimbursed. Make sure you save all records of your treatment, from the very first consultation, so you can address this question if your insurer raises it.

Watch Out!

Even if you live in a state that mandates infertility coverage, self-insurers are normally exempt from the terms of the mandate. Since large companies are generally self-insurers, the state mandates do not apply to them.

Of these 15 states, 9 have laws that mandate insurance companies *to cover* infertility treatment; 5 states have laws that mandate insurance companies *to offer coverage* for infertility treatment. While most states with laws requiring insurance companies to offer or provide coverage for infertility treatment include coverage for in-vitro fertilization, California and New York have laws that specifically exclude coverage for IVF.

For a detailed description of what the infertility insurance coverage is for each of these 15 states, see Appendix E.

It's no coincidence that the most comprehensive infertility insurance coverage laws are in Massachusetts, the birth place of RESOLVE. Founded by Barbara Eck Menning in her kitchen in 1974 in Belmont, Massachusetts, RESOLVE's national headquarters have been in that state for three decades. In 2004, they moved to Bethesda, Maryland, to be closer to the National Institutes of Health (NIH) and other influential government departments. RESOLVE has been a leading force in the fight for the rights of infertile couples to have accessible and affordable infertility treatment. Indeed, RESOLVE staff and members, members of other infertility organizations across the nation, and the ASRM have successfully lobbied in many of the states listed previously and continue to fight to change the laws so infertile men and women can get the insurance coverage they need and deserve.

A few final thoughts

Throughout this book, we have tried to illustrate the challenges faced by infertile couples, as well as their courage and fortitude to overcome those challenges. Infertile men and women often find new strengths that they never knew existed, and—as we saw in Chapter 16—many feel that they have gained something positive from their infertility trials and tribulations, whether or not they become pregnant or parents. Many of those who do become parents believe infertility helped make them better parents. Many say that they had to work so hard—and pay so much—to achieve what comes so easily for most couples, they feel they could never take their children for granted. Finding better ways to pay for infertility—especially getting insurance companies to foot more of the bill—will lessen the financial sacrifices infertile couples have to make. It will also help them pay for the costs of raising their longed-for children.

Thanks to the advancements in reproductive medicine—and the dedication and skill of reproductive endocrinologists and embryologists—most infertile couples will succeed in having their own children. And most infertile men and women, regardless of their outcome, will choose to put their infertility behind them and get on with their lives. But some—like Barbara Eck Menning—use their experiences to help other infertile couples as volunteers in support groups, or put their energies into lobbying for the rights of other infertile couples. Through their efforts, both the financial and emotional costs of infertility treatment will become more bearable.

Just the facts

- The high cost of infertility treatment is the main reason many couples who need infertility treatment don't receive it.

- Even if your insurance policy specifically denies coverage for infertility treatment, you may still be able to get many of the tests and procedures covered if you file for them separately.

- Your doctor's or program's financial office can help you decipher the complexity of your insurance policy.

- Money-back guarantees, traveling to other countries for treatment, and even moving to another state are ways infertile couples can cut the costs of treatment.

- Fifteen states currently mandate some form of infertility coverage.

Glossary

acrosome reaction test   Test used to determine if sperm heads can actually undergo the chemical changes needed to dissolve an egg's tough outer shell and penetrate it.

adhesions   Scar tissue—often found in or on the uterus, Fallopian tubes, or uterine cavity—that attaches to the surface of organs.

adrenal glands   Two small glands on the top of each kidney which produce steroids and other hormones.

AID   Artificial insemination with donor sperm. *See* artificial insemination.

AIDS (Acquired Immune Deficiency Syndrome) Immune disease caused by the human immunodeficiency virus (HIV).

AIH   Artificial insemination with husband's or partner's sperm. *See* artificial insemination.

amenorrhea   Absence of menstruation.

amniocentesis   Procedure performed around the sixteenth week of pregnancy in which a small amount of amniotic fluid is removed and studied for chromosomal abnormalities.

ampulla   Trumpet-shaped area of the Fallopian tube near the ovary; also, a widening in the upper end of the vas deferens in which sperm are stored.

androgens Male sex hormones.

andrologist M.D. or Ph.D. specifically trained in the diagnosis and treatment of male reproduction problems.

anovulation Total absence of ovulation; menses may still occur.

anteflexed uterus A uterus that is tilted forward and folds inward upon itself.

anteverted uterus A uterus that is tilted toward the front of the abdomen.

antibodies A substance produced by the body's autoimmune system to protect itself from foreign substances, such as viruses or bacteria. Antibodies can also attack parts of a person's own body.

antisperm antibodies Antibodies in men or women that react to sperm as foreign substances and attack and immobilize or kill them. They can also cause hostile cervical mucus.

artificial insemination (AI) A procedure in which sperm is placed in a cervix or uterus for the purpose of achieving a pregnancy. Also referred to as therapeutic insemination (TI). *See* also AIH and AID.

aspermia Absence of sperm.

aspiration Procedure in which eggs are retrieved from ovaries, and sperm are retrieved from the testes or epididymis by means of suction.

assisted hatching Micromanipulation procedure using chemicals, mechanical techniques, or lasers, in which the outer hard surface covering an embryo is thinned to help improve implantation.

assisted reproductive technology (ART) Treatment methods related to in-vitro fertilization (IVF) and embryo transfer.

azoospermia Absence of sperm in the seminal fluid; may be due to blockage or impaired sperm production.

basal body temperature (BBT) The body temperature of a person recorded upon arising before activity of any kind.

BBT chart Record of basal body temperature over time to detect when ovulation has likely taken place. This is a very crude test and therefore inaccurate; its main advantages are its low cost and simplicity.

beta-hCG test Blood test to determine pregnancy.

bicornate uterus A congenital malformation of the uterus in which there are two separate cavities (double uterus), with each one having just one Fallopian tube.

biochemical pregnancy (chemical pregnancy) A positive blood or urine hCG test, but one that does not continue beyond a low level, so there is no ongoing pregnancy.

biopsy Surgical removal of a tissue sample for analysis.

biphasic pattern A distinct temperature elevation seen on a basal body temperature chart.

blastocyst Early stage of embryo development, usually occurring around Day 5 after fertilization, at which time a fertilized egg loses its protective coating and is ready to attach in the uterine lining.

blastomere One cell of an early, multi-cell embryo.

capacitation Change in a sperm cell that renders it capable of fertilizing an egg.

CBC (complete blood count) Routine blood test to determine the presence or absence of infection and/or anemia.

cervical canal An opening into the uterus which produces mucus that facilitates sperm movement.

cervical mucus Secretions that are produced by the cervix that change consistency during the different phases of the menstrual cycle; during ovulation, cervical mucus becomes thin and watery to facilitate sperm movement into the uterus.

cervix The lower portion of the uterus projecting into the vagina; produces mucus that facilitates different steps during conception.

chemical pregnancy　*See* biochemical pregnancy.

Chlamydia trachomatis　Organism responsible for chlamydial infection; considered a sexually transmitted disease, which may cause infertility and neonatal infections.

chromosomal aneuploidy　Abnormal number of chromosomes.

chromosomes　Rod-shaped bodies in a cell's nucleus that carry the genetic material (DNA). Humans have 46 chromosomes—23 from the mother and 23 from the father.

cilia　Hair-like projections found in the Fallopian tubes.

cleavage　Early division of fertilized egg.

clinical pregnancy　Pregnancy in which the fetus is shown to have a heartbeat on ultrasound examination.

conception　Fertilization of an egg by a sperm resulting in an embryo.

congenital abnormality　Anatomical or other defect that is present at birth and usually not genetic in nature.

corpus luteum　Special structure that forms on the ovary from an ovulated follicle that begins to produce progesterone to help the endometrium prepare for a fertilized egg.

cryopreservation　Technique used to store cells, usually sperm, embryos, and eggs, in a frozen state for later use.

cryptorchidism　*See* undescended testes.

culdoscopy　A rarely used test in which a telescopic-like device is inserted through a small incision in the vagina to visualize the ovaries, the exterior of the Fallopian tubes, and the uterus.

DES (diethylstilbestrol)　Synthetic estrogen that had been thought to prevent miscarriage; responsible for some types of male and female infertility.

diagnostic hysteroscopy　Test in which a small telescopic-like device is inserted through the cervix into the uterus to examine the inside of the uterus.

diagnostic laparoscopy Test in which a small telescopic-like device is inserted through a small incision in or near the naval to examine the abdominal and pelvic organs.

diethylstilbestrol *See* DES.

DNA (Deoxyribonucleic acid) The chemical compound found within the nucleus of each cell that contains and transmits genetic information.

donor uteri *See* gestational carrier and surrogacy.

Down syndrome Genetic disorder, caused by a chromosomal abnormality, that causes mental retardation, facial malformations, and other medical conditions.

dysmenorrhea Painful menstruation.

dyspareunia Painful intercourse.

ectopic pregnancy Pregnancy in which the fertilized egg implants outside the uterine cavity (usually in the Fallopian tube, the ovary, or the abdominal cavity).

egg donation Third-party reproduction method in which eggs from a fertile woman are donated to an infertile woman for use in an assisted reproduction technology procedure.

egg retrieval Procedure in which eggs are removed from an ovary for fertilization in the laboratory.

ejaculate Seminal fluid (semen and sperm) expelled during orgasm and ejaculation.

ejaculation Process by which the sperm is released from the penis.

electroejaculation Process that can be used to stimulate ejaculation in men who are paralyzed below the waist.

embryo Early stage of fetal growth.

embryo donation Third-party reproduction method in which an infertile couple agrees to give extra or unneeded embryos to another infertile couple.

embryo transfer   Procedure in which an embryo produced through an assisted reproductive technology method is inserted into a woman's uterus.

endocrinologist   Medical doctor trained in the diagnosis and treatment of hormonal (endocrine) disorders.

endometrial biopsy   Procedure in which a sample of tissue is removed from the endometrium for analysis.

endometriosis   Condition in which normal endometrial tissue that should be found only within the uterine cavity is also found outside the uterus. Endometriosis can cause painful menstruation and infertility.

endometrium   Uterine lining.

epididymis   Tightly coiled, tubular structure attached to the testicle, where sperm mature and are stored.

estradiol (E_2)   Hormone released by the ovary and produced by a growing follicle.

estrogen   Major female sex hormone produced mainly by the ovaries.

Fallopian tubes   Pair of narrow tubes that carry the egg from the ovary to the uterus; the location of normal fertilization.

female-factor infertility   Used to describe infertility attributable to the female.

ferning   A fern-like pattern produced by dried cervical mucus that indicates the mucus is thin enough for sperm to pass through. It's used as an indication of impending ovulation.

fertilization   Union of an egg and sperm.

fetal loss   Miscarriage or stillbirth.

fetal reduction   Medical procedure to decrease the number of fetuses within the uterus in a multiple pregnancy.

fetus   Developing human organism after the ninth week of pregnancy until birth.

fibroid Noncancerous tumor found in the uterine wall. Also called myoma.

fimbria Fringed, finger-like outer ends of the Fallopian tubes.

FISH *See* fluorescence in situ hybridization.

fluorescence in situ hybridization (FISH) Test that helps identify chromosomal abnormalities in fertilized eggs.

follicle Tiny, fluid-filled, bubble-like structure on the ovary that usually contains and eventually releases an egg during ovulation.

follicle-stimulating hormone (FSH) Hormone produced by the pituitary gland that stimulates the ovary to develop a follicle.

follicular phase First half of the menstrual cycle during which an egg-containing follicle develops.

FSH *See* follicle-stimulating hormone.

galactorrhea Milky discharge from the breasts that may be due to excess prolactin rather than pregnancy.

gamete Male or female reproductive cell; sperm or egg, respectively.

gamete intrafallopian transfer (GIFT) Assisted reproduction technology procedure in which eggs and sperm are placed in the Fallopian tubes.

gene Structure within the nucleus of each cell that conveys hereditary characteristics and is mainly composed of DNA. *See* DNA.

genetic Determined by genes or chromosomes. Refers to heredity.

genetic abnormality A disorder which is the result of an error in the genes or chromosomes that may be inherited.

gestation Period of fetal development in the uterus until birth.

gestational carrier A woman—but not a genetic parent—who has an infertile couple's embryo implanted in her uterus and carries it to term for them. Also called surrogate host, and occasionally, donor uterus.

GIFT   *See* gamete intrafallopian transfer.

GnRH   *See* gonadotropin-releasing hormone.

gonad   Male or female sex organs; testicles or testes in men, ovaries in women.

gonadotropin   Hormone that can stimulate the testicles to produce sperm or the ovaries to produce eggs.

gonadotropin-releasing hormone (GnRH)   Hormone released from the hypothalamus that controls the production and release of FSH and LH from the pituitary gland.

gonorrhea   Sexually transmitted disease (STD) that is often asymptomatic but can cause infertility.

Graves' disease   *See* hyperthyroidism.

gynecologist   Medical doctor, board certified in the diagnosis and treatment of diseases of the female reproductive tract.

hamster (sperm) penetration assay   Test to determine whether sperm are capable of penetrating deep inside a hamster egg and fertilizing it.

high-resolution scrotal sonography or **venography**   Test to find varicoceles in the testicles too small to be felt during physical examination.

hirsutism   Overproduction or unusual body hair growth in women—such as a mustache—that gives them a masculinized appearance; frequently caused by an excess of androgens.

HIV   Human immunodeficiency virus, responsible for the development of AIDS.

host uterus   *See* gestational carrier.

hostile mucus   Cervical mucus that prevents sperm from swimming through the cervix to awaiting eggs.

HSG   *See* hysterosalpingogram.

Huhner test   *See* postcoital test.

hydrocele   Fluid buildup in the scrotum.

hyperandrogenism   *See* polycystic ovarian syndrome.

hyperprolactinemia Condition in which the pituitary gland produces an excess of prolactin. *See* galactorrhea.

hyperstimulation *See* ovarian hyperstimulation syndrome (OHSS).

hyperthyroidism (Graves' disease) A disorder that is associated with excessive thyroid activity; increases the risk of infertility and miscarriage.

hypo-osmotic swelling test Test that is used to help predict whether sperm can fertilize an egg.

hypospadias A deformity in which the urethra opens on the side of the shaft of the penis rather than the tip.

hypospermatogenisis Low sperm production.

hypothalamus A gland, located above the pituitary at the base of the brain, that sends hormonal signals to start the menstrual cycle.

hypothyroidism Deficiency in thyroid function.

hysterectomy Surgical removal of the uterus.

hysterosalpingogram (HSG) X-ray procedure using a contrast dye to evaluate the size and shape of the uterus and determine if the Fallopian tubes are open.

hysteroscopy Telescopic instrument inserted through the cervix to visualize the inside of the uterus and locate fibroids, polyps, scarring, and congenital deformities.

ICSI *See* intracytoplasmic sperm injection.

idiopathic infertility *See* unexplained infertility.

implantation Embedding of the fertilized egg in the lining of the uterus.

incompetent cervix A weakened cervix that opens prematurely, which can lead to a premature birth or pregnancy loss.

infertility Inability of a couple to achieve a successful pregnancy after one year of unprotected sexual intercourse, or after six months for a woman over 35.

intracytoplasmic sperm injection (ICSI) Micromanipulation procedure in which an individual sperm is inserted into an egg.

intrauterine insemination (IUI) Procedure in which usually washed sperm are inserted directly into the uterus through the cervical canal.

in-vitro fertilization (IVF) Assisted reproductive technology in which sperm and eggs are collected (retrieved) and are placed in a dish in the laboratory for fertilization. Any resulting embryos are gently placed in the uterine cavity (embryo transfer).

IUI *See* intrauterine insemination.

IVF *See* in-vitro fertilization.

karyotyping Genetic studies done in a lab that involve analyzing chromosomes for genetic defects.

Kleinfelter Syndrome Congenital abnormality in males that causes sterility, secondary female characteristics, and possible mental retardation.

laparoscopy Surgical procedure in which a telescopic-like device is inserted through a small incision in or near the navel to visualize the pelvic cavity, the ovaries, Fallopian tubes, and the exterior of the uterus.

laparotomy Abdominal surgery that can remove adhesions and repair Fallopian tubes; it requires a larger incision than a laparoscopy.

LH *See* luteinizing hormone.

LH surge Dramatic rise in luteinizing hormone levels that precedes and culminates in ovulation.

luteal phase Second half of the menstrual cycle, ranging from ovulation to the end of menses or embryo implantation.

luteal-phase defect Luteal phase (second half of menstrual cycle) with inadequate progesterone production.

luteinizing hormone (LH) Hormone, secreted by the pituitary gland, that causes the ovary to release a mature egg.

male-factor infertility Term to describe infertility attributable to a condition in the male partner.

meiosis Cell division that occurs during the formation of eggs and sperm that halves the number of chromosomes from 46 to 23. This prevents the number of chromosomes from doubling when fertilization takes place. After the egg is fertilized, it contains all 46 chromosomes, 23 from each parent. Compare with mitosis.

menstruation Cyclical, physiologic discharge through the vagina of blood and mucosal tissues from the nonpregnant uterus.

MESA *See* microsurgical epididymal sperm aspiration.

micromanipulation Procedures that allow working with a single sperm, egg, or embryo.

microsurgery Surgery in which microscopes, fine instruments, and microscopic sutures are used.

microsurgical epididymal sperm aspiration (MESA) Procedure in which sperm are removed from the epididymis.

miscarriage Spontaneous loss of a pregnancy.

mitosis Division of a cell into two genetically identical cells, each containing all 46 chromosomes. Most cells, except for sperm and egg cells (*see* meiosis), go through this cell division.

mittelschmerz Mild pain in the abdomen on or about the time of ovulation.

monophasic pattern No distinct temperature elevation seen on basal body temperature chart.

morphology *See* sperm morphology.

motility *See* sperm motility.

myoma *See* fibroid.

myomectomy Surgical removal of fibroid tumors from the uterus.

oligospermia Low number of sperm—below 20 million—in the semen.

oocyte   Egg, the female gamete or reproductive cell.

ovarian failure   Inability of the ovaries to respond to hormones and develop follicles.

ovarian hyperstimulation syndrome (OHSS)   Condition characterized by enlarged, painful ovaries and occasionally fluid accumulation; a possible side effect of ovulation induction.

ovary   Female sex glands in which eggs are formed.

ovulation   Release of mature egg from a follicle on the surface of an ovary.

ovulation induction   Use of fertility drugs to stimulate ovulation.

ovulatory phase   Time, usually around mid-cycle, when a mature egg is discharged from a follicle.

ovum   Egg released by the ovaries.

PCOD   Polycystic ovarian disease (*see* polycystic ovarian syndrome).

PCOS   *See* polycystic ovarian syndrome.

PCT   *See* postcoital test.

pelvic inflammatory disease (PID)   Pelvic disease usually caused by sexually transmitted or other infections; often leads to infertility.

penis   Major male reproductive organ.

percutaneous epididymal sperm aspiration (PESA)   Procedure in which sperm are extracted from the epididymis.

percutaneous testicular sperm aspiration (TESA)   Procedure in which a needle is inserted through the scrotum and sperm are aspirated from the testes.

PESA   *See* percutaneous epididymal sperm aspiration.

PID   *See* pelvic inflammatory disease.

pituitary gland   Small gland at the base of the brain beneath the hypothalamus that secretes many hormones, including follicle-stimulating hormone (FSH) and luteinizing hormone

(LH), which stimulate egg maturation and hormone production in the ovary.

polycystic ovarian syndrome (PCOS) Condition in which many cystic follicles develop in the ovaries but are not released. Sometimes referred to as polycystic ovarian disease (PCOD or hyperandrogenism), PCOS is caused by an imbalance in the FSH and LH ratio. Stein-Leventhal Syndrome is an exaggerated form of this condition.

polymerase chain reaction (PCR) Technique that replicates specific DNA sequences many times for analysis.

polyspermia Fertilization of an egg by more than one sperm.

postcoital (Sims-Huhner) test (PCT) Microscopic evaluation of cervical mucus shortly after sexual intercourse to determine sperm survival.

preimplantation genetic diagnosis (PGD) Technique that can be used during IVF procedures to test embryos for various genetic disorders prior to their transfer.

premature ejaculation Discharge of sperm from the penis prior to, or immediately after, entering the vagina.

primary infertility Infertility in a man or woman who has never had children.

progesterone Hormone secreted by the corpus luteum after ovulation that prepares the uterine lining to nourish an embryo.

progestin Synthetic hormone that has similar action as progesterone.

prolactin Pituitary hormone that stimulates breast milk production; excessive amounts can interfere with ovulation.

proliferative phase Phase of the menstrual cycle in which, under the influence of estrogen, the endometrium grows thicker.

prostate Male gland that surrounds the first portion of the urethra near the bladder and secretes a liquid that stimulates sperm movement.

retroflexed uterus Anatomic state in which the uterus tilts backward toward the spine and folds backward upon itself; a variation of a normal uterus.

retrograde ejaculation Condition in which semen flows backward into the bladder instead of forward into the urethra.

retroverted (tipped) uterus Anatomic abnormality in which the uterus tilts backward toward the spine.

salpingitis Inflammation of the Fallopian tubes.

scrotum Bag-like structure of skin and muscle that contains the testes.

secondary infertility Infertility in a man or a woman who has previously had a biological child.

selective reduction Intentional induced termination of one or more gestational sacs, usually in a multiple pregnancy.

semen Fluid containing glandular secretions and sperm discharged at ejaculation.

semen analysis Microscopic study of fresh ejaculate to determine quantity and quality of sperm.

seminiferous tubules Long, tube-like structures in the testicles where sperm are formed.

septate uterus Uterus abnormally divided by a wall of tissue. Can cause recurrent miscarriages.

sexual intercourse Sexual union.

sexually transmitted diseases (STDs) Variety of infections, including syphilis, gonorrhea, chlamydia, herpes, and AIDS, contracted through sexual activities.

Sims-Huhner test *See* postcoital test.

sonogram *See* ultrasonography.

sperm The male reproductive cell or gamete.

sperm agglutination The clumping of sperm, which can be the result of infection or antibodies.

sperm agglutination test Microscopic study to determine if sperm clump together, which impedes their ability to swim.

sperm analysis *See* semen analysis.

spermatogenesis Sperm production in the seminiferous tubules.

spermatozoa Sperm.

sperm bank Places where sperm are cryopreserved and stored for future therapeutic inseminations.

sperm count Number of sperm in an ejaculate.

spermicide Substance that can kill sperm.

sperm morphology Size and shape of sperm.

sperm motility Ability of sperm to swim forward.

sperm penetration test Using hamster eggs as a test model, it tests the ability of sperm to penetrate the outside layer of an egg and fertilize it.

sperm viscosity Thickness of the semen.

sperm washing Technique to separate sperm from seminal fluid.

spinnbarkheit Stretchability of cervical mucus.

split ejaculate Method of semen collection in which the first half of the ejaculate, which usually contains the most sperm, is caught in one container, the second in another.

spontaneous abortion *See* miscarriage.

Stein-Leventhal Syndrome *See* polycystic ovarian syndrome.

sterility Absolute inability to reproduce.

subfertile Another term for infertile. *See* infertility.

superovulation Use of fertility drugs to stimulate ovaries to produce a large number of eggs. Also called controlled ovarian hyperstimulation (COH).

surrogacy Third-party reproduction method in which a woman agrees to carry a fetus to term for another woman.

surrogate mother *See* surrogacy.

Tay-Sachs disease Deadly hereditary disease affecting young children often of Jewish heritage.

TESE *See* testicular sperm extraction.

testicles Male sex glands, located in the scrotum, which produce testosterone and sperm.

testicular biopsy Surgical procedure in which a small amount of testicular tissue is removed and then examined for microscopic structures including sperm as well as other cells.

testicular sperm extraction (TESE) Procedure in which sperm are removed directly from the testicular tissue.

testicular torsion A painful twisting of the testis inside the scrotum that can cause infertility.

testis (plural, testes) The male sex gland which is located in the scrotum and produces testosterone and sperm cells. They are also referred to as testicles.

testosterone The primary male sex hormone.

test-tube baby Popular term to describe babies conceived through assisted reproductive technologies, especially in-vitro fertilization (IVF).

TET *See* tubal embryo transfer.

therapeutic insemination *See* artificial insemination.

tubal embryo transfer (TET) Assisted reproductive technology method in which an embryo is placed in the Fallopian tubes.

tubal ligation Female sterilization procedure in which the continuity of the Fallopian tube is surgically interrupted; sometimes called "having your tubes tied."

tuboplasty Surgical procedure to repair the Fallopian tubes.

Turner Syndrome Genetic defect in which a female baby is born with only one X chromosome rather than two. This typically results in sterility.

ultrasonography Medical test that uses sound waves to visualize an organ.

undescended testes (cryptorchidism) Condition in which the testicles do not descend properly into the scrotum during fetal development.

unexplained infertility (idiopathic infertility) Term to describe a state in which no explanation for infertility is found after a couple has gone through complete testing and evaluation.

urinary luteinizing hormone (LH) test Test that measures luteinizing hormone in the urine and pinpoints more accurately the LH surge that precedes ovulation.

urologist Medical doctor, board certified in the diagnosis and treatment of disorders of the urinary tract and male sex organs.

uterus Part of the female reproductive system that holds and nourishes a fetus until birth; womb.

vagina Part of the female reproductive system that extends from the vulva to the cervix.

vaginal ultrasound An ultrasound study in which a transducer is inserted into the vagina. It is used to determine follicular development, the structure and status of the uterus, the presence of an early intrauterine pregnancy, or to guide egg retrieval.

varicocele Varicose veins around the testes.

varicocelectomy Procedure to remove varicoceles.

vas deferens Long tubelike structure that rises from the epididymis to the ejaculatory duct through which sperm travel during ejaculation.

vasectomy Male sterilization procedure in which the continuity of the vas deferens is surgically interrupted.

vasography X-ray of the vas deferens used to find a blockage in the pathway that allows sperm to be released.

washed sperm cells Sperm cells that have had the seminal plasma removed using tissue culture media and centrifugation.

ZIFT *See* zygote intrafallopian transfer.

zona pellucida   The hard outer surface of the egg, that the sperm must penetrate before fertilization can occur.

zygote   Fertilized egg; embryo in the early stages of development.

zygote intrafallopian transfer (ZIFT)   Assisted reproduction technology in which a zygote is placed into the Fallopian tubes.

Recommended Reading List

Aronson, Diane (RESOLVE). *Resolving Infertility.* HarperResource, 2001.

Ballweg, Mary Lou. *Endometriosis: The Complete Reference for Taking Charge of Your Health.* McGraw-Hill, 2003.

Bradstreet, Karen. *Overcoming Infertility Naturally.* Woodland Books, 1995.

Carter, Jean W., and Michael Carter. *Sweet Grapes: How to Stop Being Infertile and Start Living Again.* Perspectives Press, 1998.

Cooper, Susan Lewis, and Ellen Sarasohn Glazer. *Choosing Assisted Reproduction: Social, Emotional and Ethical Considerations.* Perspectives Press, 1998.

Domar, Alice D, and Alice Lesch Kelly. *Conquering Infertility: Dr. Alice Domar's Mind/Body Guide to Enhancing Fertility and Coping with Infertility.* Penguin, 2004.

Edwards, Robert. *Life Before Birth: Reflections on the Embryo Debate.* Basic Books, 1990.

Epstein, Yakov M., and Helane S. Rosenberg. *Getting Pregnant When You Thought You Couldn't.* Warner Books, 2001.

Appendix B

Glazer, Ellen Sarasohn. *The Long-Awaited Stork: A Guide to Parenting After Infertility.* Jossey-Bass, 1998.

Glazer, Ellen Sarasohn, and Evelina Weidman Sterling. *Having Your Baby Through Egg Donation.* Perspectives Press, 2005.

Henig, Robin. *Pandora's Baby: How the First Test-Tube Babies Sparked a Reproductive Revolution.* Houghton Mifflin, 2004.

Johnston, Patricia Irwin. *Adopting After Infertility.* Perspectives Press, 1994.

Lerner, Henry M., and Alice D. Domar. *Miscarriage: Why It Happens and How Best to Reduce Your Risks—A Doctor's Guide to the Facts.* Perseus Books, 2003.

Liebmann-Smith, Joan. *In Pursuit of Pregnancy.* Newmarket Press, 1989.

Lisle, Laurie. *Without Child: Challenging the Stigma of Childlessness.* Routledge, 1999.

Marsh, Margaret, and Wanda Ronner. *The Empty Cradle: Infertility in America from Colonial Times to the Present.* Johns Hopkins University Press. 1996.

May, Elaine Tyler. *Barren In the Promised Land: Childless Americans and the Pursuit of Happiness.* Basic Books, 1995.

Menning, Barbara Eck. *Infertility: A Guide for the Childless Couple.* Prentice Hall, 1977.

Robin, Peggy. *How to Be a Successful Fertility Patient.* William Morrow and Company, Inc., 1993.

Schover, Leslie R., and Anthony J. Thomas. *Overcoming Male Infertility: Understanding Its Causes and Treatments.* Wiley Publishing, Inc., 1999.

Shulgold, Barbara, and Lynne Sipiora. *Dear Barbara, Dear Lynne: The True Story of Two Women in Search of Motherhood.* Addison-Wesley, 1992.

Silber, Sherman J. *How to Get Pregnant with the New Technology.* Warner Books, 1998.

Stangel, John J. *The New Fertility and Conception: The Essential Guide for Childless Couples.* New American Library, 1993.

Thatcher, Samuel S. *PCOS: The Hidden Epidemic.* Perspectives Press. 2000.

Van Gulden, Holly, and Lisa Bartels-Rabb. *Parenting the Adopted Child.* Crossroad Classic, 1995.

Vercollone, Carol Frost, Heidi Moss, and Robert Moss. *Helping the Stork: The Choices and Challenges of Donor Insemination,* 1997.

Whitworth, Belinda. *Infertility the Natural Way.* Element Books, 1996.

Resource Guide

Medical organizations

American Association of Clinical Endocrinologists
904-353-7878
www.aace.com

American Association of Gynecologic Laparoscopists
1-800-554-AAGL (2245) or 562-946-8774
E-mail: generalmail@aagl.com
www.aagl.com

American Association of Tissue Banks (AATB)
703-827-9582
E-mail: aatb@aatb.org
www.aatb.org

The American Board of Obstetrics and Gynecology
214-871-1619
Fax: 214-871-1943
E-mail: infor@abog.org
www.abog.org

American College of Obstetricians and
Gynecologists (ACOG)
202-638-5577
www.acog.org

American Society for Reproductive Medicine (ASRM)
(formerly the American Fertility Society)
205-978-5000
www.asrm.org

American Society of Andrology (ASA)
847-619-4909
Fax: 847-517-7229
E-mail: asa@wjweiser.com
www.andrologysociety.com

American Society of Human Genetics
1-866-HUM-GENE or 301-634-7300
E-mail: society@ashg.org
www.ashg.org

American Urological Association (AUA)
301-727-1100
www.auanet.org

Association of Reproductive Health Professionals
202-466-3825
www.arph.org

Canadian Fertility and Andrology Society
514-524-9009
E-mail: info@cfas.ca
www.cfas.ca

Endocrine Society
301-941-0200
Fax: 301-941-0259
www.endo-society.org

Mental Health Professionals Group, ASRM
205-978-5000, x106
E-mail: asrm.asrm.org
www.asrm.org/Professionals/PG-SIG-Affiliated_Soc/MHPG

National Society of Genetic Counselors
215-872-7608
E-mail: fyi@nsgc.org
www.nsgc.org

Society for Assisted Reproductive Technology (SART), ASRM
205-978-5000, x109
E-mail: jzeitx@asrm.com
www.sart.org

Society for Reproductive Surgeons (SRS), ASRM
E-mail: asrm@asrm.com
www.reprodsurgery.org

Organizations for consumers

The American Fertility Association
1-888-917-3777
E-mail: info@theafa.org
www.theafa.org

American Surrogacy Center
770-426-1107
E-mail: TASC@surrogacy.com
www.surrogacy.com

Compassionate Friends
1-877-969-0010 or 630-990-0010
www.compassionatefriends.org

DES Action, USA (East Coast)
516-775-3450
www.desaction.org

DES Action, USA (West Coast)
1-800-337-9288 or 510-465-4011
Fax: 510-465-4815
www.desaction.org

Endometriosis Association
1-800-992-3636 (ENDO) or 414-355-2200
www.endometriosisassn.org

Ferre Institute
315-724-4348
Fax: 315-724-1360
E-mail: FerreInf@aol.com
www.ferre.org

InterNational Council on Infertility Information
Dissemination (INCIID)
520-544-9548
Fax: 703-379-1593
E-mail: INCIIDinfo@inciid.org
www.inciid.org

National Infertility Network Exchange (NINE)
516-794-5772
www.nine-infertility.org

Organization of Parents Through Surrogacy (OPTS)
847-782-0224
www.opts.com

Polycystic Ovarian Syndrome Association
1-877-775-PCOS
www.pcosupport.org

RESOLVE
Helpline: 617-623-0744
Business line: 617-623-1156
www.resolve.org

Turner's Syndrome Society of the U.S.
1-800-365-9944
www.turner-syndrome-us.org

Adoption resources

Adoption Network Law Center
1-800-FOR-ADOPT (1-800-367-2367)
http://adoptionnetwork.com

Alliance for Children
781-431-7148
E-mail: info@allforchildren.org
www.allforchildren.org

American Adoption Congress
1-800-274-6736
www.americanadoptioncongress.org

Committee for Single Adoptive Parents
E-mail: ncsap@hotmail.com
www.adopting.org/ncsap.html

International Children's Alliance
301-495-9710
www.adoptica.org

Latin American Parents Association (LAPA)
718-236-8689
www.lapa.com

National Adoption Information Clearinghouse
1-888-251-0075 or 703-352-3488
E-mail: naic@caliber.com
http://naic.acf.hhs.gov

National Council for Adoption
202-328-1200
www.ncfa-usa.org

National Resource Center for Special Needs Adoption
313-433-7080
www.nrcadoption.org

North American Council on Adoptable Children (NACAC)
651-644-3036
E-mail: info@nacac.org
www.nacac.org

Single Mothers by Choice
212-988-0993
E-mail: mattes@pipeline.com
http://mattes.home.pipeline.com

Alternative and complementary medicine resources

Acupuncture and Oriental Medicine Alliance
253-851-6896
www.aomalliance.org

American Academy of Medical Acupuncture
323-937-5514
www.medicalacupuncture.org

American Association of Naturopathic Physicians
1-866-538-2267 or 202-895-1392
www.naturopathic.org

American Association of Oriental Medicine
916-443-4770
www.aoom.org

American Botanical Council
512-926-4900
E-mail: abc@herbalgram.org
www.herbalgram.org

National Center for Complementary and Alternative Medicine
1-888-644-6226
E-mail: info@nccam.nih.gov
http://nccam.nih.gov

National Center for Homeopathy
703-548-7790
E-mail: info@homeopathic.org
www.homeopathic.org

National Certification Commission of Acupuncturists and
Oriental Medicine (NCCAM)
703-548-9004
E-mail: info@nccaom.org
www.nccaom.org

Other useful websites
Government and not-for-profit organizations

Centers for Disease Control and Prevention
www.cdc.gov

Infertility Resources for Consumers
www.ihr.com/infertility

La Leche League International
www.lalecheleague.org

March of Dimes
www.modimes.org

Medline
www.medlineplus.gov

National Center on Health Statistics (NCHS)
www.cdc.gov/nchs

National Institutes of Health (NIH)
www.nih.gov

National Women's Health Information Center
www.4woman.gov

U.S. Food and Drug Administration (FDA)
www.fda.gov

Pharmaceutical industry websites

Ferring Pharmaceuticals
www.ferringfertility.com

Freedom Drug/Priority Health Care
www.fertilityneighborhood.com

IVP Care, Inc.
www.ivpcare.com

Organon USA
www.fertilityjourney.com; www.follistim.com

Serono USA
www.fertilitylifelines.com

Magazines

Adoptive Families
www.adoptivefamilies.com

conceive magazine
www.conceivemagazine.com

Fertility Today
www.fertilitytoday.org

Fertility Weekly
www.fertilityweekly.com

Fertility World
www.IVFonline.com

Sample Genetic Testing Flow Sheet

Disclaimer: The following questions may help you decide whether to have pre-pregnancy genetic testing to determine carrier status. These are only guidelines and do not replace the advice and recommendations of your doctor and/or genetic counselor. There are also other genetic disorders that may be relevant in your particular case.

Ancestry	Are You or Any Blood Relatives:	Is Your Partner or Your Partner's Blood Relatives:
Mediterranean (Greek, Italian)	Yes__ No__	Yes__ No__
Ashkenazi Jewish	Yes__ No__	Yes__ No__
French Canadian	Yes__ No__	Yes__ No__
African, Caribbean, Indian, Middle Eastern, South American	Yes__ No__	Yes__ No__

Family History	Do You or Any of Your Blood Relatives Have:	Does Your Partner or Your Partner's Blood Relatives Have:
Mental retardation	Yes__ No__	Yes__ No__
Down syndrome	Yes__ No__	Yes__ No__
Cystic fibrosis	Yes__ No__	Yes__ No__
Sickle cell anemia	Yes__ No__	Yes__ No__
Thalassemia (Mediterranean anemia)	Yes__ No__	Yes__ No__
Open spine defects	Yes__ No__	Yes__ No__

If you answer yes to any of these—or are concerned about other genetic conditions—discuss having pre-pregnancy genetic testing with your doctor.

The following tests can help determine whether you or your partner are carriers for certain genetic diseases. If you are, you can evaluate the risk of having a baby with this genetic disease *before* you become pregnant.

Regardless of your ethnic or family background, you and your partner should discuss the possibility of being tested for the cystic fibrosis gene with your doctor and/or genetic counselor.

Ethnic Group*	Disorder** to Be Tested For:
Mediterranean (Greek, Italian)	Alpha and beta thalassemia
French Canadian or Cajun French	Tay-Sachs
African, Caribbean, Indian, Middle Eastern, South American	Hemoglobinopathy Alpha and beta thalassemia Sickle cell anemia
Ashkenazi Jewish	Bloom syndrome Canavan disease Cystic fibrosis Familial dysautonomia Fanconi anemia Gaucher disease Glycogen storage disease Maple syrup urine disease Mucolipidosis Niemann-Pick disease Tay-Sachs

Family History	Disorder
Mental retardation	Fragile X
Down syndrome	Trisomy 21
Cystic fibrosis	Cystic fibrosis
Sickle cell anemia	Sickle cell anemia
Thalassemia	Thalassemia

* There are other ethnic groups not listed that may be at risk of passing on certain genetic disorders to their offspring. Be sure to discuss the issue of genetic counseling with your doctor.

** This is not a complete list. There are other genetic disorders not included in this list that may be relevant in your particular case. Again, be sure to discuss genetic counseling with your doctor.

State-by-State Infertility Insurance Coverage

STATE GUIDE TO INSURANCE COVERAGE OF INFERTILITY TREATMENT
(Last Updated June 2005)
Reproduced with permission from RESOLVE, The National Infertility Association, www.resolve.org

STATE	DEFINITION OF INFERTILITY/PATIENT REQUIREMENTS	COVERAGE	EXCEPTIONS
ARKANSAS 1987 Ark. Stat. Ann Sections 23-85-137 23-86-118	• The patient and her spouse must have at least a 2-year history of unexplained infertility OR the infertility must be associated with at least one of the following: ▲ endometriosis; ▲ DES exposure; ▲ blocked or surgically removed fallopian tubes that are not the result of voluntary sterilization; ▲ abnormal male factors contributing to the infertility. • The patient must be the policyholder or the spouse of the policyholder and be covered by the policy. • The patient's eggs must be fertilized with her spouse's sperm. • The patient has been unable to obtain successful pregnancy through any less costly infertility treatments covered by insurance.	• All individual and group insurance policies that provide maternity benefits must cover In Vitro Fertilization (IVF). HMO's are exempt from the law. • Lifetime maximum of $15,000 for coverage. • IVF procedures must be performed at a facility licensed or certified by the state and conform to the American College of Obstetricians and Gynecologists'(ACOG) and the American Society of Reproductive Medicine (ASRM) guidelines. • Limits preexisting condition limitations to 12 months. • Includes cryopreservation as an IVF procedure. • The benefits for IVF shall be subject to the same deductibles, coinsurance and out-of-pocket limitations as under maternity benefit provisions. • Insurers may choose to include other infertility procedures or treatments under the IVF benefit.	
CALIFORNIA 1989 Cal. Health & Safety Code Section 1374.55 Cal. Insurance Code Section 10119.6	• Requires group insurers to offer coverage of infertility treatment, except IVF. Employers may choose whether or not to include infertility coverage as part of their employee health benefit package. • Infertility means the presence of a demonstrated condition recognized by a physician and surgeon as a cause of infertility or the inability to conceive a pregnancy or carry a pregnancy to a live birth after a year or more of regular sexual relations without contraception.	• No coverage is required. Insurers are only required to offer the following services. Employers decide if they will provide the following benefits to their employees: • Treatment includes diagnosis, diagnostic testing, medication, surgery, and Gamete Intrafallopian Transfer (GIFT).	• Only requires insurers to offer coverage. • Does not include IVF. • Does not require religious organizations to offer coverage.

STATE	DEFINITION OF INFERTILITY/PATIENT REQUIREMENTS	COVERAGE	EXCEPTIONS
CONNECTICUT **2005**	• Individual and group insurers are required to provide infertility coverage to individuals under 40 years old. • Infertility means the condition of a presumably healthy individual who is unable to conceive or sustain a successful pregnancy during a one-year period. • Limits coverage to individuals who have maintained coverage under a policy for at least 12 months. • Effective date - October 1, 2005 (pending Governor's signature)	• Lifetime maximum coverage of 4 cycles of ovulation induction. • Lifetime maximum coverage of 3 cycles of intrauterine insemination. • Lifetime maximum coverage of 2 cycles of IVF, GIFT, ZIFT or low tubal ovum transfer, with not more than 2 embryo implantations per cycle. Each fertilization or transfer is credited as one cycle towards the maximum. • Limits coverage for IVF, GIFT, ZIFT and low tubal ovum transfer to individuals who have been unable to conceive or sustain a successful pregnancy through less expensive and medically viable infertility treatment or procedures, unless the individual's physician determines that those treatments are likely to be unsuccessful. • Requires infertility treatment or procedures to be performed at facilities that conform with the American Society of Reproductive Medicine and the Society of Reproductive Endocrinology and Infertility guidelines.	• Does not require religious organizations to offer coverage.
HAWAII **1989, 2003** **Hawaii Rev. Stat** **Sections 431:10A–116.5** **432.1-604**	• Individual and group insurers are required to cover one cycle of IVF if a patient or patient's spouse has at least a 5-year history of infertility or the infertility is associated with at least one of the following conditions: ▲ endometriosis; ▲ DES exposure; ▲ blocked or surgically removed fallopian tubes; ▲ abnormal male factors contributing to the infertility.	• One cycle of IVF • The coverage shall be provided to the same extent as maternity-related benefits. • The IVF procedures must be performed at medical facilities that conform to ACOG and ASRM guidelines.	

STATE	DEFINITION OF INFERTILITY/PATIENT REQUIREMENTS	COVERAGE	EXCEPTIONS
	• The patient's eggs must be fertilized with her spouse's sperm. • Coverage is provided if the patient has been unable to obtain successful pregnancy through other infertility treatments covered by insurance.		
ILLINOIS **1991, 1997** **Ill Rev. Stat. ch 215** **Section ILCS 5/356m**	• Infertility means the inability to conceive after one year of unprotected sexual intercourse or the inability to sustain a successful pregnancy.	• Group insurers and HMOs that provide pregnancy-related coverage must provide infertility treatment including, but not limited to: ▲ diagnosis of infertility; ▲ IVF; ▲ uterine embryo lavage; ▲ embryo transfer; ▲ artificial insemination; ▲ GIFT; ▲ ZIFT; ▲ low tubal ovum transfer • Coverage for IVF, GIFT and ZIFT is provided if the patient has been unable to attain or sustain a successful pregnancy through reasonable, less costly infertility treatments covered by insurance; • Each patient is covered for up to 4 egg retrievals. However, if a live birth occurs, 2 additional egg retrievals will be covered, with a lifetime maximum of 6 retrievals covered. • The procedures must be performed at facilities that conform with ACOG and ASRM guidelines.	• Employers with fewer than 25 employees do not have to provide coverage. • Does not require religious employers to cover infertility treatment.

STATE	DEFINITION OF INFERTILITY/PATIENT REQUIREMENTS	COVERAGE	EXCEPTIONS
LOUISIANA **2001** **Louisiana State Law** **Subsection 215.23, Acts** **2001, No. 1045,** **subsection 1**	• Prohibits the exclusion of coverage for the diagnosis and treatment of a correctable medical condition, solely because the condition results in infertility.		• The law does <u>not</u> require insurers to cover fertility drugs, IVF or other assisted reproductive techniques, reversal of a tubal ligation, a vasectomy, or any other method of sterilization.
MARYLAND **2000** **MD Insurance Code Ann.** **Section 15-810** **MD Health General** **Code Ann. Section 19-701**	• The patient and the patient's spouse must have a history of infertility for 2 years or the infertility is associated with one of the following: ▲endometriosis; ▲DES exposure; ▲blocked or surgically removed fallopian tubes; ▲abnormal male factors contributing to the infertility. • The patient's eggs must be fertilized with her spouse's sperm. • The patient is the policyholder or a covered dependent of the policyholder. • The patient has been unable to obtain successful pregnancy through any less costly infertility treatments covered by insurance.	• Individual and group insurance policies that provide pregnancy-related benefits must cover the cost of 3 IVFs per live birth. • Lifetime maximum of $100,000. • IVF procedures must be performed at clinics that conform to ASRM and ACOG Guidelines.	• Does not require religious employers to cover infertility treatment. • Employers with fewer than 50 employees do not have to provide coverage.

STATE	DEFINITION OF INFERTILITY/PATIENT REQUIREMENTS	COVERAGE	EXCEPTIONS
MASSACHUSETTS 1987 **Mass Gen Laws Ann. Ch. 175, Section 47H, ch. 176A, Section 8K, ch.176B, Section 4J, ch176G, Section 4, and 211 CMR 37.00**	• Infertility means the condition of a presumably healthy individual who is unable to conceive or produce conception during a period of one year.	• All insurers providing pregnancy-related benefits shall provide for the diagnosis and treatment of infertility including the following: ▲artificial insemination; ▲IVF; ▲GIFT; ▲sperm, egg and/or inseminated egg procurement and processing, and banking of sperm or inseminated eggs, to the extent such costs are not covered by the donor's insurer, if any; ▲ICSI; ▲ZIFT • Insurers shall not impose any exclusions, limitations or other restrictions on coverage of infertility drugs that are different from those imposed on any other prescription drugs. • The law does not limit the number of treatment cycles and does not have a dollar lifetime cap.	• Insurers are not required to cover (but are not prohibited from covering) experimental infertility procedures, surrogacy, reversal or voluntary sterilization or cryopreservation of eggs.
MONTANA 1987 **Mont. Code Ann. Section 33-22-1521 Section 33-31-102(2)(v)**	• Infertility is not defined in the law or regulation.	• Requires HMOs to cover infertility services as part of basic health care services.	

STATE	DEFINITION OF INFERTILITY/PATIENT REQUIREMENTS	COVERAGE	EXCEPTIONS
NEW JERSEY **2001** **NJ Laws, Chap. 236**	• Infertility means a disease or condition that results in the abnormal function of the reproductive system such that: ▲ a male is unable to impregnate a female; ▲ a female under 35 years of age is unable to conceive after two years of unprotected sexual intercourse; ▲ a female 35 years of age and over is unable to conceive after one year of unprotected sexual intercourse; ▲ the male or female is medically sterile; or ▲ the female is unable to carry a pregnancy to live birth. • Infertility does not mean a person who has been voluntarily sterilized regardless of whether the person has attempted to reverse the sterilization. • Must be under 46 years of age. • The patient has been unable to obtain successful pregnancy through any less costly infertility treatments covered by insurance.	• Group insurers and HMOs that provide pregnancy-related coverage must provide infertility treatment including, but not limited to: ▲ artificial insemination; ▲ assisted hatching; ▲ diagnosis and diagnostic testing; ▲ fresh and frozen embryo transfers; ▲ 4 completed egg retrievals per lifetime; ▲ IVF, including IVF using donor eggs and IVF where the embryo is transferred to a gestational carrier or surrogate; ▲ ICSI; ▲ GIFT; ▲ ZIFT; ▲ medications; ▲ ovulation induction; and ▲ surgery, including microsurgical sperm aspiration. • The procedures must be performed at facilities that conform with ACOG and ASRM guidelines	• Employers with fewer than 50 employees do not have to provide coverage. • Cryopreservation is not covered. • Nonmedical costs of egg or sperm donor are not covered. • Infertility treatments that are experimental or investigational are not covered. • Does not require religious employers to cover infertility treatment.

STATE	DEFINITION OF INFERTILITY/PATIENT REQUIREMENTS	COVERAGE	EXCEPTIONS
NEW YORK 1990, 2002 NY S.B. 6257-B/A.B. 9759-B NY Insurance Law Sections 3216 (13), 3221 (6), and 4303	• Prohibits the exclusion of coverage for the diagnosis and treatment of a correctable medical condition, solely because the condition results in infertility. • The law abides by the ASRM definition of infertility. ASRM defines infertility as the inability to achieve a pregnancy after trying for 12 months if you are under 35 and 6 months if you are over 35. • Coverage is provided to patients 21 to 44 years old. • Patients must be covered under their insurance policy for at least 12 months before receiving infertility coverage.	• Group policies must provide diagnostic tests and procedures that include: ▲ hysterosalpingogram; ▲ hysteroscopy; ▲ endometrial biopsy; ▲ laparoscopy; ▲ sono–hysterogram; ▲ post coital tests; ▲ testis biopsy; ▲ semen analysis; ▲ blood tests and ▲ ultrasound • Every policy that provides for prescription drug coverage shall also include drugs (approved by the FDA) for use in the diagnosis and treatment of infertility.	• Excludes coverage for IVF, GIFT, and ZIFT; reversal of elective sterilizations; sex change procedures; cloning or experimental medical or surgical procedures.
NEW YORK DEMO 2002 A.9759-B (Budget Bill) S.6257-B (Budget Bill)	• IVF coverage is provided through a grant program to New York state residents who meet certain criteria including: ▲ must be between 21-44 years old; ▲ must be privately insured, but not covered for IVF and ▲ must have a diagnosis of infertility • The New York State Department of Health selected providers throughout the state to participate in this program. • To find out if you are eligible and if funding is still available, contact the New York State Health Department at 518-474-3368.		

STATE	DEFINITION OF INFERTILITY/PATIENT REQUIREMENTS	COVERAGE	EXCEPTIONS
OHIO 1991 Ohio Rev. Code Ann. Section 1751.01(A)(7)		• Requires HMOs to cover "basic health care services" including infertility services, when they are medically necessary. • Diagnostic and exploratory procedures are covered, including surgical procedures to correct the medically diagnosed disease or condition of the reproductive organs including, but not limited to: ▲ endometriosis; ▲ collapsed/clogged fallopian tubes; ▲ testicular failure • IVF, GIFT and ZIFT may be covered, but are not required by the law.	
RHODE ISLAND 1989 RI Gen. Laws sections 27-18-30, 27-19-23, 27-20-20, and 27-41-33	• Infertility means the condition of an otherwise presumably healthy married individual who is unable to conceive or produce conception during a period of one year.	• Insurers and HMOs that cover pregnancy benefits must provide coverage for medically necessary expenses of diagnosis and treatment of infertility. • The insurer may impose up to a 20% copayment. • The law does not specify a limit on the number of retrievals and does not impose a dollar cap.	
TEXAS 1987 Tex. Insurance Code Ann. Section 3.51-6, Sec. 3A	• Requires group insurers to offer coverage of IVF. Employers may choose whether or not to include infertility coverage as part of their employee health benefit package. • If an employer chooses to offer the benefit,	• No coverage is required. Insurers are only required to offer IVF.	• Does not require religious employers to cover infertility treatment.

STATE	DEFINITION OF INFERTILITY/PATIENT REQUIREMENTS	COVERAGE	EXCEPTIONS
	patients must meet the following: ▲the patient for the IVF procedure is the policyholder or spouse of the policyholder; ▲the patient's eggs must be fertilized with her spouse's sperm; ▲the patient and the patient's spouse have a history of infertility of at least 5 continuous years or associated with endometriosis, DES, blockage of or surgical removal of one or both fallopian tubes or oligospermia. ▲the patient has been unable to attain a pregnancy through less costly treatment covered under their policy. ▲The IVF procedures must be performed at medical facilities that conform to ACOG and ASRM guidelines.		
WEST VIRGINIA 1995 W.Va. Code Section 33-25A-2	• The law does not define "infertility"	• Requires HMOs to cover infertility services under "basic health care services."	

Index